Medical Terminology

A Short Course

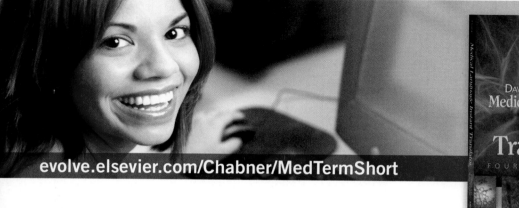
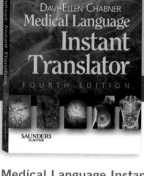

Davi-Ellen Chabner, BA, MAT

Medical Terminology

A Short Course

6th
EDITION

ELSEVIER
SAUNDERS

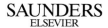

11830 Westline Industrial Drive
St. Louis, Missouri 63146

MEDICAL TERMINOLOGY: A SHORT COURSE, ISBN: 978-1-4377-3440-9
SIXTH EDITION

Notice

Library of Congress Cataloging in Publication Data

Chabner, Davi-Ellen.
  Medical terminology : a short course / Davi-Ellen Chabner.—6th ed.
    p. ; cm.
  Includes index.
  ISBN 978-1-4377-3440-9 (pbk. : alk. paper)
1. Medicine—Terminology—Programmed instruction.   I. Title.
  [DNLM: 1. Terminology as Topic—Problems and Exercises.   W 15 C427m 2009]
  R123.C434 2009
  610.1'4--dc22
2008022436

Vice-President and Publisher: Andrew Allen
Publisher: Jeanne Olson
Managing Editor: Linda Woodard
Developmental Editor: Luke Held
Publishing Services Manager: Julie Eddy
Senior Project Manager: Andrea Campbell
Senior Designer: Ellen Zanolle

Illustrations by Jim Perkins

Printed in United States of America

Last digit is the print number: 9 8 7 6 5 4 3 2 1

For Solomon, Gus, Bebe, Louisa, Amari, and Ben
These are the children whose smiles and
laughter help me relax!

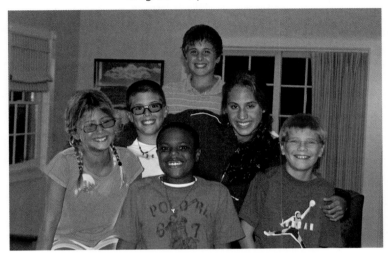

and

For Greta and Owen
These are the canine companions whose loyalty
and affection brighten my days!

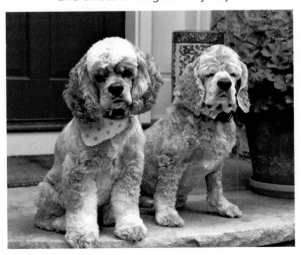

Preface to the 6th Edition

I wrote the first edition of *Medical Terminology: A Short Course* more than 20 years ago with the hope that it would fill a specific niche in the education of allied health professionals. My goal was to present a comprehensive introduction and overview of medical terminology in a straightforward and easy manner for students who had no previous background in biology or medicine.

It is gratifying to know that this book is now widely used in career schools, colleges, hospitals, and other medical settings in the United States and abroad, where allied health workers use medical language and interpret it for patients and their families. There is no doubt that the method used in *Medical Terminology: A Short Course* takes potentially complicated subject matter and makes it manageable and understandable. In this sixth edition, the text has been updated and carefully reviewed for clarity, simplicity, and practicality, but its essential elements remain. Here are its important features:

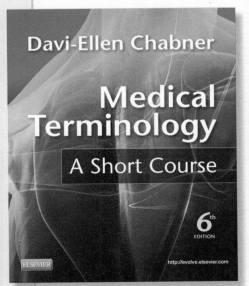

WORKBOOK-TEXT FORMAT. In this book, you learn by doing. On nearly every page you are writing and interacting with medical terminology. You complete exercises (and check your answers), label diagrams, test your understanding with review sheets, and practice pronunciation. The best path to success is to write terms and their meanings as you test yourself. I really believe this method of learning will work for you!

EASY TO READ AND UNDERSTAND. Explanations of terms are worded simply and clearly, and repetition reinforces learning throughout the text. Answers to questions are located easily so that you can check and correct your responses while gaining additional explanation of terminology.

DYNAMIC ILLUSTRATIONS AND PHOTOGRAPHS. Medical terms come alive with images on nearly every page! Learning is reinforced by seeing parts of the body, diseases, conditions and real medical procedures. At the end of each chapter, Picture Shows highlight key images and allow you to apply your knowledge of terminology.

INTRODUCTION TO BODY SYSTEMS. *Appendix 1* includes the following five sections:
- **Anatomy**—shows full-color images of each body system, labeled for easy reference with combining forms for each body part.
- **Terminology**—repeats each combining form and gives a medical term illustrating the use of the combining form. Definitions are in the *Mini-Dictionary: Glossary of Medical Terms* at the end of the book.
- **Pathology**—presents explanations of disease conditions related to each body system.
- **Diagnostic and Treatment Procedures**—explains and defines common examples for each body system.
- **Matching Exercises**—tests your understanding of the material, with answers included.

REFERENCE GUIDE FOR MEDICAL AND HOSPITAL WORK. This book is also a useful resource. Diagnostic Tests and Procedures (radiological, nuclear medicine, and clinical and laboratory tests) are found in *Appendix 2*. Abbreviations, symbols, acronyms, and eponyms are located in *Appendix 3*. The *Mini-Dictionary: Glossary of Medical Terms* helps you study each chapter and also will be a reference for you in the workplace. Each definition has been crafted carefully to explain terms using plain, nontechnical language.

PRACTICAL APPLICATIONS. Throughout the text, and on the **Student Evolve website**, you will find exciting images, medical case reports, and vignettes that illustrate terminology in the context of stories about patients and procedures. **Medical Detective** is a special feature on the Evolve website. A medical case is presented, and you answer questions to test your understanding of the situation.

CASE 10 *Neurology*

Ms. Kindrick is admitted with severe, throbbing **unilateral frontal cephalgia** that has lasted for 2 days. Light makes her cringe, and she has **nausea.** Before the onset of these symptoms, she saw zigzag lines for about 20 minutes and a **scotoma** (see Figure 5-14). Diagnosis is **acute migraine** with **aura. A vasoconstrictor** is prescribed, and Ms. Kindrick's condition is improving. [Migraine headaches are thought to be caused by sudden **dilation** of blood vessels.]

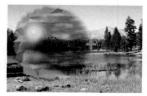

Figure 5-14 • Scotoma. This abnormal area of the visual field is both "positive" (consisting of bright flickering imagery) and "negative" (displaying a relatively dark area that obscures the visual field). It is called a scintillating scotoma. (From Yanoff M, Duker JS: Ophthalmology, ed 2, St Louis, 2004, Mosby.)

acute _____

aura _____

cephalgia _____

dilation _____

frontal _____

migraine _____

nausea _____

scotoma _____

unilateral _____

vasoconstrictor _____

New to This Edition

While the essential elements of *Medical Terminology: A Short Course* remain in place, the new sixth edition is even more dynamic and engaging.

IN PERSON

These compelling first-person narratives describe procedures and conditions from a uniquely personal perspective. After reading each story, medical terms take on new meaning as you experience intimately how it feels to be in a patient's "shoes," living through a diagnosis, disease, and treatment.

IN PERSON

This first-person narrative describes the symptoms and treatment of a 42-year-old woman with gallbladder stones.

Everyone enjoys a little dessert after dinner, but when the ice cream or a creamy tart leads to pain, most would avoid it. I loved sweets, and despite the revenge they took on my waistline, I still would not pass up an ice cream cone—until my gallbladder decided it had had enough. After several late nights spent doubled over in pain, I tried to steer clear of fatty foods but could not resist the temptation of frozen yogurt.

With one hand I pushed my cart through the supermarket; with the other hand I fed myself some delicious low-fat (not non-fat) frozen yogurt. I never dreamed that the attendant at the quick service window actually gave me soft-serve ice cream. Within 10 minutes of eating the questionable yogurt, I broke out into a sweat; a wave of nausea took me, over and a knifelike pain stabbed me in my right upper quadrant. It hurt even more when I pressed my hand on the area in an attempt to brace the pain.

Several months earlier, after a similar painful episode, I had undergone an ultrasound of my gallbladder, and the surgeon then recommended cholecystectomy. The U/S showed multiple stones in my gallbladder. Most of the stones were just the right size to lodge in the common bile duct and cause blockage of the outflow of bile that occurs after a fatty meal. When I heard the ultrasound results, I swore off all fatty foods.

I just did not imagine that ice cream masquarading as "low-fat yogurt" would be the straw that broke the camel's back! Soon enough, I abandoned my shopping cart and apologized to the manager of the store for vomiting all over aisle 4. The unrelenting pain did not cease when I vomited—it only intensified. I have no idea how I made it home and into bed, but my husband found me several hours later in a deep sweat. I managed to call my surgeon and arrange for "semiemergent" surgery the next morning.

Dr. Fernandez and his team performed a laparoscopic cholecystectomy and relayed to me as I came out of anesthesia that I no longer had a "bag of marbles" for a gallbladder. I had a gassy, distended feeling in my abdomen over the two weeks after surgery (carbon dioxide gas is injected into the abdomen before surgery to allow space between abdominal organs). I felt "tight as a drum" for the first few days and the day by day it went away. My four tiny incisions healed just fine, and in about 2 weeks I was feeling back to "normal." Now I can eat ice cream to my heart's content, only suffering the padding on my waistline, not the stabbing pain just

---

TERMINOLOGY CHECKUP

This new feature recaps and reinforces key concepts and easily confused terms in each chapter.

TERMINOLOGY CHECKUP

Before you leave this chapter, here are important concepts that you should thoroughly understand. Check the box next to each item when you know you've "got" it!

☐ 1. **Double membranes:** Remember that organs in the body are often covered and protected by double membranes. Examples are the *pleura*, a double membrane surrounding the lungs, and the *peritoneum,* a double membrane surrounding the abdominal organs. The *pericardium* is a double membrane surrounding the heart. In a later chapter, you will learn about the *meninges,* which make up the triple membrane that surrounds the brain and spinal cord.

☐ 2. **Pharynx, larynx, trachea, and esophagus:** Don't confuse these four important parts of the body. The **pharynx** is the *throat,* which is the common passageway for air and food. The **larynx** is the *voice box,* which is located in the upper portion of the *trachea,* or windpipe. Two tubes branch from the pharynx. The **trachea** (in the front) carries air to the lungs, while the **esophagus** (behind the trachea) carries food to the stomach.

☐ 3. **Planes of the body:** Distinguishing between the three planes of the body is essential to understanding images such as x-rays, as well as CT and MRI scans. The *frontal (coronal) plane* divides the body into front and back (anterior/posterior) portions. The *sagittal (lateral) plane* divides the body into right and left sides. The *transverse (axial) plane* divides the body into upper and lower portions (cross sections). Frontal and sagittal plane images are obtained from traditional x-ray procedures. The transverse plane is seen only on CT and MRI scans. Visualizing organs in all three planes is possible with CT and MRI.

☐ 4. **Mediastinum:** The mediastinum is an important area of the chest. It is the *space between the lungs* containing the heart, large blood vessels (aorta and venae cavae), trachea, bronchial tubes, esophagus, and many lymph nodes.

PRINCIPAL DIAGNOSIS

These new sections highlight the concept of **principal diagnosis,** which is essential when working with billing and coding.

PRINCIPAL DIAGNOSIS

The **principal diagnosis** is the cause, after evaluation, of the patient's admission to the hospital. Physician notes, which document clinical investigations and findings, are important for medical billing and coding. A careful reading of physician notes will identify the principal diagnosis, as in the following example.

Physician Notes

A 67-year-old man with a 2-pack-a-day h/o [history of] smoking and hypertension [high blood pressure] presents to the ED [emergency department] complaining of hemoptysis [coughing up blood], fatigue, back pain on his right side, polyuria [frequent need to urinate], and headaches. The elevated BP [blood pressure], hemoptysis, and headaches require observation in the ED. The patient is admitted and diabetes is ruled out as a cause of polyuria. A chest x-ray for hemoptysis reveals a RLL [right lower lobe] mass. Needle biopsy confirms malignancy. The patient agrees to have a lobectomy performed. He is counseled on his tobacco use during recovery and he agrees to begin therapy for tobacco cessation.

Using the information presented in the physician notes, select the principal diagnosis from the following:

A. Lung cancer—lower lobe (162.5)
B. Hemoptysis (786.30)
C. Polyuria (788.42)
D. Headache (784.0)
E. Hypertension (401.9)

PRINCIPAL DIAGNOSIS

The **principal diagnosis** is the
Physician notes, which document
billing and coding. A careful read
following example.

Physician Notes

A 45-year-old obese woman
cramping pelvic pain, dizzin
examination demonstrates m
reveals low RBCs [red blood
volume of blood], normal WB
U/S [ultrasound] of the abdo
uterine wall. Patient is admi
During the course of admission she speaks to the resident dietitian about a compulsive
eating disorder and agrees to undergo therapy at the hospital's weight loss clinic.

Using the information presented in the physician notes, select the principal diagnosis from the following:

A. Pelvic pain—female (625.9)
B. Obesity (278.00)
C. Anemia (285.9)
D. Menorrhagia (626.2)
E. Fibroid uterus (218.9)

Also Available

STUDENT EVOLVE WEBSITE (access included with text purchase)

The Evolve website included with this new edition contains additional information, images, and video clips to test and expand your understanding. Chapter by chapter, you will find case studies, games, and activities, as well as a wealth of images to illustrate medical terminology. Visit http://evolve.elsevier.com/Chabner/medtermshort to access your resources.

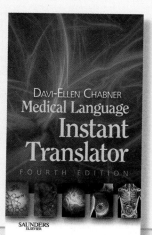

MEDICAL LANGUAGE INSTANT TRANSLATOR (for sale separately)

My *Medical Language Instant Translator* is a uniquely useful resource for all allied health professionals and students of medical terminology. It is a pocket-sized medical terminology reference with convenient information at your fingertips!

Medical Terminology: A Short Course is exactly what you need to begin your medical career—whether in an office, hospital, or other medical setting. Use this handy book in a classroom with an instructor, or study it on your own. The combination of visually reinforced hands-on learning plus easily accessible reference material will mean success for you in your allied health career.

My more comprehensive workbook-text, *The Language of Medicine, 9th edition,* may be of interest to you as you continue your study of medical terminology. It can also serve as a valuable reference in the workplace.

I still experience the thrill and joy of teaching new students. I love being in the classroom and feel privileged to continue to write this text. I am available for help at any time. Please communicate your comments, questions, and suggestions to me at MedDavi@aol.com. For technical assistance, please contact technical.support@elsevier.com.

Most of all, I hope this book brings to you excitement and enthusiasm for the medical language. It can ignite your imagination for new challenges and make your job more interesting. Work hard and have fun learning medical terminology!

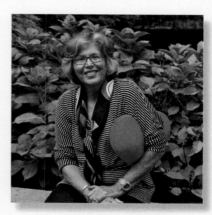

Davi-Ellen Chabner

Acknowledgments

Maureen Pfeifer, my editor extraordinaire, has once again delivered superb guidance, assistance, and painstaking attention to detail in every aspect of this edition. Her keen intelligence, willingness to tackle and solve difficult problems, and unflagging optimism helped every step of the way. With great affection and appreciation, thank you, Maureen!

Ellen Zanolle, senior book designer, Art and Design, brilliantly created the cover and interior design and skillfully executed page layouts. Ellen's superb artistic talent and keen understanding of my work continue to make her an invaluable partner with every edition. William Donnelly executed the page layout with precision and creativity.

Luke Held, developmental editor, Health Professions II Editorial, was helpful and diligent through all stages of this book.

Jim Perkins, assistant professor of medical illustration, Rochester Institute of Technology, was responsible for the excellent, first-rate individual drawings that illustrate this edition. As always, he has done an outstanding job.

Andrea Campbell, senior project manager, Book Production, coordinated production aspects with great care and thoughtful consideration of my time and work schedule. Elizabeth Galbraith did a meticulous and thoughtful job of copyediting. I appreciated her intelligent comments and questions.

My association with the Health Professions II team has always been positive. I appreciate their confidence and cooperation throughout the years. In particular, I am grateful to Andrew Allen, vice-president and publisher, Health Professions II Editorial; Jeanne Olson, publisher, Health Professions II Editorial; Linda Woodard, managing editor, Health Professions II Editorial; Peggy Fagen, director of publishing services, Book Production; Julie Eddy, publishing services manager, Book Production; Jeanne Crook, Multimedia Production; and Sharon Korn, creative director, Creative Services.

I am particularly grateful to the In Person contributors who shared their personal medical stories. Thanks so much to Ruthellen Sheldon, Cathy Ward, Elizabeth Chabner Thompson, Sidra DeKoven Ezrahi, and Nancy J. Brandwein.

I appreciate the valuable suggestions of the instructors who reviewed *Medical Terminology: A Short Course* for this new edition. They are listed with their credentials on page xiii. Their helpful comments are incorporated in this text. Kathleen A. Carbone, CPC, CHISP, a medical coding specialist, gave valuable help in creating the Principal Diagnosis feature, new to this edition.

Teachers and students continue to contact me with questions and insights. Thank you to instructors Peggy Nolan, Joyce Y. Nakano, Cindy Mason-Young, Judith Lytle, Melissa Hilker, N. Lee Price, Julie Cox, Hollie Dungan, Georgine Bills, and Dennis Cowart. Thank you to students Donna Young, Nyesha Mills, Rory Alexander, Kieran Vogel, and Jori Zama.

Special thanks to Norman Simon, MD, who contributed his expertise in reviewing Appendix 2, Diagnostic Tests and Procedures. Dr. Simon is a renowned nephrologist and internist who always has time to assist his grateful niece.

I still rely on my husband Bruce A. Chabner, MD, and my daughter, Elizabeth Chabner Thompson, MD, MPH, for expert medical advice and consultation. I am grateful for their unwavering support, patience, and availability, no matter what else is going on in their busy lives and work. During the writing of this edition, I experienced the pain and discomfort of sciatica (pressure and inflammation of the sciatic nerve in my leg) resulting from a herniated (bulging) disk (see Chapter 2, page 54). I am much improved but appreciate even more keenly the treasure of good health and absence of pain.

Enjoy every day!

Davi-Ellen Chabner

Reviewers

Debbie J. Ball, CPS, MBE
Business Systems Technology Instructor
Tennessee Technology Center
Murfreesboro, Tennessee

Kathleen Bredberg
Director, Vocational Nursing Program
Grayson County College
Denison, Texas

Bruce A. Chabner, MD
Director of Clinical Research
Massachusetts General Hospital Cancer
    Center
Professor of Medicine
Harvard Medical School
Boston, Massachusetts

Elizabeth Chabner Thompson, MD, MPH
Founder/Principal Bffl Co.
Scarsdale, New York

Karen Duckworth, RN, BSN, MHSA, IL-CSN
Highland High School - Highland, Illinois
Southwestern Illinois College – Belleville,
    Illinois

Suzanne B. Garrett, MSA, RHIA
Professor/Program Manager, Health
    Information Technology
College of Central Florida
Ocala, Florida

Rosalie Griffith, RN, MSN, MAEd
Nursing Success Coordinator
Chesapeake College
Wye Mills, Maryland

Janis Grimland, RN, BSN
Vocational Nursing Interim Coordinator
Hill College
Hillsboro, Texas

Brooke Irving Haver, CPhT
Jefferson Adult Division, Jefferson Union
    High School District
Daly City, California

Marilyn J. Lovasi, MSN, RN
Dean of Nursing
Center for Allied Health & Nursing
    Education
Hackensack, New Jersey

Anne Marie K. McCauley, RN, BS, MS
Instructor
Chester County Technical College High
    School
West Grove, Pennsylvania

Constance Phillips, MA, MPH
Director, Biomedical Laboratory &
    Clinical Sciences
City Lab Academy
Boston University
Boston, Massachusetts

(More reviewers listed on next page)

Norman M. Simon, MD
Evanston Northwestern Healthcare
Professor of Medicine
Northwestern University
Feinberg School of Medicine
Chicago, Illinois

La Tanya Young, MMsc, MPH, RMA, PA-C
Clayton State University
Morrow, Georgia

Contents

Basic Word Structure

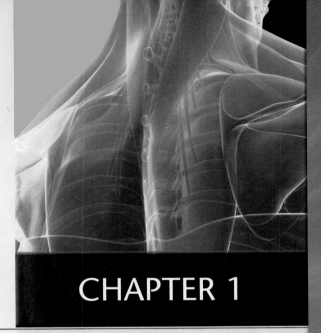

CHAPTER 1

CHAPTER OBJECTIVES

- To divide medical terms into component parts
- To analyze, pronounce, and spell medical terms using common combining forms, suffixes, and prefixes

Word Analysis

If you work in a medical setting, you use medical words every day. In addition, you hear medical terms spoken in your doctor's office, read about health issues, and make daily decisions about your own health care and the health care of your family. Terms such as arthritis, electrocardiogram, hepatitis, and anemia describe conditions and tests that are familiar. Other medical words are more complicated, but as you work in this book, you will begin to understand them even if you have never studied biology or science.

Medical words are like individual jigsaw puzzles. Once you divide the terms into their component parts and learn the meaning of the individual parts, you can use that knowledge to understand many other new terms.

For example, the term HEMATOLOGY is divided into three parts:

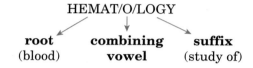

When you analyze a medical term, begin at the *end* of the word. The ending is called a **suffix.** All medical terms contain suffixes. The suffix in HEMATOLOGY is -LOGY, which means study of. Next, look at the beginning of the term. HEMAT is the word **root.** The root gives the essential meaning of the term. The root HEMAT means blood.

The third part of this term, which is the letter O, has no meaning of its own but is an important connector between the root (HEMAT) and the suffix (-LOGY). It is called a **combining vowel.** The letter O is the combining vowel usually found in medical terms.

Now put together the meanings of the suffix and the root: HEMATOLOGY means study of blood.

Another familiar medical term is ELECTROCARDIOGRAM. You probably know this term, often abbreviated as ECG (or sometimes EKG). This is how you divide it into its parts:

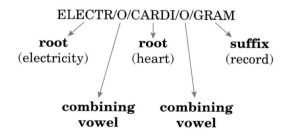

Start with the **suffix** at the end of the term. The suffix -GRAM means a record.

Now look at the beginning of the term. ELECTR is a word **root,** and it means electricity.

This medical term has two roots. The second root is CARDI, meaning heart. Whenever you see CARDI in other medical terms, you will know that it means heart.

Read the meaning of medical terms from the suffix, back to the beginning of the term, and then across. Broken down this way, ELECTROCARDIOGRAM means record of the electricity in the heart. It is the electrical current flowing within the heart that causes the heart muscle to contract, pumping blood throughout the body. The sound made by contraction and relaxation of the heart muscle is called the heartbeat.

Notice the two combining vowels in ELECTROCARDIOGRAM. Looking for the O in medical terms will help you divide the term into its parts. One combining vowel (O) lies between two roots (ELECTR and CARDI), and another between the root (CARDI) and the suffix (-GRAM).

The combining vowel *plus* the root is called a **combining form.** For example, there are *two* combining forms in the word ELECTROCARDIOGRAM. These combining forms are ELECTR/O, meaning electricity, and CARDI/O, meaning heart.

Notice how the following medical term is analyzed. Can you locate the two combining forms in this term?

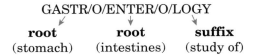

GASTR/O/ENTER/O/LOGY

root	**root**	**suffix**
(stomach)	(intestines)	(study of)

The two combining forms are GASTR/O and ENTER/O. The entire word (reading from the suffix, back to the beginning of the term, and across) means study of the stomach and the intestines. Here are other words that are divided into component parts:

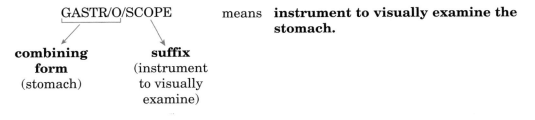

GASTR/O/SCOPE   means   **instrument to visually examine the stomach.**

combining form (stomach)   **suffix** (instrument to visually examine)

GASTR/IC   means   **pertaining to the stomach.** Notice that the combining vowel is dropped when the suffix (-IC) begins with a vowel. -IC means pertaining to. Words ending with -IC are adjectives that modify a noun (e.g., gastric pain, gastric cancer).

root (stomach)   **suffix** (pertaining to)

CARDI/AC   means   **pertaining to the heart.** Again, the combining vowel (O) is dropped when the suffix (-AC) begins with a vowel. Words ending in -AC are adjectives (e.g., cardiac care, cardiac arrest).

root (heart)   **suffix** (pertaining to)

1

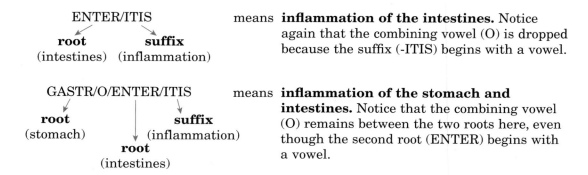

ENTER/ITIS

root   suffix
(intestines)   (inflammation)

means **inflammation of the intestines.** Notice again that the combining vowel (O) is dropped because the suffix (-ITIS) begins with a vowel.

GASTR/O/ENTER/ITIS

root   suffix
(stomach)   (inflammation)
                root
            (intestines)

means **inflammation of the stomach and intestines.** Notice that the combining vowel (O) remains between the two roots here, even though the second root (ENTER) begins with a vowel.

In addition to roots, suffixes, combining forms, and combining vowels, many medical terms have a word part attached to the *beginning* of the term. This is called a **prefix,** and it can change the meaning of a term in important ways. For example, watch what happens to the meaning of the following medical terms when the prefix changes:

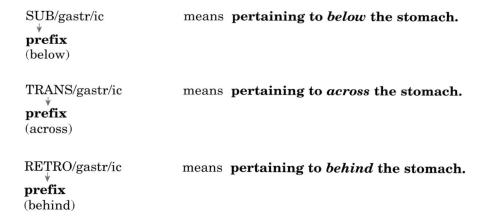

SUB/gastr/ic

prefix
(below)

means **pertaining to *below* the stomach.**

TRANS/gastr/ic

prefix
(across)

means **pertaining to *across* the stomach.**

RETRO/gastr/ic

prefix
(behind)

means **pertaining to *behind* the stomach.**

Let's **review** the important word parts:
1. **Root**—gives the essential *meaning* of the term.
2. **Suffix**—is the word *ending.*
3. **Prefix**—is a small part added to the *beginning* of a term.
4. **Combining vowel**—*connects* roots to suffixes and roots to other roots.
5. **Combining form**—is the combination of the *root* and the *combining vowel.*
Some important rules to **remember** are:
1. **Read** the meaning of medical words from the suffix to the beginning of the word and then across.
2. **Drop** the combining vowel before a suffix that starts with a vowel.
3. **Keep** the combining vowel between word roots, even if the second root begins with a vowel.

COMBINING FORMS, SUFFIXES, AND PREFIXES

Presented in this section are lists of combining forms, suffixes, and prefixes that are commonly found in medical terms. Write the meaning of the medical term on the line that is provided. Some terms will be more difficult to understand even after you know the meanings of individual word parts. For these, more extensive explanations are given in *italics*. To check your work, see the ***Mini-Dictionary: Glossary of Medical Terms*** on page 341, which contains meanings of all terms used in this book.

In your study of medical terminology, you will find it helpful to practice writing terms and their meanings many times. You'll succeed when you follow these simple steps:

1. Complete **Exercises** beginning on page 23 for this chapter and faithfully check your answers on pages 31 to 32.
2. Fill in the meanings in the **Pronunciation of Terms** list on pages 33 to 36.
3. Apply your knowledge in the **Practical Applications** and **Picture Show** features beginning on page 37.
4. Complete the **Review** of word parts beginning on page 43 and check your answers.
5. Make sure you understand the key medical terminology concepts in the **Terminology CheckUp** on page 46.

COMBINING FORMS

Notice that the **combining form** is in **bold** type, while the <u>root</u> in the medical term is <u>underlined</u>.

COMBINING FORM	MEANING	MEDICAL TERM	MEANING
aden/o	gland	<u>adenoma</u> _____ -OMA *means tumor or mass.*	
		<u>adenitis</u> _____ -ITIS *means inflammation.*	
arthr/o	joint	<u>arthritis</u> _____	
bi/o	life	<u>biology</u> _____ -LOGY *means study of.*	
		<u>biopsy</u> _____ -OPSY *means (process of) viewing. Living tissue is removed and viewed under a microscope.*	
carcin/o	cancer, cancerous	<u>carcinoma</u> _____	
cardi/o	heart	<u>cardiology</u> _____	

cephal/o   head   cephalic _____

                                        -IC *means pertaining to. If an infant is born with the head delivered first, it is a* **cephalic** *presentation.*

cerebr/o   cerebrum, largest   cerebral _____
                    part of the brain
                                        -AL *means pertaining to. Figure 1-1 shows the cerebrum and its functions.*

                                        cerebrovascular accident (CVA) _____

                                        -VASCULAR *means pertaining to blood vessels; a CVA is commonly known as a* **stroke**.

What happens in a stroke?

Blood is prevented from reaching areas of the cerebrum. Depending on the location and extent of reduced blood flow, signs and symptoms may include loss of movement (paralysis), loss of speech (aphasia), weakness, and changes in sensation.

1

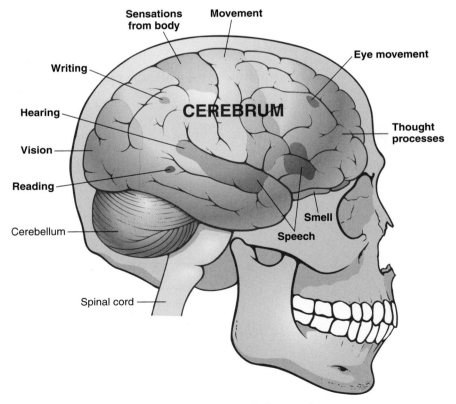

Figure 1-1 • **Functions of the cerebrum.**

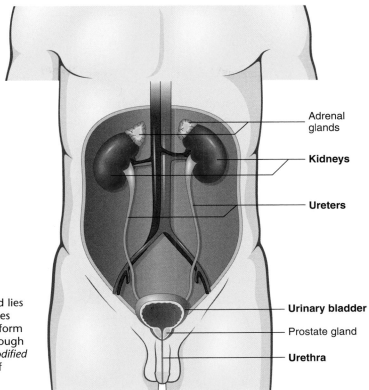

Figure 1-2 • The male urinary tract. Note that the prostate gland lies below the urinary bladder. It secretes fluid that combines with sperm to form semen. Semen leaves the body through the urethra during ejaculation. *(Modified from Chabner D-E: The Language of Medicine, ed 9, Philadelphia, 2011, Saunders.)*

Adrenal glands
Kidneys
Ureters
Urinary bladder
Prostate gland
Urethra

cyst/o	urinary bladder	cystoscope

-SCOPE *means instrument to visually examine. Figure 1-2 shows the urinary bladder and urinary tract in a male. A cystoscope is placed through the urethra into the urinary bladder. See Figure 1-3.*

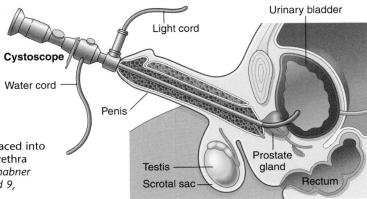

Light cord
Urinary bladder
Cystoscope
Water cord
Penis
Testis
Scrotal sac
Prostate gland
Rectum

Figure 1-3 • A **cystoscope** is placed into the urinary bladder through the urethra within the penis. *(Modified from Chabner D-E: The Language of Medicine, ed 9, Philadelphia, 2011, Saunders.)*

cyt/o	cell	cytology _____
derm/o	skin	dermal _____
dermat/o	skin	dermatitis _____
electr/o	electricity	electrocardiogram (ECG) _____

-GRAM *means record. EKG is an older abbreviation for this test.*

1

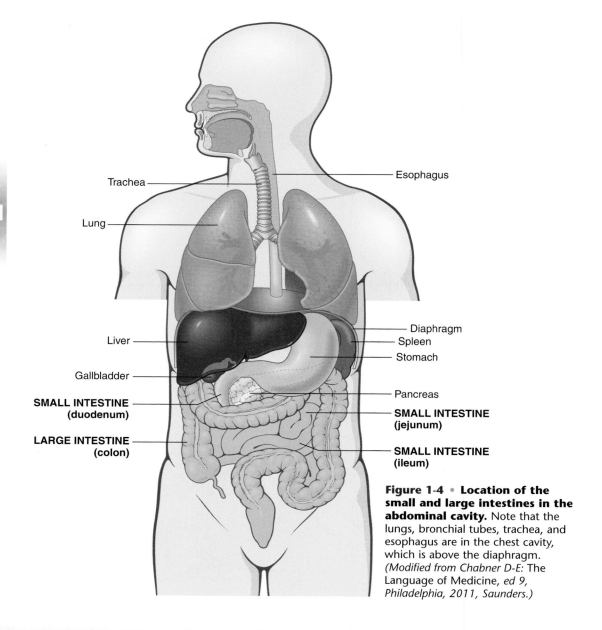

Trachea — — Esophagus

Lung —

Liver —

— Diaphragm
— Spleen
— Stomach

Gallbladder —

SMALL INTESTINE
(duodenum) —

— Pancreas

— **SMALL INTESTINE**
(jejunum)

LARGE INTESTINE —
(colon)

— **SMALL INTESTINE**
(ileum)

Figure 1-4 • Location of the small and large intestines in the abdominal cavity. Note that the lungs, bronchial tubes, trachea, and esophagus are in the chest cavity, which is above the diaphragm. *(Modified from Chabner D-E:* The Language of Medicine, *ed 9, Philadelphia, 2011, Saunders.)*

encephal/o	brain	electroencephalogram (EEG) _____
		This record is helpful in determining whether a patient has a seizure disorder, such as epilepsy.
enter/o	intestines (often the small intestine)	enteritis _____
		Figure 1-4 shows the small and large intestines. ENTER/O describes the small intestine and sometimes intestines in general. COL/O and COLON/O are combining forms for the large intestine (colon).
erythr/o	red	erythrocyte _____
		-CYTE means cell. Figure 1-5 shows the three major types of blood cells.

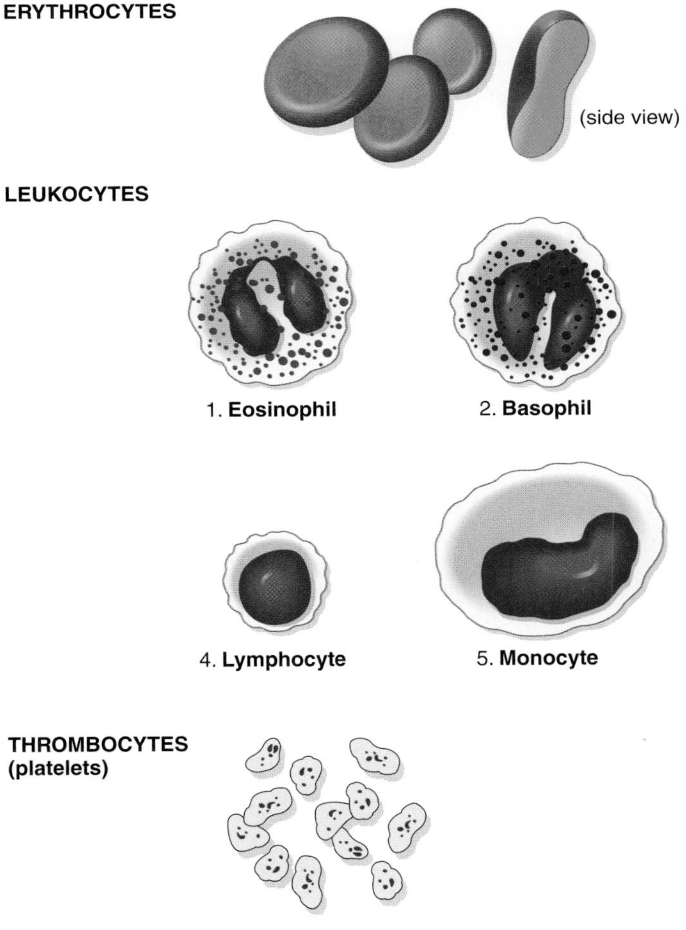

ERYTHROCYTES

(side view)

LEUKOCYTES

1. **Eosinophil**   2. **Basophil**   3. **Neutrophil**

4. **Lymphocyte**   5. **Monocyte**

THROMBOCYTES
(platelets)

Figure 1-5 • **Blood cells:** *erythrocytes* (carry oxygen), *leukocytes* (five different types help fight disease), **and** *thrombocytes* or *platelets* (help blood to clot). *(Modified from Chabner D-E: The Language of Medicine, ed 9, Philadelphia, 2011, Saunders.)*

gastr/o	stomach	gastroscopy ————————————————

-SCOPY *means process of visual examination using an instrument, or "scope."*

gnos/o	knowledge	diagnosis ————————————————

-SIS *means state of;* DIA- *means complete. A diagnosis is the complete knowledge gained after testing and examining the patient. The plural of diagnosis is diagnoses. Table 1-1 shows other plural formations.*

prognosis ————————————————

PRO- *means before. A prognosis is a prediction (before knowledge) that is made after the diagnosis. It forecasts the outcome of treatment.*

Table 1-1 FORMATION OF PLURALS

Consult the *Mini-Dictionary: Glossary of Medical Terms* on page 341 for pronunciations of all terms.

1. Words ending in **a** retain the **a** and add **e**:

Singular	Plural	Meaning
vertebr**a**	vertebra**e**	Backbones
burs**a**	bursa**e**	Sacs of fluid near a joint

2. Words ending in **is** drop the **is** and add **es**:

Singular	Plural	Meaning
diagnos**is**	diagnos**es**	Determinations of the nature and cause of diseases
psychos**is**	psychos**es**	Abnormal conditions of the mind

3. Words ending in **ex** or **ix** drop the **ex** or **ix** and add **ices**:

Singular	Plural	Meaning
ap**ex**	ap**ices**	Pointed ends of organs
cort**ex**	cort**ices**	Outer parts of organs
var**ix**	var**ices**	Enlarged, swollen veins

4. Words ending in **on** drop the **on** and add **a**:

Singular	Plural	Meaning
gangli**on**	gangli**a**	Groups of nerve cells; benign cysts near a joint (such as the wrist)

5. Words ending in **um** drop the **um** and add **a**:

Singular	Plural	Meaning
bacteri**um**	bacteri**a**	Types of one-celled organisms
ov**um**	ov**a**	Egg cells

6. Words ending in **us** drop the **us** and add **i***:

Singular	Plural	Meaning
bronch**us**	bronch**i**	Tubes leading from the windpipe to the lungs
calcul**us**	calcul**i**	Stones

*Exceptions to this rule are viruses and sinuses.

gynec/o	woman, female	gynecology _____
hem/o, hemat/o	blood	hemoglobin _____ -GLOBIN *means protein. Hemoglobin is the protein in red blood cells (erythrocytes) that helps carry oxygen in the blood.* hematoma _____ -OMA *means mass or tumor. In this term, -oma indicates a mass or swelling containing blood.*
hepat/o	liver	hepatitis _____

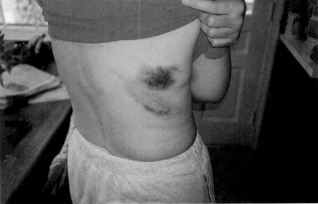

Be careful about spelling this term!

The combining form is **gynec**/o. A gynecologist specializes in diseases of the female reproductive organs. Gynecology involves both surgical and internal medicine expertise and is often practiced with **obstetrics** (care of pregnant women and delivery of a fetus).

Hematoma

A **hematoma** is a mass of blood trapped in tissues of the skin or in an organ. It often results from trauma and is commonly called a bruise or "black-and-blue" mark. Figure 1-6, *A* and *B* shows hematomas.

1

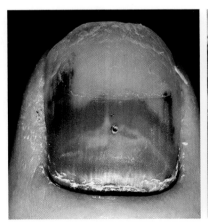

Figure 1-6 • **A,** Subungual hematoma. This collection of blood under (SUB-) a nail (UNGU/O = nail) resulted from trauma to the toe. **B,** Hematoma from broken ribs. (**A,** *From Habif TP:* Clinical Dermatology, *ed 4, St Louis, 2004, Mosby.)*

lapar/o	abdomen (area between the chest and hip)	laparotomy _____ -TOMY *means cutting into. In an* **exploratory** **laparotomy** *the surgeon makes a large incision in the abdominal wall to inspect organs for evidence of disease. See Figure 1-7. Another combining form for abdomen is* ABDOMIN/O, *as in abdominal.*
leuk/o	white	leukocyte _____ *Figure 1-5 on page 9 shows five different types of leukocytes.*
nephr/o	kidney	nephrectomy _____ -ECTOMY *means cutting out—an excision or resection of an organ or other part of the body.*
neur/o	nerve	neurology _____
onc/o	tumor	oncologist _____ -IST *means a specialist.*

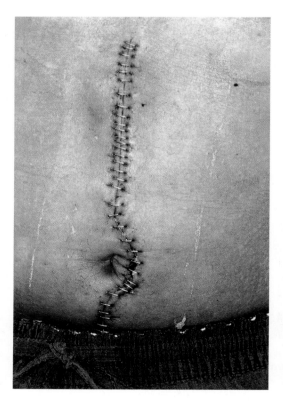

Figure 1–7 • **Laparotomy.** This incision was closed with surgical staples.

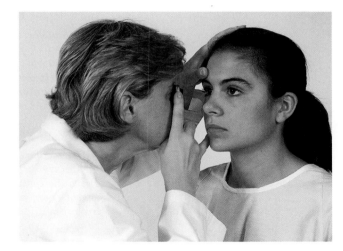

Figure 1-8 • **Ophthalmoscope.** This instrument allows the ophthalmologist to view the outer and inner areas of the eye. *(From Jarvis C: Physical Examination and Health Assessment, ed 3, Philadelphia, 2000, Saunders.)*

ophthalm/o	eye	ophthalmoscope _____

*Figure 1-8 shows an **ophthalmologist,** a medical doctor, examining a patient's eyes with an **ophthalmoscope.***

oste/o	bone	osteoarthritis _____

Figure 1-9 shows a normal knee joint and a knee joint with osteoarthritis. Degenerative changes and thinning and loss of cartilage occur. Inflammation of the joint membrane occurs late in the disease.

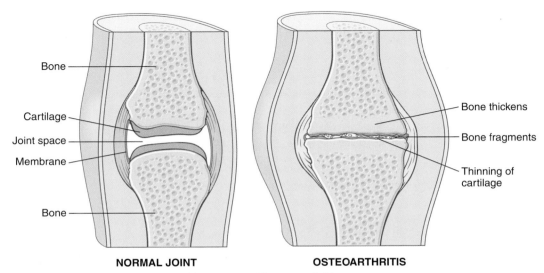

NORMAL JOINT   OSTEOARTHRITIS

Bone
Cartilage
Joint space
Membrane
Bone

Bone thickens
Bone fragments
Thinning of cartilage

Figure 1-9 • Normal knee joint and knee joint with osteoarthritis.

path/o	disease	pathologist _____

A pathologist is a medical doctor who views biopsy samples to make a diagnosis and examines dead bodies (in an autopsy) to determine the cause of death. AUT- means self, and -OPSY means (process of) viewing. Thus, an autopsy is an opportunity to see for oneself what caused a patient's death.

psych/o   mind   psychosis _____

*-OSIS means abnormal condition. In this serious mental condition, the patient loses touch with reality. Psychotic symptoms include **hallucinations** (unreal sensory perceptions, such as hearing voices when none are present) and **delusions** (fixed, false beliefs that can't be changed by logical reasoning).*

ren/o   kidney   renal _____

Sometimes there are two combining forms for the same part of the body. Often, one comes from Latin, and the other from Greek. (REN- is the Latin root meaning "kidney," and NEPHR- is the Greek root meaning "kidney.") The Greek root describes abnormal conditions and procedures, whereas the Latin root is used with -AL, meaning "pertaining to."

rhin/o   nose   rhinitis _____

sarc/o   flesh   sarcoma _____

Sarcomas and carcinomas are cancerous tumors. Sarcomas grow from the fleshy tissues of the body, such as muscle, fat, bone, and cartilage, whereas carcinomas arise from skin tissue and the linings of internal organs.

thromb/o   clotting   thrombocyte _____

*A thrombocyte **(platelet)** is a small cell that helps blood to clot. Platelets are shown in Figure 1-5 (see page 9).*

thrombosis _____

*Formation of a **thrombus** (blood clot) occurs when thrombocytes and other clotting factors combine. **Thrombosis** describes the condition of forming a clot (thrombus).*

Pathologist/Medical examiner/Coroner

A **medical examiner (M.E.)** is a **pathologist** who specializes in forensic (legal) medicine related to criminal issues. A **coroner**, however, is an elected official (administrator) who investigates any suspicious death. This official may or may not be a medical examiner.

SUFFIXES

Each suffix is in **bold** type in the Suffix column and <u>underlined</u> in the Medical Term column.

SUFFIX	MEANING	MEDICAL TERM	MEANING
-al	pertaining to	neur<u>al</u> _____	
		Other suffixes meaning pertaining to are listed on page 375 in the Mini-Dictionary: Glossary of Word Parts.	
-algia	pain	arthr<u>algia</u> _____	
-cyte	cell	leuko<u>cyte</u> _____	
-ectomy	cutting out; removal, excision	gastr<u>ectomy</u> _____	
		In a partial or subtotal gastrectomy, only a portion of the stomach is removed.	
-emia	blood condition	leuk<u>emia</u> _____	
		Large numbers of immature, cancerous cells are found in the bloodstream and bone marrow (inner part of bone that makes blood cells).	
-globin	protein	hemo<u>globin</u> _____	
-gram	record	arthro<u>gram</u> _____	
		This is an x-ray record of a joint.	
-ia	condition	neural<u>ia</u> _____	
-ic	pertaining to	gastr<u>ic</u> _____	
-ism	condition, process	hyperthyroid<u>ism</u> _____	
		HYPER- means excessive. The thyroid gland is in the neck. It secretes the hormone thyroxine, which helps cells burn food to release energy. See Figure 1-10.	
-itis	inflammation	gastroenter<u>itis</u> _____	
-logist	specialist in the study of	neuro<u>logist</u> _____	
-logy	study of	nephro<u>logy</u> _____	
		See Table 1-2 on page 16 for a list of other terms using -LOGY.	
-oma	tumor, mass	hepat<u>oma</u> _____	
		This is a cancerous (malignant) tumor, also called ***hepatocellular carcinoma.***	

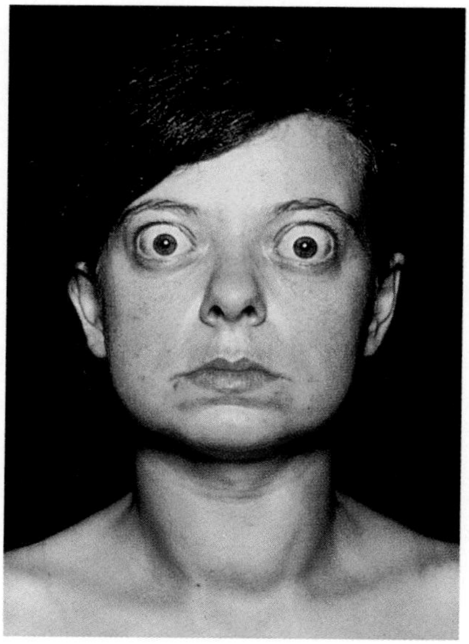

Figure 1-10 • Hyperthyroidism (Graves disease). The thyroid gland produces too much hormone, which causes signs and symptoms such as rapid pulse, nervousness, excessive sweating, and swelling of tissue behind the eyeball (resulting in exophthalmos, or "bulging" of the eyes). *(Modified from Seidel H, et al:* Mosby's Guide to Physical Examination, *ed 4, St Louis, 1998, Mosby.)*

-opsy	to view	bio<u>psy</u> _____
-osis	abnormal condition	nephr<u>osis</u> _____
		leukocyt<u>osis</u> _____

This is an increase in numbers of normal white blood cells as a response to infection.

Table 1-2 TERMS USING -LOGY (STUDY OF)

cardiology	Study of the heart
dermatology	Study of the skin
endocrinology	Study of the endocrine glands
gastroenterology	Study of the stomach and intestines
gynecology	Study of women and women's diseases
hematology	Study of the blood
neurology	Study of the nerves and the brain and spinal cord
oncology	Study of tumors (cancerous or malignant diseases)
ophthalmology	Study of the eye
pathology	Study of disease
psychology	Study of the mind and mental disorders
rheumatology	Study of joint diseases (RHEUMAT/O = flow or watery discharge, which was once thought to cause aches and pains, especially in joints)

-scope	instrument to visually examine	gastro<u>scope</u> _____
		laparo<u>scope</u> _____
-scopy	process of visual examination	laparo<u>scopy</u> _____

Small incisions are made near the navel, and instruments are inserted into the abdomen for viewing organs and performing procedures such as tying off the fallopian or uterine tubes. See Figure 1-11.

arthro<u>scopy</u> _____

See Figure 1-12 (page 18).

-sis	state of	progno<u>sis</u> _____
-tomy	process of cutting into; incision	neuro<u>tomy</u> _____

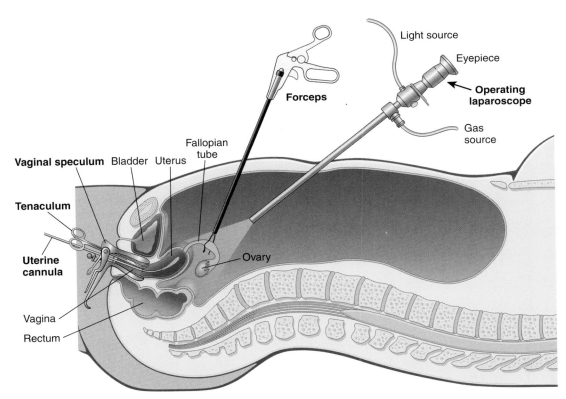

Figure 1-11 • **Laparoscopy for tubal ligation** (interruption of the continuity of the fallopian tubes) as a means of preventing future pregnancy. The **vaginal speculum** keeps the vaginal cavity open. The **uterine cannula** is a tube placed into the uterus to manipulate the uterus during the procedure. **Forceps** and **tenaculum** are used for grasping or manipulating tissue. *(Modified from Chabner D-E: The Language of Medicine, ed 9, Philadelphia, 2011, Saunders.)*

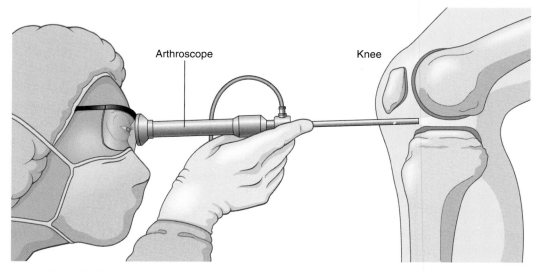

Figure 1-12 • Arthroscopy of the knee. A surgeon (orthopedist) performs an arthroscopic examination to make a diagnosis or treat disease of the joints.

PREFIXES

Each prefix is in **bold** type in the Prefix column and <u>underlined</u> in the Medical Term column.

PREFIX	MEANING	MEDICAL TERM	MEANING
a-, an-	no, not	<u>a</u>nemia	
		Literally, anemia means a condition of "no blood." Actually, it is a decrease in the number of red blood cells or a decrease in their ability to carry oxygen resulting from less hemoglobin, a protein that helps carry oxygen in red blood cells.	
aut-	self	<u>aut</u>opsy	
		Viewing and examining a dead body with one's own (self) eyes. Here the root OPS- (viewing) is embedded in the suffix -OPSY (process of viewing).	

Where is the root?

Some suffixes can contain roots. In the term anemia, notice that the root EM- (from HEM, meaning blood) is embedded in the suffix -EMIA.

dia-	complete, through	diagnosis _____
		In this term, DIA- means complete.
		diameter _____
		The suffix -METER means measurement. DIA- means through in this term.
dys-	bad, painful, difficult, abnormal	dysentery _____
		The suffix -Y means condition or process.
endo-	within	endocrine glands _____
		*CRIN/O means to secrete (to form and give off). Examples of endocrine glands are the thyroid gland, pituitary gland, adrenal glands, ovaries, and testes. All of these glands secrete hormones **within** the body and into the bloodstream.*
		endocardium _____
		The valves and chambers within the heart are lined with endocardium. The suffix -UM indicates a structure.
exo-	outside	exocrine glands _____
		*Examples of exocrine glands are sweat, tear, and mammary (breast) glands, which secrete substances to the **outside** of the body.*
hyper-	excessive, more than normal, too much	hyperglycemia _____
		GLYC/O means sugar. Hyperglycemia may be a sign of diabetes mellitus. Mellitus means "sweet."
hypo-	below, less than normal, under	hypoglycemia _____
		This condition results from too much insulin in the bloodstream. Symptoms are weakness, headache, and hunger.
peri-	surrounding	pericardium _____

Hyperglycemia and diabetes

People with hyperglycemia lack insulin (**type 1 diabetes**) or have ineffective insulin (**type 2 diabetes**). Insulin is a hormone normally released by the pancreas, an endocrine gland near the stomach. Insulin allows sugar to leave the bloodstream and enter cells. When insulin is either absent or not working, sugar remains in the blood, resulting in hyperglycemia and diabetes.

pro- before, forward <u>pro</u>state gland _____

This exocrine gland "stands" (-STATE) before or in front of the urinary bladder (see Figure 1-2, page 7) in males.

re- back <u>re</u>section _____

-SECTION means cutting into an organ, but RESECTION means removing some or all of an organ in the sense of cutting back or away. The Latin resectio means "a trimming or pruning."

retro- behind <u>retro</u>gastric _____

sub- below, under <u>sub</u>hepatic _____

trans- across, through <u>trans</u>dermal _____

<u>trans</u>urethral _____

The urethra is a tube that leads from the urinary bladder to the outside of the body. See Figure 1-2 (page 7).

1

Transurethral resection of the prostate gland (TURP)

This is a surgical procedure to remove noncancerous (benign) growth of the prostate gland. Pieces of the enlarged gland are removed through the urethra.

IN PERSON

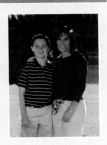

The following first-person narrative describes the reality of living with a particular medical condition—type 1 diabetes in a teenager. In each of the subsequent chapters, you'll find other first-person accounts of diseases and procedures that will make your study of medical terminology more relevant to real-life situations.

Jake Sheldon is a 14-year-old boy who has type 1 diabetes mellitus, which was diagnosed when he was 8. The following narrative was written by his mother, Ruthellen Sheldon.

On school days, I wake Jake up at 6:30 AM. He tests his blood sugar by pricking his finger until it bleeds, and then sticks a test strip into the drop of blood. Then he inserts the strip into a small hand-held glucometer and waits 3 to 5 seconds for a reading of his blood sugar. If this is 120 mg/dL or higher, he gives himself insulin 10 to 15 minutes before breakfast. I calculate how many carbohydrates (by reading labels and measuring food quantities precisely) he will have in his breakfast so that he can bolus [give himself enough insulin to cover the food he will eat] correctly. He has an insulin pump, so he types in the amount of carbohydrates he will eat, plus his current blood sugar reading. The pump calculates how much insulin he needs to cover the carbs and any extra insulin he may need to bring down a high blood sugar. If Jake's blood sugar is less than 120 mg/dL when he wakes up, he will wait until he takes his first bite of food to give himself his insulin to avoid hypoglycemia.

As I make his lunch, I count carbs and place an index card in his lunch to help him calculate his lunchtime bolus. Before lunch, Jake checks his blood sugar in the classroom and self-administers his insulin via his insulin pump.

Throughout the school day, if his blood sugar is high or low, he visits the nurse. I worry about his exposure to all the sick kids at school when he visits the nurse. If it's high, he gives himself an insulin bolus, or correction, by pump, he drinks water and then checks his urine for ketones, which may indicate ketoacidosis. If it is positive for ketones, he is sent home from school. If his blood sugar is low or less than 70, he eats or drinks some fast-acting sugar (Skittles, Smarties, or Sprite) and waits in the healthroom for his blood sugar to rise so he can return to class. He misses a lot of classroom time to manage his diabetes.

During the night, his dad and I set an alarm to wake up around 3 hours after bedtime. If his blood sugar is high while he sleeps, we use his pump to give him extra insulin, "a correction." If it is low, we wake him and have him drink Sprite or eat Smarties. If his blood sugars are high or low, we often check him again a few hours later until his numbers are in range. Even if his numbers are stable, it's not a guarantee that he won't drop suddenly and have a seizure (this happened once after we had tested him at 11 PM and 2 AM and he was steady). The pump is connected to his body with a small cannula [tube]. It is inserted manually through a needle into his hip region. The needle is then removed and the tiny Teflon cannula remains in his body, delivering fast-acting insulin under the skin. His pump is always connected to him with plastic tubing, and he carries it with him in his pants pocket. When he

1

bathes, he can disconnect the pump, and when he sleeps, he places it on the mattress next to his body.

His body naturally rejects the Teflon cannula, so after 2 days Jake must change his pump site, or his blood sugar numbers will start to rise. Although changing the pump site is time-consuming and expensive, a bad site means that not enough insulin is getting into his body, which can quickly spiral into stomach pains and DKA [diabetic ketoacidosis].

When Jake is playing sports, he times his meals with the start of the activity so his blood sugar is around 150 mg/dL. He disconnects his pump during sports, and at halftime he tests his blood sugar. If it is low, he needs to eat. If it is high, he needs to reconnect his pump and administer more insulin. After sports, his blood sugar usually spikes because of an adrenaline rush and then may crash 3 to 10 hours later. This is unpredictable, so it takes guesswork to keep his blood sugar in range after a sports game or practice. If he has an evening practice, sometimes his blood sugar can even be low at school the next day.

In general, Jake's diabetes doesn't disrupt his life other than for his nighttime checks, wearing an insulin pump, and paying attention to how many carbs he eats. We encourage him to make good nutritional choices and to limit certain foods (doughnuts, Slurpees, candy) to special occasions. He also must carry a glucometer with him at all times and a sugar to take when his blood glucose is low.

Having a child with diabetes forces me to carefully plan the preparation and timing of meals. I always have certain foods and medical supplies in the house, and I also carry snacks and sugar sources wherever I go. I am always available to Jake and to the school nurse. My husband and I hope that keeping Jake's blood sugar in tight control will help avoid many of the complications frequently encountered later in life by people with type 1 diabetes.

1

? EXERCISES AND ANSWERS

These exercises give you practice writing and understanding the terms presented in the chapter. An important part of your work is to check your answers with the Answers to Exercises beginning on page 31. If you cannot answer a question, then please look at the answer key and copy the correct answer. You may want to photocopy some of the exercises before you complete them so that you can practice doing them many times. **Remember the 3 "Rs"—wRite, Review, Repeat—and you will succeed!**

Visit the Evolve website (http://evolve.elsevier.com/Chabner/medtermshort) for additional information, images, games, videos, and interactive activities.

A **Using slashes (/), divide the following terms into their component parts and give the meaning for the whole term. The first term is completed as an example.**

1. aden/oma *tumor of a gland*

2. arthritis

3. biopsy

4. cardiology

5. dermal

6. cytology

7. cystoscope

8. cerebral

9. cephalic

10. adenitis

B Complete the following sentences using the medical terms given below.

diagnosis   erythrocyte   hepatitis
electrocardiogram   gynecology   prognosis
electroencephalogram hematoma
enteritis   hemoglobin

1. A mass of blood, or "black-and-blue" mark, is a/an _____.

2. A red blood cell is a/an _____.

3. Inflammation of the small intestine is _____.

4. The prediction about the outcome of an illness is a/an _____.

5. The record of electricity in the brain is a/an _____.

6. The study of women and women's diseases is _____.

7. The record of electricity in the heart is a/an _____.

8. Complete knowledge of a patient's illness on the basis of tests and other

   information is a/an _____.

9. A protein found in red blood cells is _____.

10. Inflammation of the liver is _____.

C Name the tissue or part of the body described in the following terms and give the meaning of the entire term.

TISSUE/BODY PART	MEANING OF TERM
1. laparotomy _____	_____
2. nephrectomy _____	_____
3. neuritis _____	_____
4. ophthalmoscope _____	_____
5. osteotomy _____	_____
6. renal _____	_____
7. rhinitis _____	_____
8. sarcoma _____	_____

D Give the meanings of the following terms.

1. oncologist _____

2. pathologist _____

3. psychosis _____

4. leukocyte _____

5. thrombocyte _____

6. gastritis _____

7. adenoma _____

8. thrombosis _____

E Give the meanings of the following suffixes.

1. -cyte _____

2. -ism _____

3. -ectomy _____

4. -al _____

5. -emia _____

6. -gram _____

7. -algia _____

8. -itis _____

9. -globin _____

10. -ic _____

F Complete the following medical terms to end each sentence.

1. Nerve pain is **neur**_____.

2. Presence of large numbers of immature, cancerous white blood cells is a blood

   condition known as **leuk**_____.

3. An x-ray record of a joint is **arthro**_____.

4. Study of the kidney is **nephro**_____.

5. Tumor of the liver is **hepat**_____.

6. Visual examination of the abdomen is **laparo**_____.

7. An incision of a joint is called **arthro**_____.

8. Abnormal condition of the skin is **dermat**_____.

9. Inflammation of the skin is **dermat**_____.

10. A specialist in the study of blood is a **hemato**_____.

G Give the meanings of the following prefixes.

1. hyper- _____

2. sub- _____

3. dys- _____

4. trans- _____

5. retro- _____

6. dia- _____

7. exo- _____

8. aut- _____

9. hypo- _____

10. endo- _____

11. peri- _____

H Give the meanings of the following medical terms.

1. autopsy _____

2. hyperthyroidism _____

3. anemia _____

4. dysentery _____

5. endocrine glands _____

6. hypoglycemia _____

7. exocrine glands _____

8. resection _____

9. transdermal _____

10. hyperglycemia _____

I Complete the following medical terms related to the stomach.

1. _____gastric   **Pertaining to under** the stomach

2. gastr_____   **Pain** in the stomach

3. gastr_____   **Inflammation** of the stomach

4. _____gastric   Pertaining to **across** or **through** the stomach

5. gastr_____   **Process of visually examining** the stomach

6. _____gastric   Pertaining to **behind** the stomach

7. gastr_____   **Study of** the stomach and intestines

8. gastr_____   **Incision** of the stomach

9. gastr_____   **Excision** of the stomach

10. gastr_____   **Instrument to visually examine** the stomach

1

J On the line provided, give the meaning of the term in **bold**.

1. An **oncologist** treats abnormal conditions such as sarcomas and carcinomas.

   _____

2. After explaining the diagnosis, Dr. Jones outlined the treatment and assured the

   patient that the **prognosis** was hopeful. _____

   _____

3. Elderly Mrs. Scott has constant arthralgia in her knees and hips. Her physician

   prescribes anti-inflammatory drugs and aspirin to treat her **osteoarthritis** but

   advises that joint replacement may be necessary. _____

   _____

4. A **pathologist** is a medical doctor who performs autopsies and examines biopsy

   samples. _____

5. **Thrombosis** is a serious condition that may result in blockage of blood vessels.

   _____

6. **Hyperglycemia** results from lack of insulin (hormone) secretion from the pancreas

   (endocrine gland near the stomach). Without insulin, sugar cannot enter cells and

   remains in the blood. _____

7. Schizophrenia is an example of a **psychosis,** in which the patient loses touch with

   reality and displays abnormal behavior (delusions and hallucinations may occur).

   _____

8. Minimally invasive surgery of the abdomen may be performed using **laparoscopy.**

   For example, a gallbladder or appendix can be removed with instruments inserted

   through small incisions. _____

   _____

9. Clinical signs of **hyperthyroidism** include an enlarged thyroid gland and protruding eyeballs (exophthalmos). _____

_____

10. Sally's diagnosis of **dysentery** was made after she returned from a trip to Mexico with abdominal pain, fever, and severe diarrhea (loose, watery stools).

_____

11. Mr. Smith died of a **cerebrovascular accident.** Confirmation at autopsy revealed a thrombus blocking one of his cerebral arteries. _____

_____

12. **Erythrocytes** contain hemoglobin, which enables them to carry oxygen throughout the body. _____

13. **Leukemia** was confirmed after a bone marrow biopsy and high white blood cell counts. _____

14. Certain types of bleeding or clotting disorders may be caused by reduced numbers of thrombocytes, also known as **platelets.** _____

15. An example of **anemia** is iron deficiency anemia. _____

_____

16. **Transdermal** delivery by patch is used for administering drugs such as nicotine, nitroglycerin, and scopolamine (for motion sickness). _____

_____

17. When Bill had difficulty urinating (urinary retention), his doctor discovered that his **prostate gland** was enlarged. _____

_____

1

18. To relieve his symptoms related to urinary retention, Bill's urologist performed a

   transurethral resection of his enlarged prostate gland. _____

   _____

19. Although the small intestine is longer (20 feet) than the large intestine (5 feet), the

   diameter of the large intestine (colon) is greater. _____

   _____

K Refer to Table 1-1, page 10, to form the plurals of the following terms.

1. psychosis _____

2. ovum _____

3. vertebra _____

4. bronchus _____

5. spermatozoon _____

6. apex _____

L In the following medical vignettes, circle the **bold** term that best completes the meaning of the sentences.

1. Selma ate a spicy meal at an Indian restaurant. Later that night she experienced **(osteoarthritis, dermatitis, gastroenteritis).** Fortunately the cramping and diarrhea subsided by morning.

2. Christina was feeling very sluggish, both physically and mentally. Her hair seemed coarse, she had noticed weight gain in the past weeks, and she had hot and cold intolerance. Her internist ordered a blood test that revealed low levels of a hormone normally secreted from a gland in the neck. She was referred to a specialist, a/an **(gynecologist, endocrinologist, pathologist).** The physician ordered a blood test that confirmed low levels of the hormone. The diagnosis of **(hypothyroidism, hyperthyroidism, psychosis)** was thus made, and proper treatment prescribed.

3. Dr. Fischer examined the lump in Bruno's thigh. An imaging technique using magnetic waves and radio signals (MRI scan) revealed a suspicious mass in the soft connective tissue of the thigh. Suspecting a cancerous mass of flesh tissue, or **(hematoma, carcinoma, sarcoma),** Dr. Fischer ordered a/an **(prognosis, biopsy, autopsy)** of the mass.

4. On her seventh birthday, Susie fell down during her birthday party. Her mother noticed bruises on Susie's knees and elbows that seemed to "come up overnight." Her pediatrician ordered a blood test, which demonstrated a decreased platelet count and an elevated **(leukocyte, erythrocyte, thrombocyte)** count at 40,000 cells. Susie was referred to a/an **(dermatologist, nephrologist, oncologist),** who made a diagnosis of **(hepatitis, anemia, leukemia).**

5. When Mr. Saluto collapsed and died while eating dinner, the family requested a/an **(laparotomy, gastroscopy, autopsy)** to determine the cause of death. The **(hematologist, pathologist, gastroenterologist)** discovered that Mr. Saluto had died of a **(cardiovascular accident, dysentery, cerebrovascular accident),** otherwise known as a stroke.

ANSWERS TO EXERCISES

A
1. Tumor of a gland
2. Inflammation of a joint
3. Process of viewing living tissue under a microscope
4. Study of (process of study of) the heart
5. Pertaining to the skin
6. Study of (process of study of) cells
7. Instrument to visually examine the urinary bladder
8. Pertaining to the cerebrum (largest part of the brain)
9. Pertaining to the head
10. Inflammation of a gland

B
1. hematoma
2. erythrocyte
3. enteritis
4. prognosis
5. electroencephalogram
6. gynecology
7. electrocardiogram
8. diagnosis
9. hemoglobin
10. hepatitis

C
1. abdomen: incision of the abdomen (this is also called exploratory surgery)
2. kidney: excision (removal, resection) of the kidney
3. nerve: inflammation of a nerve
4. eye: instrument to visually examine the eye
5. bone: incision (to cut into, section) of a bone
6. kidney: pertaining to the kidney
7. nose: inflammation of the nose
8. flesh tissue: tumor (cancerous or malignant) of flesh tissue

D
1. Specialist in the study of tumors (cancerous or malignant tumors)
2. Specialist in the study of disease (examines biopsy samples and performs autopsies)
3. Abnormal condition of the mind
4. White blood cell
5. Clotting cell or platelet
6. Inflammation of the stomach
7. Tumor of a gland (this is a benign or harmless tumor). An adenocarcinoma is a malignant tumor (CARCIN/O means cancerous).
8. Abnormal condition of clotting (occurring in a blood vessel)

E
1. cell
2. condition, process
3. process of cutting out, excision, resection, removal
4. pertaining to
5. condition of blood (blood condition)
6. record
7. pain; condition of pain
8. inflammation
9. protein
10. pertaining to

1

F
1. neuralgia
2. leukemia
3. arthrogram
4. nephrology
5. hepatoma or hepatocellular carcinoma
6. laparoscopy
7. arthrotomy
8. dermatosis
9. dermatitis
10. hematologist

G
1. excessive, above, more than normal
2. under, below
3. abnormal, bad, difficult, painful
4. across, through
5. behind, back
6. complete, through
7. out, outside
8. self
9. below, deficient, less than normal
10. within, in, inner
11. surrounding

H
1. Examination of a dead body to determine the cause of death
2. Excessive activity of the thyroid gland
3. Deficiency of hemoglobin or numbers of red blood cells; literally "no" (AN-) "blood" (-EMIA)
4. Condition of painful intestines; marked by inflammation, abdominal pain, and frequent and bloody stools and often caused by bacteria
5. Organs that produce (secrete) hormones directly into the bloodstream
6. Blood condition of decreased sugar (lower than normal levels)
7. Organs that produce (secrete) chemicals to the outside of the body (through tubes or ducts)
8. Removal (excision) of an organ or structure
9. Pertaining to through the skin
10. Blood condition of increased sugar (higher than normal levels)

I
1. subgastric or hypogastric
2. gastralgia
3. gastritis
4. transgastric
5. gastroscopy
6. retrogastric
7. gastroenterology
8. gastrotomy
9. gastrectomy
10. gastroscope

J
1. Specialist in the study (and treatment) of tumors
2. Prediction of the outcome of an illness or treatment
3. Inflammation of bones and joints (including degeneration of joints)
4. Specialist in the study of disease
5. Abnormal condition of clotting (clot formation)
6. Blood condition of increased sugar (high blood sugar)
7. Abnormal condition of the mind
8. Visual examination of the abdomen
9. Condition of increased secretion of hormone from the thyroid gland
10. Condition of painful intestines
11. Stroke; trauma to blood vessels of the brain (cerebrum)
12. Red blood cells
13. Increase in cancerous (malignant) white blood cells in blood and bone marrow
14. Clotting cells
15. Deficiency of hemoglobin and/or numbers of red blood cells; results in reduced oxygen to cells
16. Pertaining to through the skin
17. Gland in males located in front of the urinary bladder (the prostate is an exocrine gland)
18. Removal of portions of the prostate gland through the urethra (procedure is called TURP)
19. Measurement of the width across a circle

K
1. psychoses (drop -is and add -es)
2. ova (drop -um and add -a)
3. vertebrae (add -e)
4. bronchi (drop -us and add -i)
5. spermatozoa (drop -on and add -a)
6. apices (drop -ex and add -ices)

L
1. gastroenteritis
2. endocrinologist, hypothyroidism
3. sarcoma, biopsy
4. leukocyte, oncologist, leukemia
5. autopsy, pathologist, cerebrovascular accident

PRONUNCIATION OF TERMS

The terms that you have learned in this chapter are presented here with their pronunciations. The capitalized letters in **BOLDFACE** *indicate the accented syllable. Pronounce each word out loud; then write the meaning in the space provided. All meanings of terms are found in the* **Mini-Dictionary: Glossary of Medical Terms** *on page 341 and on the audio section of the Evolve site (http://evolve. elsevier.com/Chabner/medtermshort). After you write all of the meanings, it is a good idea to cover the Term column and write each term from its meaning.*

TERM	PRONUNCIATION	MEANING
adenitis	ad-eh-**NI**-tis	
adenoma	ah-deh-**NO**-mah	
anemia	ah-**NE**-me-ah	
arthralgia	ar-**THRAL**-jah	
arthritis	ar-**THRI**-tis	
arthrogram	**AR**-thro-gram	
arthroscope	**AR**-thro-skop	
arthroscopy	ar-**THROS**-ko-pe	
autopsy	**AW**-top-se	
biology	bi-**OL**-o-je	
biopsy	**BI**-op-se	
carcinoma	kar-sih-**NO**-mah	
cardiac	**KAR**-de-ak	
cardiology	kar-de-**OL**-o-je	
cephalic	seh-**FAL**-ik	
cerebral	seh-**RE**-bral	
cerebrovascular accident	seh-re-bro-**VAS**-ku-lar **AK**-sih-dent	
cystoscope	**SIS**-to-skop	

1

cystoscopy	sis-**TOS**-ko-pe _____
cytology	si-**TOL**-o-je _____
dermal	**DER**-mal _____
dermatitis	der-mah-**TI**-tis _____
dermatosis	der-mah-**TO**-sis _____
diagnosis	di-ag-**NO**-sis _____
diameter	di-**AM**-eh-ter _____
dysentery	**DIS**-en-teh-re _____
electrocardiogram	e-lek-tro-**KAR**-de-o-gram _____
electroencephalogram	e-lek-tro-en-**SEF**-ah-lo-gram _____
endocardium	en-do-**KAR**-de-um _____
endocrine glands	**EN**-do-krin glanz _____
endocrinology	en-do-krih-**NOL**-o-je _____
enteritis	en-teh-**RI**-tis _____
erythrocyte	eh-**RITH**-ro-site _____
exocrine glands	**EK**-so-krin glanz _____
gastrectomy	gas-**TREK**-to-me _____
gastric	**GAS**-trik _____
gastritis	gas-**TRI**-tis _____
gastroenteritis	gas-tro-en-teh-**RI**-tis _____
gastroenterology	gas-tro-en-ter-**OL**-o-je _____
gastroscope	**GAS**-tro-skop _____
gastroscopy	gas-**TROS**-ko-pe _____
gastrotomy	gas-**TROT**-o-me _____

gynecologist	gi-neh-**KOL**-o-jist _____
gynecology	gi-neh-**KOL**-o-je _____
hematoma	he-mah-**TO**-mah _____
hemoglobin	**HE**-mo-glo-bin _____
hepatitis	hep-ah-**TI**-tis _____
hepatoma	hep-ah-**TO**-mah _____
hyperglycemia	hi-per-gli-**SE**-me-ah _____
hyperthyroidism	hi-per-**THI**-royd-izm _____
hypoglycemia	hi-po-gli-**SE**-me-ah _____
hypothyroidism	hi-po-**THI**-royd-izm _____
laparoscope	**LAP**-ah-ro-skop _____
laparoscopy	lap-ah-**ROS**-ko-pe _____
laparotomy	lap-ah-**ROT**-o-me _____
leukemia	loo-**KE**-me-ah _____
leukocyte	**LOO**-ko-site _____
leukocytosis	loo-ko-si-**TO**-sis _____
nephrectomy	neh-**FREK**-to-me _____
nephrology	neh-**FROL**-o-je _____
nephrosis	neh-**FRO**-sis _____
neural	**NOO**-ral _____
neuralgia	nu-**RAL**-jah _____
neuritis	nu-**RI**-tis _____
neurology	nu-**ROL**-o-je _____
neurotomy	nu-**ROT**-o-me _____

1

oncologist	ong-**KOL**-o-jist _____
ophthalmoscope	of-**THAL**-mo-skop _____
osteitis	os-te-**I**-tis _____
osteoarthritis	os-te-o-ar-**THRI**-tis _____
pathologist	pah-**THOL**-o-jist _____
pericardium	peh-reh-**KAR**-de-um _____
platelet	**PLAYT**-let _____
prognosis	prog-**NO**-sis _____
prostate gland	**PROS**-tate gland _____
psychosis	si-**KO**-sis _____
renal	**RE**-nal _____
resection	re-**SEK**-shun _____
retrogastric	reh-tro-**GAS**-trik _____
rhinitis	ri-**NI**-tis _____
rhinotomy	ri-**NOT**-o-me _____
sarcoma	sar-**KO**-mah _____
subgastric	sub-**GAS**-trik _____
subhepatic	sub-heh-**PAT**-ik _____
thrombocyte	**THROM**-bo-site _____
thrombosis	throm-**BO**-sis _____
transdermal	trans-**DER**-mal _____
transgastric	trans-**GAS**-trik _____
transurethral	trans-u-**RE**-thral _____

1

MEDICAL CONDITIONS AND PROCEDURES

Match the conditions listed below with the correct procedure used to diagnose or treat each. Answers begin on page 39.

- adenocarcinoma of an endocrine gland in the neck
- epilepsy (seizure disorder)
- heart attack
- leukemia
- osteogenic sarcoma (bone cancer)
- renal cell carcinoma
- stomach ulcer
- urinary bladder carcinoma

PROCEDURE	CONDITION
1. Below-knee leg resection (amputation) _____	
2. Bone marrow biopsy _____	
3. Electrocardiogram _____	
4. Cystoscopy _____	
5. Nephrectomy _____	
6. Thyroid gland resection _____	
7. Gastroscopy _____	
8. Electroencephalogram _____	

1

PRINCIPAL DIAGNOSIS

The **principal diagnosis** *is the cause,* after *evaluation, for the patient's admission to the hospital. The patient's physician documents the findings during evaluation. These physician notes are important for medical billing and coding, as you will see from the following example.*

Physician Notes

This seven-year-old boy presents with fever, sore throat, runny nose, and persistent fatigue [feeling of being tired all the time]. Physical examination reveals multiple bruises [contusions] of his lower extremities and arms, an erythematous [red] pharynx [throat] with white plaques on the tonsils, and pale gums, lips, and nailbeds. CBC [complete blood count] was performed. Increasing fever prompted immediate admission to the children's ward of the hospital.

During the course of admission, the patient's pharyngitis was monitored and subsided. Tonsillitis was ruled out. Fatigue and contusions on his arms and legs were noted and addressed with the parents while taking his social history. A lab hematologist reviews the high WBC [white blood cell] count, and a WBC differential [percentages of the various types of these cells] shows immature cells. A bone marrow biopsy confirms the diagnosis of WBC malignancy.

Using the information presented in these notes, select the principal diagnosis from the following:

    A. Pharyngitis (462)

    B. Leukemia (208.90)

    C. Fever (780.60)

    D. Contusions—arms/legs (923.8/924.4)

    E. Leukocytosis (288.60)

(The numbers in parentheses are medical codes as given in the *International Classification of Diseases, Ninth Revision [ICD-9] Coding Handbook 2011.*)

ANSWERS TO PRACTICAL APPLICATIONS

Medical Conditions and Procedures

1. osteogenic sarcoma (bone cancer)
2. leukemia
3. heart attack
4. urinary bladder carcinoma
5. renal cell carcinoma
6. adenocarcinoma of an endocrine gland in the neck
7. stomach ulcer
8. epilepsy (seizure disorder)

Principal Diagnosis

Answer: B. Leukemia
A. Pharyngitis is a **POA (present on admission) diagnosis.***
C. Fever is an **admitting diagnosis**† but not the major diagnosis after evaluation.
D. Contusions—arms/legs is a **POA diagnosis.**
E. Leukocytosis is a **POA diagnosis.**

*A **POA (present on admission) diagnosis** reflects incidental conditions that are noted and treated if necessary but are not a cause for hospital admission. Such conditions are not life-threatening (at the time of admission) but may require treatment and monitoring during the patient's stay.
†An **admitting diagnosis** is a cause, before further evaluation, for admission to the hospital. Such conditions may not resolve in the ED and can become life-threatening without proper treatment.

PICTURE SHOW

Answer the questions that follow each image. Answers are found on page 42.

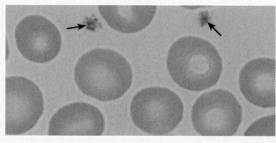

Blood smear. *(Modified from Carr JH, Rodak BF: Clinical Hematology Atlas, Philadelphia, 1999, Saunders.)*

1. The *arrows* in this photo of a blood smear are pointing to cells that are necessary in blood clotting. These cells are:
   a. leukocytes
   b. thrombosis
   c. platelets
   d. erythrocytes

2. The other blood cells in the photo contain a protein that helps the cell carry oxygen. These cells are:
   a. leukocytes
   b. thrombosis
   c. platelets
   d. erythrocytes

3. The protein contained in the cells is:
   a. hemoglobin
   b. anemia
   c. sarcoma
   d. carcinoma

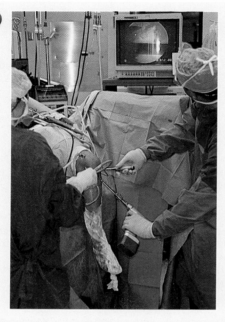

(From Miller MD, Howard RF, Plancher KD: Surgical Atlas of Sports Medicine, *Philadelphia, 2003, Saunders.)*

1. The image shows a minimally invasive procedure used to visually examine the knee. This procedure is:
   a. laparotomy
   b. arthroscopy
   c. laparoscopy
   d. arthrectomy

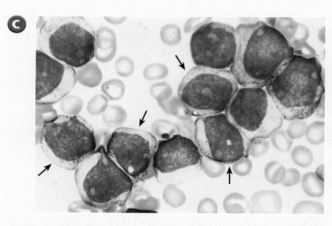

Blood smear. *(Courtesy Dr. Robert W. McKenna, Department of Pathology, University of Texas Southwestern Medical School, Dallas, Texas; from Kumar V, Cotran RS, Robbins SL, editors:* Basic Pathology, *ed 7, Philadelphia, 2003, Saunders.)*

1. In this blood smear, the arrows point to an increased number of large, immature cells (that would normally fight infection). These cells are:
   a. hepatocytes
   b. erythrocytes
   c. thrombocytes
   d. leukocytes

2. The name of the abnormal condition in which these cells predominate is:
   a. iron deficiency anemia
   b. sickle cell anemia
   c. leukemia
   d. hyperglycemia

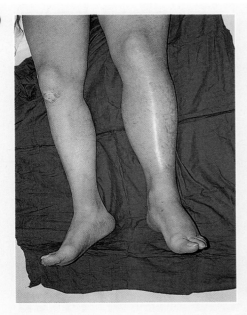

(From Forbes CD, Jackson WF: Color Atlas and Text of Clinical Medicine, *ed 3, London, 2003, Mosby.)*

1. Notice that the left leg of the patient is swollen (edema), resulting from blood flow that is slow and sluggish. Fluid seeps out of tiny vessels into tissue spaces. The abnormal condition often associated with this problem is caused by a blood clot in a blood vessel. The condition is called:
   a. hyperglycemia
   b. deep vein thrombosis
   c. cerebrovascular accident
   d. hematoma

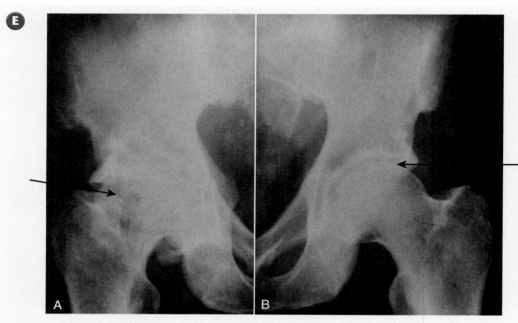

E

(Courtesy American Rheumatism Association; from Noble J: Textbook of Primary Care Medicine, *ed 3, St Louis, 2001, Mosby.)*

1

1. The image in *A* shows degeneration of the hip (pelvic) joint with narrowed joint spaces (see *arrow*). The image in *B* shows a normal hip for comparison (see *arrow*). The patient with the hip changes has arthralgia, stiffness, and joint tenderness. Your diagnosis?
   a. osteoarthritis
   b. gastroenteritis
   c. hyperthyroidism
   d. osteogenic sarcoma

ANSWERS TO PICTURE SHOW

A	1. c	2. d	3. a
B	1. b		
C	1. d	2. c	
D	1. b		
E	1. a		

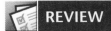 **REVIEW**

Here is your chance to test your understanding of all the **combining forms, suffixes,** *and* **prefixes** *that you have studied in this chapter. Write the meaning of each term in the space provided and* **check** *your answers with the Answers to Review section on page 45. All of the meanings for word parts are found in the* **Glossary of Word Parts** *beginning on page 375.* **Remember the 3 "Rs"—wRite, Repeat, Review.**

COMBINING FORMS

COMBINING FORM	MEANING	COMBINING FORM	MEANING
1. aden/o		18. gnos/o	
2. arthr/o		19. gynec/o	
3. bi/o		20. hem/o, hemat/o	
4. carcin/o		21. hepat/o	
5. cardi/o		22. lapar/o	
6. cephal/o		23. leuk/o	
7. cerebr/o		24. nephr/o	
8. crin/o		25. neur/o	
9. cyst/o		26. onc/o	
10. cyt/o		27. ophthalm/o	
11. derm/o, dermat/o		28. oste/o	
12. electr/o		29. path/o	
13. encephal/o		30. psych/o	
14. enter/o		31. rhin/o	
15. erythr/o		32. sarc/o	
16. gastr/o		33. thromb/o	
17. glyc/o			

SUFFIXES

SUFFIX	MEANING	SUFFIX	MEANING
1. -al	_____	11. -logist	_____
2. -algia	_____	12. -logy	_____
3. -cyte	_____	13. -oma	_____
4. -ectomy	_____	14. -opsy	_____
5. -emia	_____	15. -osis	_____
6. -globin	_____	16. -scope	_____
7. -ia	_____	17. -scopy	_____
8. -ic	_____	18. -sis	_____
9. -ism	_____	19. -tomy	_____
10. -itis	_____		

PREFIXES

PREFIX	MEANING	PREFIX	MEANING
1. a-, an-	_____	8. hypo-	_____
2. aut-	_____	9. peri-	_____
3. dia-	_____	10. pro-	_____
4. dys-	_____	11. re-	_____
5. endo-	_____	12. retro-	_____
6. exo-	_____	13. sub-	_____
7. hyper-	_____	14. trans-	_____

ANSWERS TO REVIEW

COMBINING FORMS

1. gland
2. joint
3. life
4. cancer, cancerous
5. heart
6. head
7. cerebrum
8. secrete
9. urinary bladder
10. cell
11. skin
12. electricity
13. brain
14. intestines (often small intestine)
15. red
16. stomach
17. sugar
18. knowledge
19. woman, female
20. blood
21. liver
22. abdomen
23. white
24. kidney
25. nerve
26. tumor
27. eye
28. bone
29. disease
30. mind
31. nose
32. flesh
33. clotting

SUFFIXES

1. pertaining to
2. pain
3. cell
4. cutting out; removal; excision
5. blood condition
6. protein
7. condition
8. pertaining to
9. condition; process
10. inflammation
11. specialist in the study of
12. study of
13. tumor, mass
14. to view (process of viewing)
15. abnormal condition
16. instrument to visually examine
17. process of visual examination
18. state of
19. cutting into; incision

PREFIXES

1. no, not
2. self
3. complete, through
4. bad, painful, difficult, abnormal
5. within
6. out, outside
7. excessive, more than normal, too much
8. below, less than normal, under
9. surrounding
10. before
11. back
12. behind
13. below, under
14. across, through

1

✓ TERMINOLOGY CHECKUP

Before you leave this chapter, make sure you are able to distinguish between the following terms. Check the box next to each item when you know you've "got" it!

☐ 1. **Endocrine and exocrine glands:** Both of these types of glands *secrete* chemicals. **Endocrine glands,** such as the thyroid, pituitary, and adrenal glands, *secrete hormones* that travel *within* the body to affect other organs and tissues. **Exocrine glands,** such as the sweat, tear, and salivary glands, *secrete chemicals* through ducts to the *outside* of the body.

☐ 2. **Diagnosis and prognosis:** A **diagnosis** is *complete knowledge* gained after examining and performing tests on the patient. A **prognosis,** however, is a *prediction* made *after the diagnosis.* It forecasts and describes the likely outcome of an illness.

☐ 3. **Carcinoma and sarcoma:** These are both examples of *malignant tumors.* A **carcinoma** is a cancerous tumor arising from *cells that line the internal organs* of the body. An example is an adenocarcinoma. A sarcoma, however, arises, from *connective tissues* (bone, cartilage, fat). An example is an *osteosarcoma.*

☐ 4. **Anemia, leukemia, and leukocytosis:** All of these are conditions of the blood. **Anemia** involves an abnormality (deficiency) of *red blood cells (erythrocytes)* or the *hemoglobin* within the red cells. **Leukemia** is a cancerous condition involving an increase in numbers of *abnormal white blood cells.* **Leukocytosis,** however, is a slight increase in numbers of *normal white blood cells* as a response to infection.

☐ 5. **Laparotomy and laparoscopy:** Both of these procedures involve the abdomen! A **laparotomy** is a large *incision* to explore or remove organs and tissues. **Laparoscopy** is *visual examination* of the abdomen using small incisions and the insertion of instruments including a laparoscope to view and operate on organs and tissues.

1

Organization of the Body

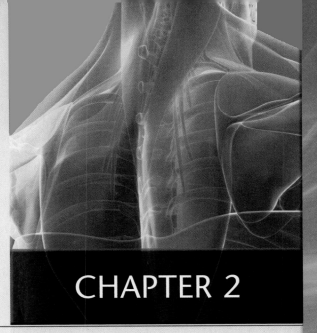

CHAPTER 2

CHAPTER OBJECTIVES

- To name the body systems and their functions
- To identify body cavities and specific organs within them
- To list the divisions of the back
- To identify three planes of the body
- To analyze, pronounce, and spell new terms
- To apply medical terms in real-life situations

Body Systems

All the parts of your body are composed of individual units called **cells.** Examples are muscle, nerve, skin (epithelial), and bone cells.

Similar cells grouped together are **tissues.** Groups of muscle cells are muscle tissue, and groups of epithelial cells are epithelial tissue.

Collections of different tissues working together are **organs.** An organ, such as the stomach, has specialized tissues, such as muscle, epithelial (lining of internal organs and outer layer of skin cells), and nerve, that help the organ function.

Groups of organs working together are the **systems** of the body. The digestive system, for example, includes the mouth, throat (pharynx), esophagus, stomach, and intestines, which bring food into the body, break it down, and deliver it to the bloodstream.

Figure 2-1 reviews the differences between cells, tissues, organs, and systems. There are 11 systems of the body, and each plays an important role in the way the body works.

The **circulatory system** (heart, blood, and blood vessels such as arteries, veins, and capillaries) transports blood (containing all types of blood cells) throughout the body. The **lymphatic system** includes lymph vessels, and nodes that carry a clear fluid called lymph. Lymph contains white blood cells called lymphocytes that fight against disease and play an important role in immunity.

The **digestive system** brings food into the body and breaks it down so that it can enter the bloodstream. Food that cannot be broken down is then removed from the body at the end of the system as waste.

The **endocrine system,** composed of glands, sends chemical messengers called hormones into the blood to act on other glands and organs.

The **female and male reproductive systems** produce the cells (eggs and sperm) that join to form the embryo. Male (testis) and female (ovary) sex organs produce hormones as well.

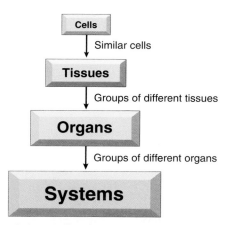

Figure 2-1 • **Cells, tissues, organs, and systems.**

The **musculoskeletal system,** including muscles, bones, joints, and connective tissues, supports the body and allows it to move.

The **nervous system** carries electrical messages to and from the brain and spinal cord.

The **respiratory system** controls breathing, a process by which air enters and leaves the body.

The **skin and sense organ system,** including the skin and eyes and ears, receives messages from the environment and sends them to the brain.

The **urinary system** produces urine and sends it out of the body through the kidneys, ureters, bladder, and urethra.

Table 2-1 lists selected organs and structures and the systems to which they belong.

At the end of the book you will find useful and important reference information. ***Appendix 1,*** page 211, contains diagrams of each body system with combining forms for body parts; examples of terminology, pathology, and laboratory tests; and diagnostic and treatment procedures. ***Appendix 2,*** page 291, names and explains common diagnostic tests and procedures, and ***Appendix 3,*** page 311, defines medical abbreviations, acronyms, and symbols. ***Appendix 4,*** page 331, provides health careers information. The ***Mini-Dictionary: Glossary of Medical Terms,*** page 341, and the ***Glossary of Word Parts,*** page 375, contain definitions of terms and meanings of word parts, respectively. Use these valuable references as you work through this book.

Table 2-1 ORGANS/STRUCTURES AND SYSTEMS

Organ/Structure	System
1. Bronchial tubes	Respiratory
2. Cerebrum	Nervous
3. Coccyx (tailbone)	Musculoskeletal
4. Colon (large intestine)	Digestive
5. Esophagus (food tube)	Digestive
6. Kidneys	Urinary
7. Larynx (voice box)	Respiratory
8. Lungs	Respiratory
9. Ovaries	Female reproductive/endocrine
10. Pharynx (throat)	Digestive/respiratory
11. Pituitary gland	Endocrine
12. Prostate gland	Male reproductive
13. Spinal cord	Nervous
14. Trachea (windpipe)	Respiratory
15. Ureters	Urinary
16. Urethra	Urinary
17. Uterus	Female reproductive
18. Vertebrae (backbones)	Musculoskeletal

2

2

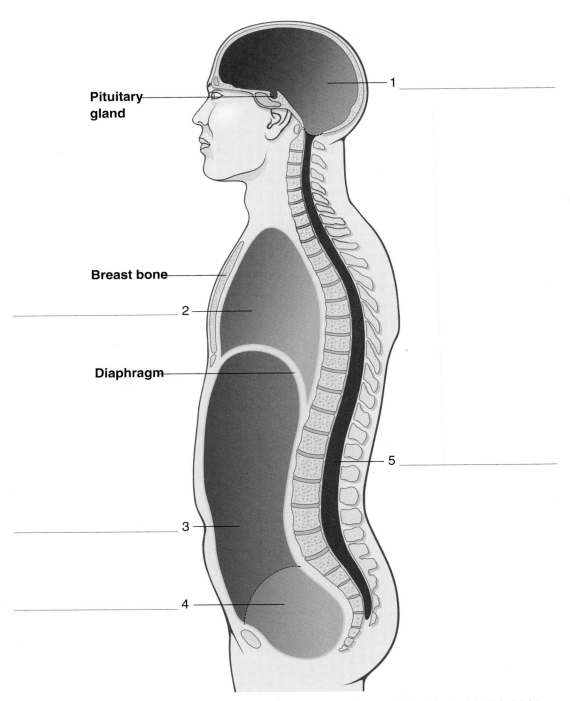

Pituitary gland

Breast bone

Diaphragm

1

2

3

4

5

Figure 2-2 • **Body cavities.** *(Modified from Chabner D-E:* The Language of Medicine, *ed 9, Philadelphia, 2011, Saunders.)*

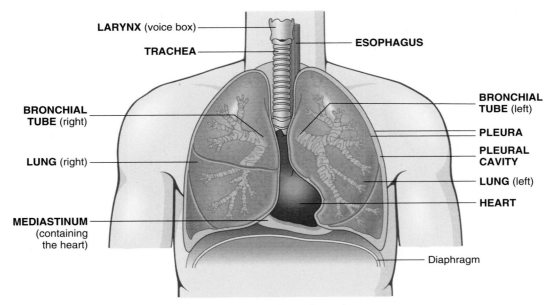

LARYNX (voice box)

TRACHEA

ESOPHAGUS

BRONCHIAL TUBE (right)

LUNG (right)

MEDIASTINUM (containing the heart)

BRONCHIAL TUBE (left)

PLEURA

PLEURAL CAVITY

LUNG (left)

HEART

Diaphragm

Figure 2-3 • Thoracic cavity.

Body Cavities

Figure 2-2 shows the five body cavities. A body cavity is a space that contains organs. Label the figure in the spaces provided as you read the following paragraphs.

The **cranial cavity** (1) is located in the head and surrounded by the skull (CRANI/O means skull). The cranial cavity contains the brain and other organs, such as the pituitary gland (an endocrine gland located below the brain).

The **thoracic cavity** (2), also known as the chest cavity (THORAC/O means chest), is surrounded by the breastbone and ribs. The lungs, heart, windpipe (trachea), bronchial tubes (leading from the trachea to the lungs), and other organs are in this cavity.

Figure 2-3 shows a front view of the thoracic cavity. The lungs are each surrounded by a double membrane known as the **pleura.** The space between the pleural membranes is the **pleural cavity.** The large area between the lungs (*yellow* in Figure 2-3) is the **mediastinum.** The heart, esophagus (food tube), trachea, and bronchial tubes are organs within the mediastinum.

In Figure 2-2, the **abdominal cavity** (3) is the space below the thoracic cavity. The **diaphragm** is the muscle that separates the abdominal and thoracic cavities. Organs in the abdomen include the stomach, liver, gallbladder, and small and large intestines.

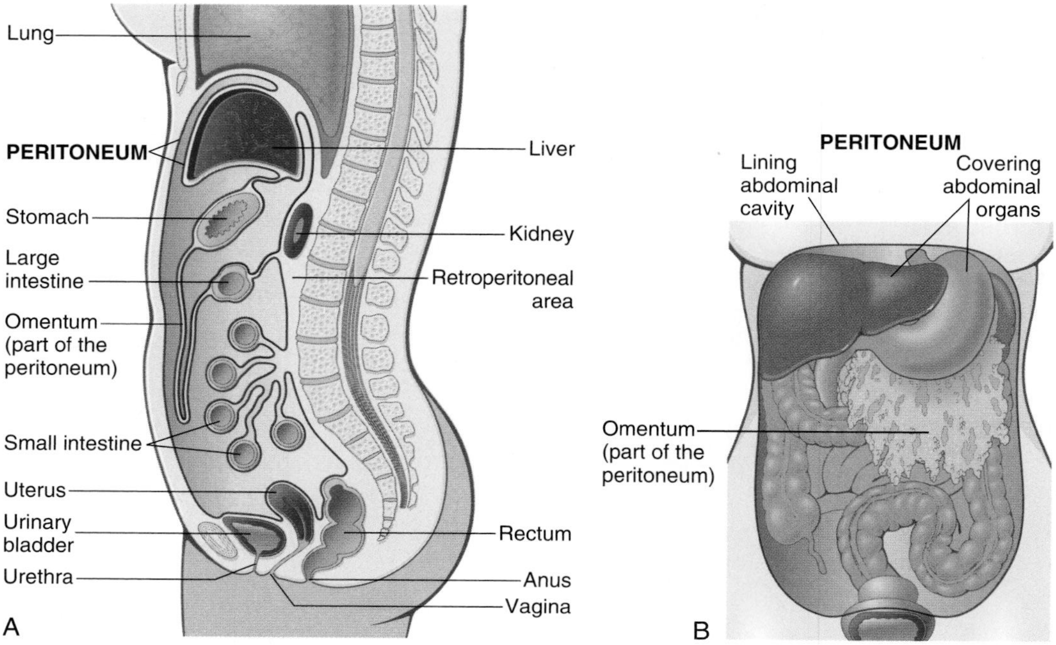

Lung

PERITONEUM

Liver

Stomach

Kidney

Large
intestine

Retroperitoneal
area

Omentum
(part of the
peritoneum)

Small intestine

Uterus

Urinary
bladder

Rectum

Urethra

Anus

Vagina

A

PERITONEUM

Lining
abdominal
cavity

Covering
abdominal
organs

Omentum
(part of the
peritoneum)

B

Figure 2-4 • **A,** The **peritoneum** (side view) surrounds the organs in the abdomen. **B,** Frontal view of the peritoneum.

2

The organs in the abdomen are covered by a double membrane called the **peritoneum** (Figure 2-4). The peritoneum attaches the abdominal organs to the abdominal muscles and surrounds each organ to hold it in place.

Turn back to Figure 2-2 and locate the **pelvic cavity** (4), below the abdominal cavity. The pelvic cavity is surrounded by the **pelvis** (bones of the hip). The major organs located within the pelvic cavity are the urinary bladder, ureters (tubes from the kidneys to the bladder), urethra (tube from the bladder to the outside of the body), rectum, and anus, and the uterus (muscular organ that nourishes the developing embryo and fetus) in females.

Label the spinal cavity (5) on Figure 2-2. This is the space surrounded by the **spinal column** (backbones). The **spinal cord** is the nervous tissue within the spinal cavity. Nerves enter and leave the spinal cord and carry messages to and from all parts of the body.

Double membrane

You can visualize the way organs are surrounded by a double membrane by imagining your fist pushing deep into a soft balloon. The balloon is then in two layers folded over your fist, just the way membranes such as the pleura and peritoneum surround an internal organ. Double wrapping around organs provides protection and cushioning as well as attachment to muscles. In the event of inflammation or disease to organs or membranes, fluid may collect in the space between the membranes and surrounding the organs. This collection of fluid in the pleural cavity is called a **pleural effusion**. The collection of fluid in the peritoneal cavity is called **ascites** (see page 62).

As a quick review of the terms presented in this section, match the term with its meaning and write it in the space provided.

TERM	MEANING

Abdominal cavity

1. Membrane surrounding the lungs _____

Cranial cavity

2. Space between the lungs, containing the heart

Diaphragm

_____

Mediastinum

3. Bones of the hip _____

Pelvic cavity

4. Space containing the liver, gallbladder, and stomach;

Pelvis

also called the abdomen _____

Peritoneum

5. Space within the backbones, containing the spinal cord

Pleura

_____

Spinal cavity

6. Membrane surrounding the organs in the abdomen

Thoracic cavity

_____

7. Space within the skull, containing the brain

_____

8. Space below the abdominal cavity, containing the

urinary bladder _____

9. Muscle between the thoracic and abdominal cavities

_____

10. Entire chest cavity, containing the lungs, heart, trachea,

esophagus, and bronchial tubes _____

2

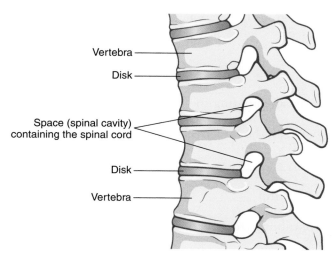

Vertebra —

Disk —

Space (spinal cavity)
containing the spinal cord

Disk —

Vertebra —

**Figure 2-5 • Vertebrae and disks
(discs).**

Divisions of the Back

The **spinal column** is a long row of bones from the neck to the tailbone. Each bone in the spinal column is called a **vertebra** (backbone). Two or more bones are called **vertebrae.**

A piece of flexible connective tissue, called a **disk** (or **disc**), lies between each backbone. The disk, composed of **cartilage,** is a cushion between the bones. If the disk slips or moves out of its place, it can press on the nerves that enter or leave the spinal cord, causing pain. Figure 2-5 shows a side view of vertebrae and disks.

The divisions of the spinal column are pictured in Figure 2-6. Label them according to the following list:

DIVISION	BONES	ABBREVIATION
1. **Cervical** (neck) region	7 bones	C1-C7
2. **Thoracic** (chest) region	12 bones	T1-T12
3. **Lumbar** (loin or waist) region	5 bones	L1-L5
4. **Sacral** (sacrum or lower back) region	5 fused bones	S1-S5
5. **Coccygeal** (coccyx or tailbone) region	4 fused bones	

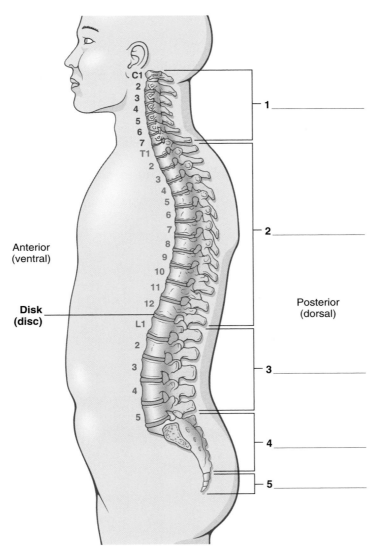

Anterior
(ventral)

Disk
(disc)

Posterior
(dorsal)

1 _____

2 _____

3 _____

4 _____

5 _____

Figure 2-6 • **Divisions of the back (spinal column).** *(Modified from Chabner D-E:* The Language of Medicine, *ed 9, Philadelphia, 2011, Saunders.)*

Planes of the Body

A plane is an imaginary flat surface. Organs appear in different relationships to one another according to the plane of the body in which they are viewed.

Figure 2-7 shows three planes of the body. Label them as you read the following descriptions:

1. **Frontal (coronal) plane**

   A vertical plane that divides the body, or body part such as an organ, into front and back portions.

   Anatomically, *anterior* means the front portion and *posterior* means the back portion.

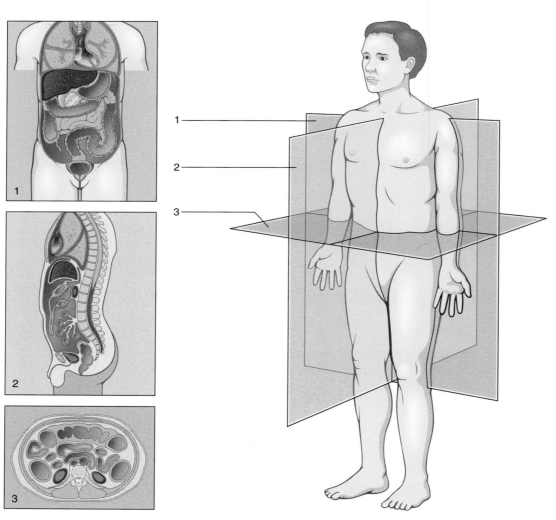

Figure 2-7 • Planes of the body.

2. **Sagittal (lateral) plane**   A vertical plane that divides the body or organ into right and left sides. The **midsagittal plane** divides the body vertically into right and left **halves.**

3. **Transverse (axial) plane**   A horizontal plane that divides the body or organ into upper and lower portions, as in a **cross section.** (Think of cutting a long loaf of French bread into circular sections.)

Knowing the planes of the body is helpful in looking at imaging studies such as x-ray films (radiographs) and computed tomography (CT) scans. See Figure 2-8.

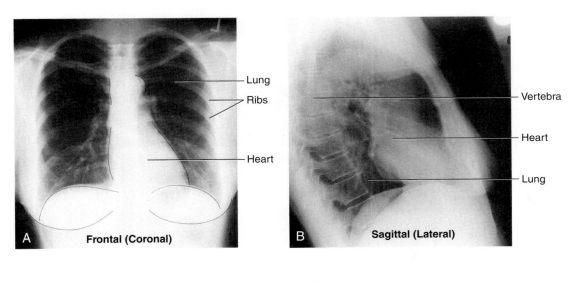

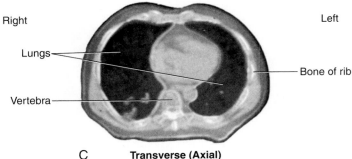

Figure 2-8 • X-ray views of the chest. A, Frontal (coronal) plane. X-ray is an anterior-posterior view of the chest. **B, Sagittal (lateral) plane.** This is a lateral (side) x-ray view of the chest. **C, Transverse (axial) plane.** This CT image is a snapshot of structures at a specific level of the body. (**A,** *Modified from Black JM, Matassarin-Jacobs E:* Medical-Surgical Nursing: Clinical Management for Continuity of Care, *ed 5, Philadelphia, 1997, Saunders.* **B,** *Modified from Weir J, Abrahams PH:* An Imaging Atlas of Human Anatomy, *ed 2, London, 2000, Mosby.* **C,** *From Chabner D-E:* The Language of Medicine, *ed 9, Philadelphia, 2011, Saunders.)*

Magnetic resonance imaging (MRI) is another technique for producing images of the body. With **MRI,** magnetic waves instead of x-rays are used to create the images, which show organs and other structures in specialized detail and in all three planes of the body (Figure 2-9). Figure 2-10 shows a patient undergoing MRI.

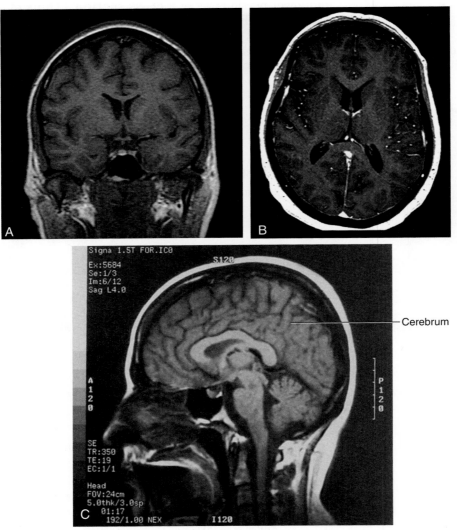

Figure 2-9 • **Magnetic resonance images.** Basic views are coronal, axial (transverse plane), and sagittal. **A, Frontal (coronal) plane** of the head. **B, Transverse plane (axial view, from top to bottom)** of the head. **C, Sagittal plane (lateral view)** showing the head and side of the brain. (**A** *and* **B,** *From Frank ED, et al:* Merrill's Atlas of Radiographic Positioning and Procedures, *ed 12, St Louis, 2012, Elsevier.* **C,** *Modified from Black JM, Matassarin-Jacobs E:* Medical-Surgical Nursing: Clinical Management for Continuity of Care, *ed 5, Philadelphia, 1997, Saunders.)*

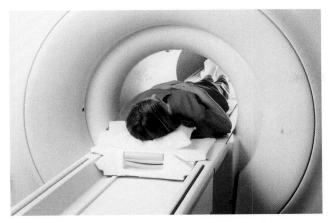

Figure 2-10 • Patient is inside an MRI unit, surrounded by a superconducting 1.5-tesla magnet. Magnetic field changes are picked up by the surrounding machine and processed by a computer to create images. For this examination, the patient must lie very still and have no metal objects on or within the body. *(Courtesy GE Medical Systems, Milwaukee, Wisconsin. From Frank ED, et al:* Merrill's Atlas of Radiographic Positions and Radiologic Procedures, *ed 11, St Louis, 2007, Mosby.)*

Terminology

Write the meanings of the medical terms on the line provided. Check your answers with the ***Mini-Dictionary Glossary of Medical Terms,*** page 341.

COMBINING FORMS

COMBINING FORM	MEANING	MEDICAL TERM	MEANING
abdomin/o	abdomen	abdominal _____	
anter/o	front	anterior _____ *The suffix* -IOR *means pertaining to.*	
bronch/o	bronchial tubes (leading from the windpipe to the lungs)	bronchoscopy _____	
cervic/o	*neck* of the body or *neck* (cervix) of the uterus	cervical _____ *You must decide from the context of what you are reading whether* **cervical** *means pertaining to the neck of the body or pertaining to the uterine cervix (lower portion of the uterus). Figure 2-11 shows the uterus and the cervix.*	

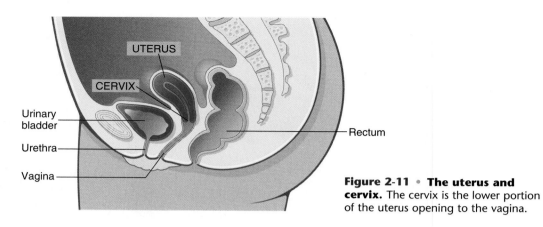

Figure 2-11 • **The uterus and cervix.** The cervix is the lower portion of the uterus opening to the vagina.

chondr/o   cartilage   hypochondriac _____

This term refers to the regions of the abdominopelvic cavity under the cartilage of the ribs. (Figure A on page 77 shows the abdominopelvic regions.) It also describes a person who experiences unusual anxiety about his or her health and has symptoms that cannot be explained. The Greeks thought that organs (liver and spleen) in the hypochondriac regions of the abdomen were the origin of imaginary illnesses.

coccyg/o   coccyx, tailbone   coccygeal _____
                                    -EAL means pertaining to.

crani/o   skull   craniotomy _____

epitheli/o skin, surface   epithelial _____
                tissue
*The term **epithelial** was first used to describe the surface (EPI means upon) of the breast nipple (THELI/O actually means nipple). More correctly, it describes the cells on the outer layer (surface) of the skin as well as the lining of the internal organs that lead to the outside of the body.*

esophag/o   esophagus (tube   esophageal _____
                from the throat
                to the stomach)

hepat/o   liver   hepatitis _____

lapar/o   abdomen   laparoscopy _____

laryng/o   larynx (voice   laryngeal _____
                box)   *The larynx (pronounced **LAR**-inks) is found in the upper part of the trachea.*

                laryngectomy _____

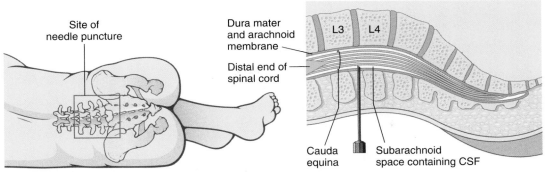

Site of needle puncture

Dura mater and arachnoid membrane

L3 L4

Distal end of spinal cord

Cauda equina

Subarachnoid space containing CSF

Figure 2-12 • **Lumbar puncture ("spinal tap").** The patient lies on his side with his knees drawn up to the abdomen and the chin brought down to the chest. This position increases the spaces between the vertebrae. The physician inserts a needle between the third and fourth (or fourth and fifth) lumbar vertebrae, and cerebrospinal fluid (CSF) is withdrawn, or medication can be injected. The distal end of the spinal cord is where the spinal nerves begin to fan out toward the legs. Performing a lumbar puncture below this level avoids injury to the spinal cord. *(Modified from Chabner D-E:* The Language of Medicine, *ed 9, Philadelphia, 2011, Saunders.)*

later/o	side	lateral _____
lumb/o	loin (waist)	lumbar _____

-AR *means pertaining to. A lumbar puncture ("spinal tap") is the placement of a needle within the membranes in the lumbar region of the spinal cord to inject or withdraw fluid. See Figure 2-12.*

lymph/o	lymph (clear fluid in tissue spaces and lymph vessels)	lymphocyte _____

Lymphocytes are white blood cells that fight disease. One type of lymphocyte (B cell) produces disease-fighting proteins called **antibodies.**

mediastin/o	mediastinum (space between the lungs)	mediastinal _____
pelv/o	pelvis (bones of the hip)	pelvic _____
peritone/o	peritoneum (membrane surrounding the abdominal organs)	peritoneal _____

Peritoneal fluid, produced by the peritoneal membrane, lubricates the surfaces of the peritoneum to prevent friction. With inflammation of the peritoneum or disease affecting abdominal organs, fluid may accumulate in the peritoneal cavity. This accumulation of fluid is called **ascites** *(see Figure 2-13).*

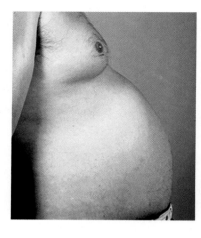

Figure 2-13 • **Ascites.** Abnormal intraperitoneal fluid can result from conditions such as liver disease, peritonitis, and ovarian cancer. *(From Lewis SM, Heitkemper MM, Dirksen SR:* Medical-Surgical Nursing, *ed 6, St Louis, 2004, Mosby.)*

pharyng/o	pharynx (throat)	pharyngeal _____

*The pharynx (pronounced **FAR**-inks) is the common passageway for food from the mouth and air from the nose. See Figure 2-14.*

pleur/o	pleura	pleuritis _____
poster/o	back, behind	posterior _____

2

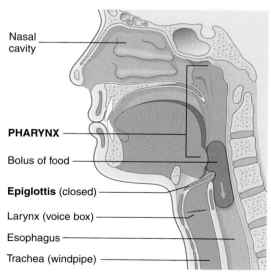

Nasal cavity

PHARYNX

Bolus of food

Epiglottis (closed)

Larynx (voice box)

Esophagus

Trachea (windpipe)

Figure 2-14 • **Pharynx.** Notice that the **epiglottis** (a flap of cartilage) closes over the trachea during swallowing so that the bolus (mass) of food travels down the esophagus and not the windpipe. *(Modified from Chabner D-E:* The Language of Medicine, *ed 9, Philadelphia, 2011, Saunders.)*

sacr/o	sacrum (five fused bones in the lower back)	sacral _____
spin/o	spine (backbone)	spinal _____
thorac/o	chest	thoracotomy _____
		thoracic _____
trache/o	trachea (windpipe)	tracheotomy _____ *See Figure 2-15.*
vertebr/o	vertebra (backbone)	vertebral _____

Don't confuse sacr/o and sarc/o

Notice the difference in spelling! Sacr/o always refers to the sacrum, a part of the back, while sarc/o means flesh and is used in **sarcoma**, a malignant tumor of connective or fleshy tissue of the body.

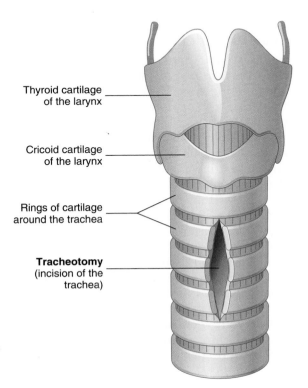

Thyroid cartilage of the larynx

Cricoid cartilage of the larynx

Rings of cartilage around the trachea

Tracheotomy (incision of the trachea)

Figure 2-15 • **Tracheotomy.** This procedure may be performed to open the trachea below a blockage from a foreign body or tumor. For an emergency procedure, any available instrument, even the barrel of a ballpoint pen, with the inner part removed, can be used to keep the airway open.

IN PERSON

The following first-person narrative provides a detailed look at two common diagnostic procedures—CT and MRI—from the perspective of the patient. It was written by a 77-year-old woman with head and neck cancer.

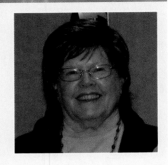

CT—Computed Tomography

Before an upcoming surgical procedure, I was told that I would need to have a CT scan. The doctors wanted to see if the cancer on my scalp had spread into the bones in my skull. They explained that these images of my head would be in thin "slices," taken as the CT camera rotated around me.

When I arrived in the room, I saw the CT machine. It was a large, circular hollow tube about 18 inches wide. There was a narrow table through the center. It was clear to me immediately that I would not have to worry about feeling "closed in." I lay down on the table, and the technician explained he would add contrast through an intravenous (IV) line halfway through the procedure.

The table was rolled into the machine to a specific spot where a series of pictures were taken. There were several short periods when I was asked to stay as still as possible and hold my breath. The noise was minimal, just soft whirring and clicking. Halfway through the procedure, I was slid out of the machine on the table so that the contrast could be added to the IV line. Once I was back in the machine, more pictures were taken and the test was completed with a minimum of discomfort, much to my grateful surprise.

MRI—Magnetic Resonance Imaging

Before yet another surgery procedure, my doctors requested an MRI exam. This time, they wanted to get the best possible image of my malignant tumor and the surrounding area. They explained that the MRI and CT procedures are similar in that they both produce images in thin slices, but that MRI shows more detail, especially of soft tissue.

The technician confirmed I had nothing metal (such as a pacemaker or surgical screws) inside or on my body. The magnet that is used in the MRI machine is so strong that it could cause any metal objects to shift. This movement could disrupt the imaging process or cause damage to tissue in my body.

The MRI machine is a 6-foot-long round tube, open on both ends. Because the body part to be examined was my head, a rubber shield was placed over and very close to my face to hold me in the correct position. I was then rolled inside to the middle of the tube. This was really uncomfortable for me because I have mild claustrophobia. I took deep breaths to relax myself.

Although the technicians had told me the procedure would be loud, I was still taken aback by just how loud it was inside the tube. Even though I was wearing earplugs, the sound was like the pounding of huge hammers held by giant arms, or of heavy-duty jackhammers. At the same time, there was an abrupt shaking of the entire machine from side to side. I knew immediately that this could be an overwhelming experience, so I used the "relax-substitution" method to replace these

2

violent sounds with more familiar ones. I remembered a very loud time as my family and I made our way to Nantucket Island on a ferry for a brief vacation. Now the previously strident and threatening sound was replaced by the welcoming sound of the ferry horn bellowing a happy welcome to the visitors' smiling faces as they came onto the ferry with straw hats, sunscreen, backpacks, and duffel bags. This relaxation method was extremely effective for me. I was then rolled out of the machine for addition of the IV contrast, and the process was repeated.

I am still amazed that the doctors could get such detailed information on what was going on inside my body using these two tests.

? EXERCISES AND ANSWERS

Complete these exercises and check your answers. An important part of your success in learning medical terminology is checking your answers carefully with the Answer to Exercises on page 71. Be sure to visit the Evolve website which has additional information, images, games, videos, and interactive activities.

Ⓐ   Match the following systems of the body with their functions.

circulatory	musculoskeletal	respiratory
digestive	nervous	skin and sense organs
endocrine	reproductive	urinary

1. Produces urine and sends it out of the body _____

2. Secretes hormones that are carried by blood to other organs _____

3. Supports the body and helps it move _____

4. Takes food into the body and breaks it down to be absorbed into the bloodstream

_____

5. Transports food, gases, and other substances through the body _____

_____

6. Moves air into and out of the body _____

7. Produces the cells that unite to form a new baby _____

8. Receives messages from the environment and sends them to the brain _____

_____

9. Carries electrical messages to and from the brain and spinal cord _____

_____

B Select from the following body systems to match the organ or tissue that is found within the system.

cardiovascular	digestive	endocrine
female reproductive	lymphatic	male reproductive
musculoskeletal	nervous	respiratory
skin and sense organs	urinary	

1. brain _____

2. cartilage _____

3. kidney _____

4. liver _____

5. heart _____

6. bronchial tubes _____

7. cervix _____

8. epidermis _____

9. adrenal glands _____

10. testes _____

C Use the following terms to complete the chart below. Give the name of the cavity and an organ that is contained within the cavity.

abdominal	lungs	stomach
brain	pelvic	thoracic
cranial	spinal	urinary bladder
heart	spinal cord	uterus

	CAVITY	ORGAN
1. Space located within the bones of the hip	_____	_____
2. Space located within the skull	_____	_____
3. Space located within the chest	_____	_____
4. Space located within the abdomen	_____	_____
5. Space located within the backbones	_____	_____

D Complete the following sentences using the terms listed below.

abdomen (abdominal   mediastinum   spinal column
   cavity)   pelvis   spinal cord
diaphragm   peritoneum   vertebra
disk (disc)   pleura

1. The bones of the hip are the _____.

2. The muscle separating the chest and the abdomen is the _____.

3. The membrane surrounding the organs in the abdomen is the_____.

4. The membrane surrounding the lungs is the_____.

5. The space between the lungs in the chest is the_____.

6. The space that contains organs such as the stomach, liver, gallbladder, and

   intestines is the _____.

7. The backbones are the _____.

8. The nerves running down the back form the _____.

9. A single backbone is a _____.

10. A piece of cartilage in between two backbones is a _____.

E Name the five divisions of the spinal column from the neck to the tailbone.

1. c ___ ___ ___ ___ ___ ___ ___

2. t ___ ___ ___ ___ ___ ___ ___

3. l ___ ___ ___ ___ ___

4. s ___ ___ ___ ___ ___

5. c ___ ___ ___ ___ ___ ___ ___ ___

2

F Match the following terms with their meanings below.

anterior	frontal (coronal) plane	sagittal plane
cartilage	MRI	transverse (axial) plane
CT scan	posterior	

1. Pertaining to the back _____

2. Pertaining to the front _____

3. A plane that divides the body into an upper and a lower part _____

4. An image of the body using magnetic waves; all three planes of the body are

   viewed _____

5. A plane that divides the body into right and left parts _____

6. Flexible connective tissue found between bones at joints _____

7. A plane that divides the body into front and back parts _____

8. Series of cross-sectional x-ray images_____

G Give meanings for the following terms.

1. craniotomy _____

2. abdominal _____

3. pelvic _____

4. thoracic _____

5. mediastinal _____

6. epithelial _____

7. tracheotomy _____

8. peritoneal _____

9. hepatitis _____

10. cervical _____

11. lymphocyte _____

12. lateral _____

13. bronchoscopy _____

14. diaphragm _____

15. pleura _____

16. hypochondriac _____

H **Match the following terms with their meanings below.**

coccygeal	laparotomy	pleuritis
epithelial	laryngeal	sacral
esophageal	lumbar	thoracotomy
laparoscopy	pharyngeal	vertebral

1. Pertaining to the loin (waist) region below the thoracic vertebrae _____

2. Pertaining to skin (lining or surface) cells _____

3. Incision of the abdomen _____

4. Pertaining to the tube from the throat to stomach _____

5. Pertaining to the voice box _____

6. Inflammation of the membrane surrounding the lungs _____

7. Pertaining to the throat _____

8. Pertaining to the sacrum _____

9. Incision of the chest _____

10. Pertaining to the tailbone _____

11. Visual examination of the abdomen _____

12. Pertaining to backbones _____

I **Circle the boldface term that best completes the meaning of the sentences in the following medical vignettes.**

1. After her car accident, Cathy had severe neck pain. An MRI study revealed a protruding (**diaphragm, disk, uterus**) between C6 and C7. The doctor asked her to wear a (**sacral, cervical, cranial**) collar for several weeks.

2. Mr. Sellar was a heavy smoker all his adult life. He began coughing and losing weight and became very lethargic (tired). His physician suspected a tumor of the **(musculoskeletal, urinary, respiratory)** system. A chest CT scan showed a **(lung, pharyngeal, spinal)** mass. Dr. Baker performed **(laparoscopy, craniotomy, bronchoscopy)** to biopsy the lesion.

3. Grace had never seen a gynecologist. She had pain in her **(cranial, pelvic, thoracic)** cavity and increasing **(abdominal, vertebral, laryngeal)** girth (size). Dr. Hawk suspected a/an **(esophageal, ovarian, mediastinal)** tumor after palpating (examining by touch) a mass.

4. Mr. Cruise worked in the shipyards for several years during World War II. Now, many years later, his doctor encouraged him to stop smoking because of a recently discovered link between asbestos, smoking, and the occurrence of mesothelioma (malignant tumor of cells of the pleura or the membrane surrounding the lungs). A routine chest x-ray film had shown thickening of the **(esophagus, pleura, trachea)** on both sides of Mr. Cruise's **(abdominal, spinal, thoracic)** cavity.

5. Kelly complained of headaches, together with nausea, disturbances of vision, and loss of coordination in her movements. Also, she had generalized weakness and stiffness on one side of her body. Dr. Brown suspected a tumor of the central **(circulatory, digestive, nervous)** system. Treatment involved a **(thoracotomy, craniotomy, laryngectomy)** to remove the lesion (mass) in her brain.

6. Mr. Smith experienced increasing weakness and loss of movement in his left arm and left leg. He saw his family doctor, who immediately referred him to a **(neurologist, cardiologist, rheumatologist).** This specialist examined him and sent him to **(pathology, hematology, radiology)** for x-ray imaging. (Results are shown in Figure 2-16.) This image is a/an **(MRI, CT scan, AP film).** The imaging clearly showed a large white region in the brain, indicating an area of dead tissue. Mr. Smith's doctor informed him that he had had a stroke, which also is known as a **(pituitary gland tumor, myocardial infarction, CVA or cerebrovascular accident).**

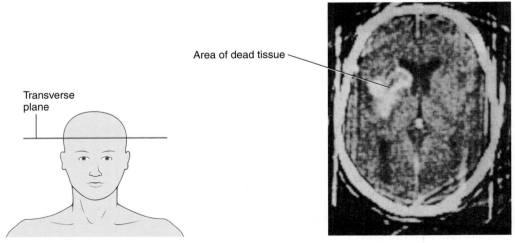

Figure 2-16 • Cross-sectional x-ray image of Mr. Smith's head.

ANSWERS TO EXERCISES

A
1. urinary
2. endocrine
3. musculoskeletal
4. digestive
5. circulatory
6. respiratory
7. reproductive
8. skin and sense organs
9. nervous

B
1. nervous
2. musculoskeletal
3. urinary
4. digestive
5. cardiovascular
6. respiratory
7. female reproductive
8. skin and sense organs
9. endocrine
10. male reproductive

C
1. pelvic (urinary bladder, uterus)
2. cranial (brain)
3. thoracic (lungs, heart)
4. abdominal (stomach)
5. spinal (spinal cord)

D
1. pelvis
2. diaphragm
3. peritoneum
4. pleura
5. mediastinum
6. abdomen (abdominal cavity)
7. spinal column
8. spinal cord
9. vertebra
10. disk (disc)

E
1. cervical   2. thoracic   3. lumbar   4. sacral   5. coccygeal

F
1. posterior
2. anterior
3. transverse (axial) plane
4. MRI
5. sagittal plane
6. cartilage
7. frontal (coronal) plane
8. CT scan

G
1. incision of the skull
2. pertaining to the abdomen
3. pertaining to the pelvis (bones of the hip)
4. pertaining to the chest
5. pertaining to the mediastinum (the space between the lungs)
6. pertaining to skin (lining or surface) cells
7. incision of the trachea (windpipe)
8. pertaining to the peritoneum (the membrane surrounding the organs in the abdomen)
9. inflammation of the liver
10. pertaining to the neck of the body, or neck (cervix) of the uterus
11. lymph cell (a type of white blood cell)
12. pertaining to the side
13. visual examination of bronchial tubes using an endoscope
14. muscle separating the abdomen from the chest
15. membrane surrounding the lungs
16. pertaining to under the cartilage of the rib (two upper lateral areas of the abdomen); or describing a person with unusual anxiety about symptoms that cannot be explained

H
1. lumbar
2. epithelial
3. laparotomy
4. esophageal
5. laryngeal
6. pleuritis
7. pharyngeal
8. sacral
9. thoracotomy
10. coccygeal
11. laparoscopy
12. vertebral

I
1. disk, cervical
2. respiratory, lung, bronchoscopy
3. pelvic, abdominal, ovarian
4. pleura, thoracic
5. nervous, craniotomy
6. neurologist, radiology, CT scan, CVA or cerebrovascular accident (stroke)

2

PRONUNCIATION OF TERMS

The terms that you have learned in this chapter are presented here with their pronunciations. The capitalized letters in **BOLDFACE** *represent the accented syllable. Pronounce each word out loud; then write the meaning in the space provided. Meanings of terms are found in the* ***Mini-Dictionary: Glossary of Medical Terms,*** *beginning on page 341, and on the audio section of the Evolve website (http://evolve.elsevier.com/Chabner/medtermshort).*

TERM	PRONUNCIATION	MEANING
abdomen	**AB**-do-men	
abdominal cavity	ab-**DOM**-in-al **KAV**-ih-te	
anterior	an-**TE**-re-or	
bronchial tubes	**BRON**-ke-al tubz	
bronchoscopy	bron-**KOS**-ko-pe	
cartilage	**KAR**-tih-lij	
cervical	**SER**-vih-kal	
circulatory system	**SER**-ku-lah-tor-e **SIS**-tem	
coccygeal	kok-sih-**JE**-al	
coccyx	**KOK**-siks	
cranial cavity	**KRA**-ne-al **KAV**-ih-te	
craniotomy	kra-ne-**OT**-o-me	
diaphragm	**DI**-ah-fram	
digestive system	di-**JES**-tiv **SIS**-tem	
disk (disc)	disk	
endocrine system	**EN**-do-krin **SIS**-tem	
epithelial	ep-ih-**THE**-le-al	
esophageal	eh-sof-ah-**JE**-al	
esophagus	eh-**SOF**-ah-gus	

female reproductive system	**FE**-mal re-pro-**DUK**-tiv **SIS**-tem _____
frontal plane	**FRUN**-tal plan _____
hepatitis	hep-ah-**TI**-tis _____
hypochondriac	hi-po-**KON**-dre-ak _____
laparoscopy	lap-ah-**ROS**-ko-pe_____
laparotomy	lap-ah-**ROT**-o-me _____
laryngeal	lah-**RIN**-je-al _or_ lah-rin-**JE**-al _____
laryngectomy	lah-rin-**JEK**-to-me _____
larynx	**LAR**-inks _____
lateral	**LAT**-er-al _____
lumbar	**LUM**-bar_____
lymphocyte	**LIMF**-o-site _____
mediastinal	me-de-ahs-**TI**-nal _____
mediastinum	me-de-ahs-**TI**-num _____
musculoskeletal system	mus-ku-lo-**SKEL**-eh-tal **SIS**-tem _____
nervous system	**NER**-vus **SIS**-tem _____
ovary	**O**-vah-re _____
pelvic cavity	**PEL**-vik **KAV**-ih-te _____
pelvis	**PEL**-vis_____
peritoneal	per-ih-to-**NE**-al _____
peritoneum	per-ih-to-**NE**-um _____
pharyngeal	fah-**RIN**-je-al _or_ fah-rin-**JE**-al_____
pharynx	**FAR**-inks _____

2

pituitary gland	pih-**TOO**-ih-teh-re gland
pleura	**PLOO**-rah
pleuritis	ploo-**RI**-tis
posterior	pos-**TER**-e-or
respiratory system	**RES**-pir-ah-tor-e **SIS**-tem
sacral	**SA**-kral
sacrum	**SA**-krum
sagittal plane	**SAJ**-ih-tal plan
spinal cavity	**SPI**-nal **KAV**-ih-te
spinal column	**SPI**-nal **KOL**-um
spinal cord	**SPI**-nal kord
thoracic cavity	tho-**RAS**-ik **KAV**-ih-te
thoracotomy	tho-rah-**KOT**-o-me
trachea	**TRAY**-ke-ah
tracheotomy	tray-ke-**OT**-o-me
transverse plane	trans-**VERS** plan
ureter	**YOOR**-eh-ter *or* u-**RE**-ter
urethra	u-**RE**-thrah
urinary system	**UR**-in-air-e **SIS**-tem
uterus	**U**-ter-us
vertebra	**VER**-teh-brah
vertebrae	**VER**-teh-bray
vertebral	**VER**-teh-bral

2

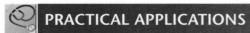

PRACTICAL APPLICATIONS

PROCEDURES

Select one of the procedures listed below to identify the descriptions in the following paragraphs. Answers are found on page 76.

bronchoscopy	laparotomy	thoracotomy
craniotomy	laryngectomy	tracheotomy
laparoscopy (peritoneoscopy)		

1. A skin incision is made, and muscle is stripped away from the skull. Four or five burr (or bur) holes are drilled into the skull. The bone between the holes is cut using a craniotome (bone saw). The bone flap is turned down or completely removed. After the bone flap is secured, the membrane surrounding the brain is incised and the

   brain is exposed. This procedure is a _____.

2. A major surgical incision is made into the chest for diagnostic or therapeutic purposes. One type of incision is a medial sternotomy (the sternum is the breastbone). A straight incision is made from the upper part of the sternum (suprasternal notch) to the lower end of the sternum (xiphoid process). The sternum must be cut with an electric or air-driven saw. The procedure is done to perform a biopsy or to locate sources of bleeding or injury. It often is performed to remove all

   or a portion of a lung. This procedure is a _____.

3. A needle is inserted below the umbilicus (navel) to inject carbon dioxide (a gas) into the abdomen. The gas distends (expands) the abdomen, permitting better visualization of the organs. A trocar (sharp-pointed instrument used to puncture the wall of a body cavity) within a cannula (tube) is inserted into an incision under the umbilicus. After the cannula is in place in the abdominal cavity, the trocar is removed and an endoscope is inserted through the cannula. The surgeon can then visualize the abdominopelvic cavity and reproductive organs. This procedure is a

   _____.

4. A flexible, fiberoptic endoscope is inserted through the mouth and down the throat and trachea to assess the tracheobronchial tree for tumors and obstructions, to obtain biopsy specimens, and to remove secretions and foreign bodies. This

   procedure is a _____.

2

PRINCIPAL DIAGNOSIS

The **principal diagnosis** *is the cause, after evaluation, of the patient's admission to the hospital. The patient's physician documents the finding during evaluation. After reading the following physician notes, you will be asked to identify the principal diagnosis for the case. Accurate assessment of the principal diagnosis is important for medical billing and coding.*

Physician Notes

A 67-year-old man with a 2-pack-a-day h/o [history of] smoking and hypertension [high blood pressure] presents to the ED [emergency department] complaining of hemoptysis [coughing up blood], fatigue, back pain on his right side, polyuria [frequent need to urinate], and headaches. The elevated BP [blood pressure], hemoptysis, and headaches require observation in the ED. The patient is admitted and diabetes is ruled out as a cause of polyuria. A chest x-ray for hemoptysis reveals a RLL [right lower lobe] mass. Needle biopsy confirms malignancy. The patient agrees to have a lobectomy performed. He is counseled on his tobacco use during recovery and he agrees to begin therapy for tobacco cessation.

Using the information presented in the physician notes, select the principal diagnosis from the following:

    A. Lung cancer—lower lobe (162.5)

    B. Hemoptysis (786.30)

    C. Polyuria (788.42)

    D. Headache (784.0)

    E. Hypertension (401.9)

(The numbers in parentheses are medical codes as given in the *International Classification of Diseases, Ninth Revision [ICD-9] Coding Handbook 2011.*)

ANSWERS TO PRACTICAL APPLICATIONS

Procedures

    1. craniotomy   3. laparoscopy (peritoneoscopy)
    2. thoracotomy   4. bronchoscopy

Principal Diagnosis

    Answer: A. Lung cancer—lower lobe
                     B. Hemoptysis is an **admitting diagnosis.***
                     C. Polyuria is a **POA (present on admission) diagnosis.**†
                     D. Headache is an **admitting diagnosis.**
                     E. Hypertension is an **admitting diagnosis.**

*An **admitting diagnosis** is a cause, before further evaluation, for admission to the hospital. Such conditions may not resolve in the ED and can become life-threatening without proper treatment.

†A **POA (present on admission) diagnosis** reflects incidental conditions that are noted and treated if necessary but are not a cause for hospital admission. Such conditions are not life-threatening (at the time of admission) but may require treatment and monitoring during the patient's stay.

PICTURE SHOW

Answer the questions that follow each image. Answers are found on page 79.

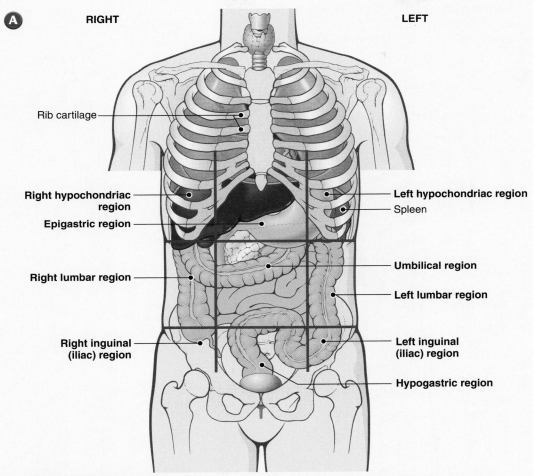

Abdominopelvic regions. *(Modified from Chabner D-E:* The Language of Medicine, *ed 9, Philadelphia, 2011, Saunders.)*

1. Which abdominopelvic regions are the middle lateral regions?
   a. epigastric
   b. lumbar (right and left)
   c. hypochondriac (right and left)
   d. inguinal (right and left)

2. Which abdominopelvic region lies above the stomach?
   a. epigastric
   b. inguinal (right and left)
   c. umbilical
   d. hypogastric

3. Which abdominopelvic regions lie under the cartilage of the ribs?
   a. hypogastric
   b. hypochondriac (right and left)
   c. umbilical
   d. inguinal (right and left)

4. Which lateral abdominopelvic regions are in the area of the groin (depression between the thigh and the trunk of the body)?
   a. umbilical
   b. hypochondriac (right and left)
   c. lumbar (right and left)
   d. inguinal (right and left)

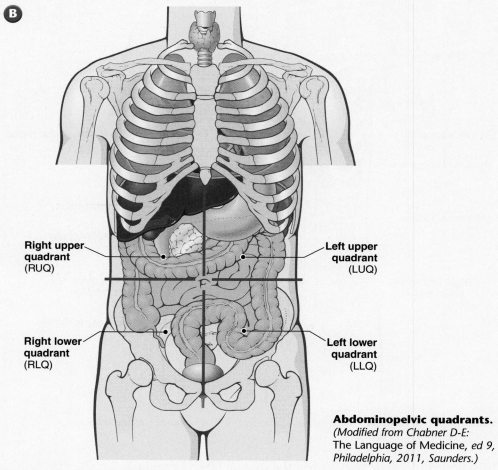

Abdominopelvic quadrants.
(Modified from Chabner D-E: The Language of Medicine, ed 9, Philadelphia, 2011, Saunders.)

1. A large organ in the RUQ is the:
   a. stomach
   b. lung
   c. heart
   d. liver

2. The spleen is located in which quadrant?
   a. LUQ
   b. RUQ
   c. RLQ
   d. LLQ

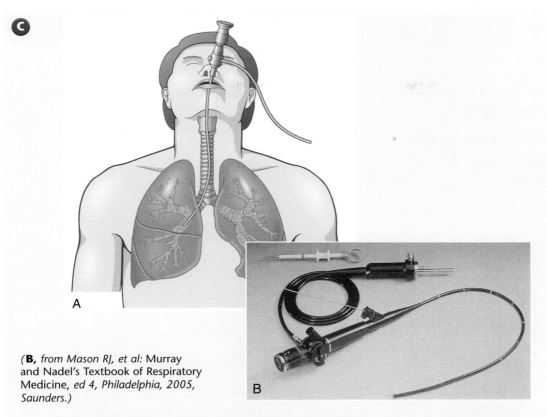

A

(**B,** *from Mason RJ, et al:* Murray and Nadel's Textbook of Respiratory Medicine, *ed 4, Philadelphia, 2005, Saunders.)*

B

1. In the procedure shown, an endoscope (pictured in **B**) is inserted into the mouth to visualize tubes leading to the lungs. This procedure is:
   a. laryngoscopy
   b. laparoscopy
   c. mediastinoscopy
   d. esophagoscopy
   e. bronchoscopy

2. The instrument is a/an:
   a. mediastinoscope
   b. laparoscope
   c. bronchoscope
   d. esophagoscope
   e. laryngoscope

ANSWERS TO PICTURE SHOW

A 1. b   2. a   3. b   4. d

B 1. d   2. a

C 1. e. This procedure is used for removing material (sputum) from the bronchial tubes, obtaining a biopsy specimen, or removing foreign bodies.
   2. c. This flexible bronchoscope permits passage of various instruments to obtain specimens from airways and lungs.

2

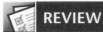

REVIEW

Write the meanings of the following combining forms and suffixes in the spaces provided. Check your answers with the Answers to Review on page 81. Meanings for word parts also are listed in the **Glossary of Word Parts** *beginning on page 375.* **Remember: The key to success is wRite, Repeat, Review!**

COMBINING FORMS

COMBINING FORM	MEANING	COMBINING FORM	MEANING
1. abdomin/o		14. lumb/o	
2. anter/o		15. lymph/o	
3. bronch/o		16. mediastin/o	
4. cervic/o		17. pelv/o	
5. chondr/o		18. peritone/o	
6. coccyg/o		19. pharyng/o	
7. crani/o		20. pleur/o	
8. epitheli/o		21. poster/o	
9. esophag/o		22. sacr/o	
10. hepat/o		23. spin/o	
11. lapar/o		24. thorac/o	
12. laryng/o		25. trache/o	
13. later/o		26. vertebr/o	

SUFFIXES

SUFFIX	MEANING	SUFFIX	MEANING
1. -ac _____		7. -ic _____	
2. -al _____		8. -itis _____	
3. -ar _____		9. -logy _____	
4. -cyte _____		10. -oma _____	
5. -eal _____		11. -scopy _____	
6. -ectomy _____		12. -tomy _____	

2

ANSWERS TO REVIEW

COMBINING FORMS

1. abdomen
2. front
3. bronchial tubes
4. neck
5. cartilage
6. tailbone
7. skull
8. skin
9. esophagus
10. liver
11. abdomen
12. voice box
13. side
14. loin, waist region
15. lymph
16. mediastinum
17. bones of the hip region
18. peritoneum
19. throat
20. pleura
21. back, behind
22. sacrum
23. backbone
24. chest
25. windpipe
26. backbone

SUFFIXES

1. pertaining to
2. pertaining to
3. pertaining to
4. cell
5. pertaining to
6. cutting out, removal, excision, resection
7. pertaining to
8. inflammation
9. study of
10. tumor, mass
11. process of visual examination
12. cutting into, incision, to cut into

✓ TERMINOLOGY CHECKUP

Before you leave this chapter, here are important concepts that you should thoroughly understand. Check the box next to each item when you know you've "got" it!

☐ 1. **Double membranes**: Remember that organs in the body are often covered and protected by double membranes. Examples are the ***pleura,*** a double membrane surrounding the lungs, and the ***peritoneum,*** a double membrane surrounding the abdominal organs. The ***pericardium*** is a double membrane surrounding the heart. In a later chapter, you will learn about the ***meninges,*** three membranes that surround the brain and spinal cord.

☐ 2. **Pharynx, larynx, trachea, and esophagus:** Don't confuse these four important parts of the body. The **pharynx** is the ***throat,*** which is the common passageway for air and food. The **larynx** is the ***voice box,*** which is located in the upper portion of the **trachea,** or ***windpipe.*** Two tubes branch from the pharynx. The **trachea** (in the front) carries air to the lungs, while the **esophagus** (behind the trachea) carries food to the stomach.

☐ 3. **Planes of the body:** Distinguishing among the three planes of the body is essential to understanding images such as x-rays, as well as CT and MRI scans. The ***frontal (coronal) plane*** divides the body into front and back (anterior/posterior) portions. The ***sagittal (lateral) plane*** divides the body into right and left sides. The ***transverse (axial) plane*** divides the body into upper and lower portions (cross sections). Frontal and sagittal plane images are obtained from traditional x-ray procedures. The transverse plane is seen only on CT and MRI scans. Visualizing organs in all three planes is possible with CT and MRI.

☐ 4. **Mediastinum:** The mediastinum is an important area of the chest. It is the ***space between the lungs*** containing the heart, large blood vessels (aorta and venae cavae), trachea, bronchial tubes, esophagus, and many lymph nodes.

☐ 5. **Spinal cord and spinal column:** The **spinal cord** is a bundle of ***nerves*** surrounded by the **spinal column,** a series of ***bones*** extending down the back. The sections of the spinal column and spinal cord are ***cervical, thoracic, lumbar, sacral,*** and ***coccygeal.*** The spinal cord ends in the lower lumbar region where the spinal nerves begin to fan out toward the legs.

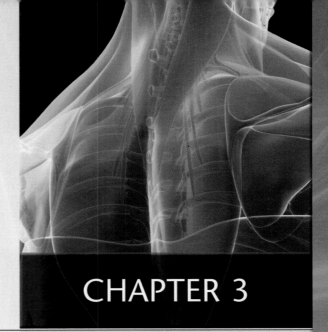

Suffixes

CHAPTER 3

CHAPTER OBJECTIVES

- To identify and define useful diagnostic and procedural suffixes
- To analyze, spell, and pronounce medical terms that contain diagnostic and procedural suffixes
- To apply medical terms in real-life situations

Introduction

This chapter reviews the suffixes that you have learned in the first two chapters and also introduces new suffixes and medical terms. The combining forms used in the chapter are listed below. Refer to this list as you write the meanings of the terms in the Suffixes and Terminology section that follows (beginning on page 85). Be faithful about completing all of the Exercises (page 105), and remember to check your answers on page 112 and 113! These exercises will help you spell terms correctly and understand their meanings. Test yourself by completing the Pronunciation of Terms on pages 114 to 117 and Review (page 123 and 124) and. Remember the 3 "Rs"—wRite, Review, Repeat—and you will succeed!

COMBINING FORMS

COMBINING FORM	MEANING
aden/o	gland
amni/o	amnion (sac of fluid surrounding the embryo)
angi/o	vessel (usually a blood vessel)
arteri/o	artery
arthr/o	joint
ather/o	plaque (a yellow, fatty material)
axill/o	armpit (underarm)
bronch/o	bronchial tube
bronchi/o	bronchial tube
carcin/o	cancerous
cardi/o	heart
chem/o	drug; also chemical
cholecyst/o	gallbladder
chron/o	time
col/o	colon (large intestine or bowel)
crani/o	skull
cry/o	cold
cyst/o	urinary bladder; also a sac of fluid or a cyst
electr/o	electricity
encephal/o	brain
erythr/o	red
esophag/o	esophagus (tube leading from the throat to the stomach)
hem/o	blood
hemat/o	blood
hepat/o	liver
hyster/o	uterus
inguin/o	groin (area in which the thigh meets the trunk of the body)
isch/o	to hold back
lapar/o	abdomen (abdominal wall)
laryng/o	voice box (larynx)

3

leuk/o	white
mamm/o	breast (use with -ARY, -GRAPHY, -GRAM, and -PLASTY)
mast/o	breast (use with -ECTOMY and -ITIS)
men/o	menses (menstruation); month
mening/o	meninges (membranes around the brain and spinal cord)
my/o	muscle
myel/o	spinal cord (nervous tissue connected to the brain, located within the spinal column. MYEL/O can also mean bone marrow (soft, inner part of bones, where blood cells are made)
necr/o	death (of cells)
nephr/o	kidney (use with all suffixes, except -AL and -GRAM; use REN/O with -AL and -GRAM)
neur/o	nerve
oophor/o	ovary
oste/o	bone
ot/o	ear
pelv/o	hip area
peritone/o	peritoneum (membrane surrounding organs in the abdomen)
phleb/o	vein
pneumon/o	lung
pulmon/o	lung
radi/o	x-rays
ren/o	kidney (use with -AL and -GRAM)
rhin/o	nose
salping/o	fallopian (uterine) tube
sarc/o	flesh
septic/o	pertaining to infection
thorac/o	chest
tonsill/o	tonsil
trache/o	windpipe; trachea
ur/o	urine or urea (a waste material); urinary tract
vascul/o	blood vessel

Suffixes and Terminology

Suffixes are divided into two groups: those that describe **diagnoses** and those that describe **procedures.**

DIAGNOSTIC SUFFIXES

Diagnostic suffixes describe disease conditions or their symptoms. Use the list of combining forms in the previous section to write the meaning of each term. You will find it helpful to check the meanings of the terms with the *Mini-Dictionary: Glossary of Medical Terms,* beginning on page 341.

NOUN SUFFIX	MEANING	TERMINOLOGY	MEANING
-algia	condition of pain, pain	arthralgia _____	
		otalgia _____	
		myalgia _____	
		neuralgia _____	
-emia	blood condition	leukemia _____	
		Increase in numbers of leukocytes; cells are malignant (cancerous).	
		septicemia 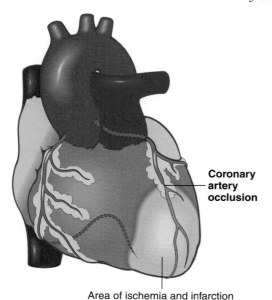 _____	
		Blood infections result when pathogens enter the blood from a wound.	
		ischemia _____	
		Figure 3-1 illustrates ischemia of heart muscle caused by blockage of a coronary (heart) artery.	

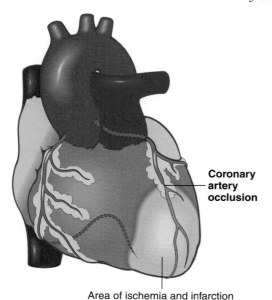

Coronary artery occlusion

Area of ischemia and infarction

Figure 3-1 • Ischemia of heart muscle. Blood is held back from an area of the heart muscle by an occlusion (blockage) of a coronary (heart) artery. The muscle then loses its supply of oxygen and nutrition and, if the condition persists, dies. The death of the affected part of the heart muscle is a myocardial infarction (heart attack). *(From Chabner D-E:* The Language of Medicine, *ed 9, Philadelphia, 2011, Saunders.)*

Septicemia and bacteremia

Bacteremia is bacterial invasion of the blood without or without symptoms. Septicemia (sepsis), however, is a more serious bacteremia that moves rapidly and may be life-threatening.

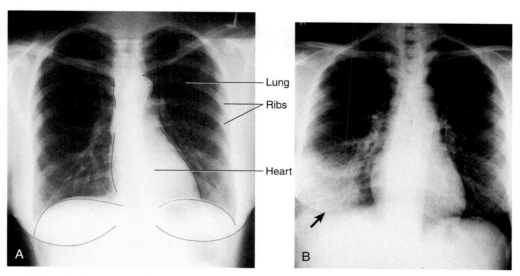

Figure 3-2 • **A, Chest x-ray** film showing **normal lungs. B,** Chest x-ray showing pneumonia in the right lower lobe of the lung (see arrow). (**A,** *From Mason RJ, et al:* Murray and Nadel's Textbook of Respiratory Medicine, *ed 4, Philadelphia, 2005, Saunders;* **B,** *from Mettler FA:* Essentials of Radiology, *ed 2, Philadelphia, 2005, Saunders.)*

		uremia _____
		Uremia occurs when the kidneys fail to function and urea (a waste material) accumulates in the blood.
-ia	condition	pneumonia _____
		The lung is inflamed, causing fluid and material to collect in the air sacs of the lung. See Figure 3-2.
-itis	inflammation	bronchitis _____
		Bronchial tubes are inflamed, with hypersecretion of mucus.
		esophagitis _____
		laryngitis _____
		meningitis _____
		The meninges are membranes that surround and protect the brain and spinal cord. See Figure 3-3.
		cystitis _____
		phlebitis _____
		colitis _____
		Table 3-1 lists other common inflammatory conditions with their meanings.

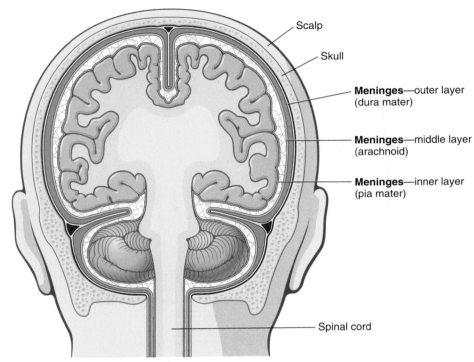

Figure 3-3 • **Meninges** (frontal view) are the membranes surrounding the brain and spinal cord.

Table 3-1 **INFLAMMATIONS**	
appendicitis	Inflammation of the appendix (hangs from the colon in the lower right abdomen)
bursitis	Inflammation of a small sac of fluid (bursa) near a joint
cellulitis	Inflammation of soft tissue under the skin
dermatitis	Inflammation of the skin
endocarditis	Inflammation of the inner lining of the heart (endocardium)
epiglottitis	Inflammation of the epiglottis (cartilage at the upper part of the windpipe)
gastritis	Inflammation of the stomach
hepatitis	Inflammation of the liver
myositis	Inflammation of muscle (MYOS/O means muscle)
nephritis	Inflammation of the kidney
osteomyelitis	Inflammation of bone and bone marrow
otitis	Inflammation of the ear
peritonitis	Inflammation of the peritoneum
pharyngitis	Inflammation of the throat
thrombophlebitis	Inflammation of a vein with formation of clots

3

-megaly	enlargement	cardiomegaly _____
		hepatomegaly _____
-oma	tumor, mass	adenoma _____

This is a benign (noncancerous) tumor.

adenocarcinoma _____

Carcinomas are malignant (cancerous) tumors of epithelial (skin or lining) tissue in the body. Glands and the linings of internal organs are composed of epithelial tissue. See Figure 3-4.

myoma _____

*This is a benign tumor. Myomas commonly occur in the uterus and are known as **fibroids**. See Figure 3-5.*

myosarcoma _____

Sarcomas are cancerous tumors of connective (flesh) tissue. Muscle, bone, cartilage, fibrous tissue, and fat are examples of connective tissues. See Table 3-2.

myeloma _____

*MYEL/O means bone marrow in this term. Also called **multiple myeloma,** this is a malignant tumor of cells (called plasma cells) in the bone marrow. See Table 3-3 for names of other malignant tumors that do not contain the combining forms CARCIN/O and SARC/O.*

3

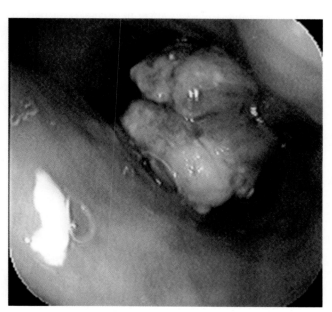

Figure 3-4 • **Esophageal adenocarcinoma.** *(Courtesy Dr. Erik-Jan Wamsteker: Gastroenterology. In Rakel RE, editor:* Textbook of Family Medicine, *ed 7, Philadelphia, 2007, Saunders.)*

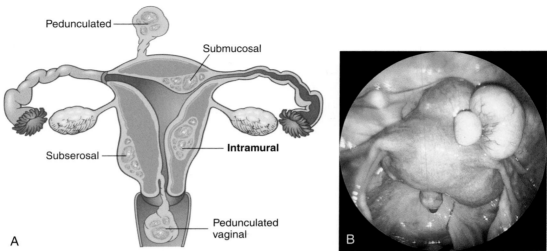

Figure 3-5 • **A, Location of uterine fibroids (leiomyomas). Pedunculated** growths protrude on stalks. A **subserosal** mass lies under the serosal (outermost) layer of the uterus. A **submucosal** leiomyoma grows under the mucosal (innermost) layer. **Intramural** (mural means wall) masses arise within the muscular uterine wall. **B, Multiple myomas viewed laparoscopically. (A,** *From Damjanov I:* Pathology for the Health-Related Professions, *ed 3, Philadelphia, 2006, Saunders;* **B,** *from Hunt RB:* Text and Atlas of Female Infertility Surgery, *ed 3, St Louis, 1999, Mosby.)*

Table 3-2 SARCOMAS

chondrosarcoma	Cancer of cartilage tissue (CHONDR/O means cartilage)
fibrosarcoma	Cancer of fibrous tissue (FIBR/O means fibrous tissue)
leiomyosarcoma	Cancer of visceral (attached to internal organs) muscle (LEIOMY/O means visceral or "smooth" muscle)
liposarcoma	Cancer of fatty tissue (LIP/O means fat)
osteogenic sarcoma	Cancer of bone
rhabdomyosarcoma	Cancer of skeletal (attached to bones) muscle (RHABDOMY/O means skeletal muscle)

Table 3-3 MALIGNANT TUMORS WHOSE NAMES DO NOT CONTAIN THE COMBINING FORMS *CARCIN/O* AND *SARC/O*

hepatoma	Malignant tumor of the liver *(hepatocellular carcinoma)*
lymphoma	Malignant tumor of lymph nodes (previously called lymphosarcoma)
melanoma	Malignant tumor of pigmented (MELAN/O means black) cells in the skin
mesothelioma	Malignant tumor of pleural cells (membrane surrounding the lungs)
multiple myeloma	Malignant tumor of bone marrow cells
thymoma	Malignant tumor of the thymus gland (located in the mediastinum)

-osis	condition, abnormal condition	nephrosis _____
		necrosis _____
		erythrocytosis _____
		When -OSIS is used with blood cell words, it means a slight increase in numbers of cells.
		leukocytosis _____
-pathy	disease condition	encephalopathy _____
		Pronunciation is en-sef-ah-**LOP**-ah-the.
		cardiomyopathy _____
		Pronunciation is kar-de-o-mi-**OP**-ah-the.
		nephropathy _____
		Pronunciation is neh-**FROP**-ah-the. *Table 3-4 lists other disease conditions.*

Leukocytosis versus leukemia

Leukocytosis—slight increase in normal white blood cells (WBCs)—is the body's response to bacterial infection. Leukemia is a malignant condition marked by dramatic increase in cancerous WBCs.

Cardiomyopathy and myocardial infarction

Cardiomyopathy is chronic (ongoing) disease of heart muscle with inflammation and weakness. A myocardial infarction (MI) is an area of heart muscle that has died as a result of ischemia. MI is also known as a heart attack.

Table 3-4 DISEASE CONDITIONS *(-PATHIES)*

adenopathy	Disease condition of lymph nodes ("glands"); lymphadenopathy
adrenopathy	Disease condition of the adrenal glands
hepatopathy	Disease condition of the liver
lymphadenopathy	Disease condition of the lymph nodes (previously called glands)
myopathy	Disease condition of muscles
neuropathy	Disease condition of nerves
osteopathy	Disease condition of bones
retinopathy	Disease condition of the retina of the eye

-rrhea	flow, discharge	rhino<u>rrhea</u> _____
		meno<u>rrhea</u> _____ _Normal menstrual flow._
-rrhage _or_ **-rrhagia**	excessive discharge of blood	hemo<u>rrhage</u> _____
		meno<u>rrhagia</u> _____ _Excessive bleeding during menstruation._
-sclerosis	hardening	arterio<u>sclerosis</u> _____ **Atherosclerosis** _is the most common type of_ _arteriosclerosis. A fatty plaque (atheroma) collects on the_ _lining of arteries. See Figure 3-6._
-uria	condition of urine	hemat<u>uria</u> _____ _Bleeding into the urinary tract can cause this sign of_ _kidney disease or of disorders of the urinary and genital_ _tracts._

All of the following **adjective suffixes** mean _pertaining to_ and describe a part of the body, process, or condition. Don't worry about which suffix (-al, -eal, -ar, -ary, or -ic) to use with a particular organ or root. Just identify the suffix as meaning "pertaining to" in each term.

-al _or_ **-eal**	pertaining to	periton<u>eal</u> _____
		inguin<u>al</u> _____
		ren<u>al</u> _____
		esophag<u>eal</u> _____
		myocardi<u>al</u> _____ _Don't forget that a heart attack is a_ **myocardial** **infarction (MI).** _An infarction is an area of dead tissue_ _caused by_ **ischemia** _(a condition in which blood supply_ _is held back from a part of the body)._

 Menorrhea and menorrhagia

Menorrhea is the normal discharge of blood and tissue from the lining of the uterus; menorrhagia is abnormally heavy or long menstrual periods. Chronic menorrhagia can result in anemia. Menorrhagia is a common complication of uterine myomas or fibroids.

 Hematuria and uremia

Hematuria is blood in the urine, whereas uremia is high levels of urea in the blood.

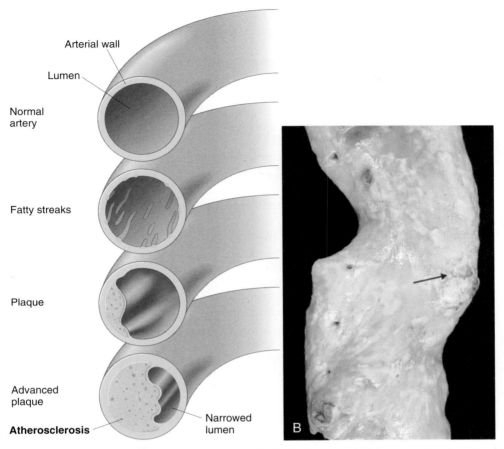

Figure 3-6 • **Atherosclerosis** (a type of arteriosclerosis). **A,** A fatty material (cholesterol) collects in an artery, narrowing it and eventually blocking the flow of blood. **B,** Photo of resected aorta with mild atherosclerotic disease.

-ar	pertaining to	vascular _____
		*A **cerebrovascular accident (CVA)** is a stroke.*
-ary	pertaining to	axillary _____
		mammary _____
		pulmonary _____
-ic	pertaining to	chronic _____
		*Chronic conditions occur over a long period of time, as opposed to **acute** conditions, which are sharp, sudden, and brief.*
		pelvic _____

PROCEDURAL SUFFIXES

The following suffixes describe *procedures* used in patient care.

SUFFIX	MEANING	TERMINOLOGY	MEANING
-centesis	surgical puncture to remove fluid	thoracentesis _____ *This term is a shortened form of thoracocentesis. See Figure 3-7.*	
		amniocentesis _____ *See Figure 3-8.*	
		arthrocentesis _____	
-ectomy	removal, resection, excision	tonsillectomy _____ *Tonsils and adenoids are lymph tissue in the pharynx (throat). Lymph is composed of white blood cells that fight infection. See Figure 3-9.*	
		hysterectomy _____ *In a **total hysterectomy,** the entire uterus, including the cervix, is removed. If only a portion of the uterus is removed, the procedure is a partial or **subtotal hysterectomy.** See Figure 3-10 on page 96.*	

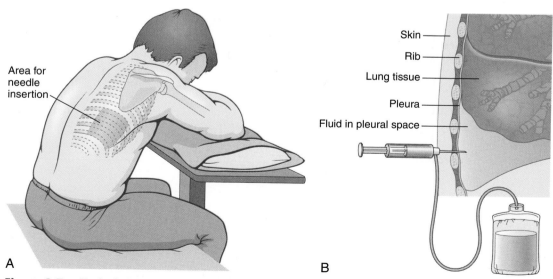

Area for needle insertion

Skin
Rib
Lung tissue
Pleura
Fluid in pleural space

A

B

Figure 3-7 • Technique of thoracentesis. A, The patient is sitting in the correct position for the procedure. **B,** The needle is advanced, and the fluid (pleural effusion) is drained.

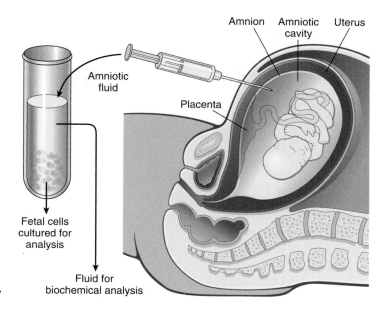

Figure 3-8 • **Amniocentesis.**

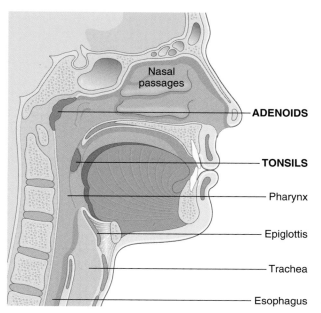

Figure 3-9 • **Tonsils and adenoids.**
Removal of the tonsils and adenoids is called
**tonsillectomy and adenoidectomy
(T&A).**

3

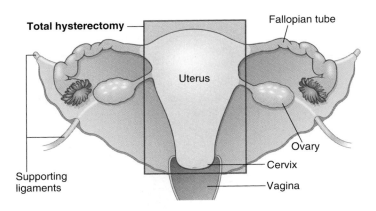

Figure 3-10 • **Total hysterectomy.** In a total abdominal hysterectomy (TAH), the uterus is removed through the abdomen. A TAH-BSO is a total abdominal hysterectomy with bilateral salpingectomy and oophorectomy. Laparoscopic hysterectomy can be performed as well.

oophorectomy _____

Figure 3-11 shows a laparoscopic oophorectomy.

salpingectomy _____

cholecystectomy _____

See Figure 3-12. Laparoscopic cholecystectomy is performed whenever possible, instead of an open (more invasive) procedure.

mastectomy _____

Table 3-5 lists additional resection procedures.

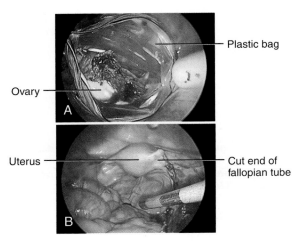

Figure 3-11 • **Laparoscopic oophorectomy. A,** Notice the ovary within a plastic bag. The bag was inserted through the laparoscope and then opened, and the ovary was placed inside. **B,** Both are extracted through the laparoscope, leaving the uterus and the cut end of the fallopian tube. *(Courtesy Dr. A. K. Goodman, Massachusetts General Hospital, Boston.)*

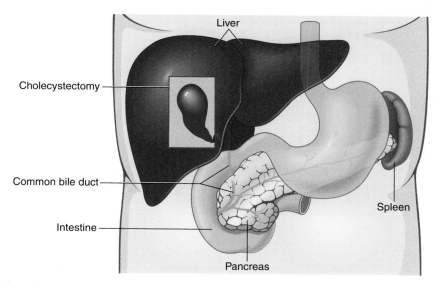

Figure 3-12 • Cholecystectomy. The liver is lifted up to show the gallbladder underneath. The pancreas is a long, thin gland located behind and to the left of the stomach, toward the spleen. The common bile duct carries bile from the liver and gallbladder to the intestine. After cholecystectomy, the liver continues to produce bile and release it, via the common bile duct, into the intestine.

Table 3-5 RESECTIONS	
adenectomy	Excision of a gland
adenoidectomy	Excision of the adenoids
appendectomy	Excision of the appendix
colectomy	Excision of the colon
gastrectomy	Excision of the stomach
laminectomy	Excision of a piece of backbone (lamina) to relieve pressure on nerves from a (herniating) disk
myomectomy	Excision of a muscle tumor (commonly a fibroid of the uterus)
pneumonectomy	Excision of lung tissue: total pneumonectomy (an entire lung) or lobectomy (a single lobe)
prostatectomy	Excision of the prostate gland
splenectomy	Excision of the spleen

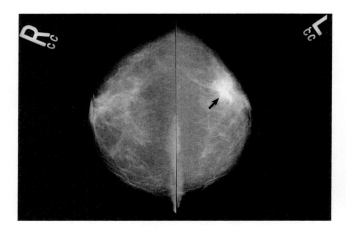

Figure 3-13 • Mammograms from a 63-year-old woman. The right breast is normal, and the left breast contains a carcinoma (breast cancer) *(arrow)*. *(From Frank ED, et al:* Merrill's Atlas of Radiographic Positions and Radiologic Procedures, *ed 11, vol 2, St Louis, 2007, Mosby.)*

-gram   record   myelo<u>gram</u> _____

MYEL/O *means spinal cord in this term. Contrast material is injected into the membranes around the spinal cord (by lumbar puncture), and then x-ray pictures are taken of the spinal cord. This procedure is performed less frequently now that MRI is available.*

                                    mammo<u>gram</u> _____
                                    See Figure 3-13.

-graphy   process of recording   electroencephalo<u>graphy</u> _____

                                    mammo<u>graphy</u> _____
                                    See Figure 3-14.

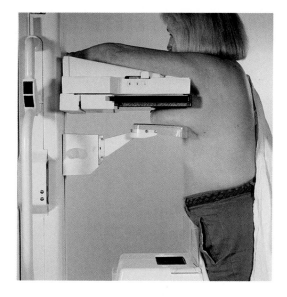

Figure 3-14 • **Mammography.** The breast is compressed, and x-ray images, craniocaudal (top to bottom) and lateral, are taken. *(From Frank ED, et al:* Merrill's Atlas of Radiographic Positions and Radiologic Procedures, *ed 11, St Louis, 2007, Mosby.)*

angiography _____

Contrast material (such as iodine) is injected into an artery or vein, and x-ray images are taken.

-lysis   separation, breakdown, destruction

dialysis _____

The root (LYS, meaning to loosen) in this term is embedded in the suffix (-LYSIS). **Hemodialysis** *is the removal of blood for passage through (DIA means through or complete) a kidney machine to filter out waste materials, such as urea. Another form of dialysis is* **peritoneal dialysis.** *A special fluid is put into the peritoneum through a tube in the abdomen. The wastes seep into the fluid from the blood during a period of time. The fluid and wastes are then drained from the peritoneum. See Figure 3-15.*

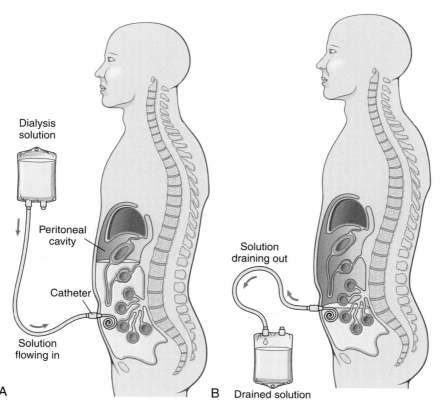

Dialysis solution

Peritoneal cavity

Catheter

Solution flowing in

Solution draining out

A   B   Drained solution

Figure 3-15 • Peritoneal dialysis. This procedure (or the alternative method of hemodialysis) is necessary when the kidneys are not functioning to remove waste materials (such as urea) from the blood. Without dialysis or kidney transplantation, uremia can result. *(From Chabner D-E: The Language of Medicine, ed 9, Philadelphia, 2011, Saunders.)*

-plasty	surgical repair, or surgical correction	mammoplasty _____
		rhinoplasty _____
		angioplasty _____

*Balloon angioplasty is performed on narrowed, blocked coronary arteries that surround the heart. A wire with a collapsed balloon is placed in a clogged artery. Opening of the balloon widens the vessel, allowing more blood to flow through. A **stent** (mesh tube) is placed in the artery to hold it open. See Figure 3-16.*

-scopy	process of visual examination	bronchoscopy _____
		laparoscopy _____
		laryngoscopy _____

See Figure 3-17.

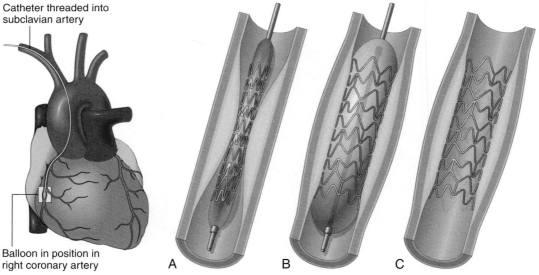

Catheter threaded into subclavian artery

Balloon in position in right coronary artery

A   B   C

Figure 3-16 • **Angioplasty and placement of an intracoronary artery stent. A,** The stent is positioned at the site of the lesion. **B,** The balloon is inflated, expanding the stent. **C,** The balloon is then deflated and removed, and the implanted stent is left in place. Coronary artery stents are stainless steel mesh, tubelike devices that help hold arteries open. Drug-eluting stents release chemicals to dissolve plaque.

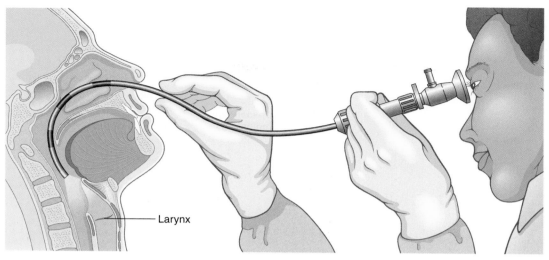

Figure 3-17 • **Laryngoscopy.**

-stomy	opening	colostomy _____

A -STOMY *procedure is the creation of a permanent or semipermanent opening (stoma) from an organ to the outside of the body. See Figure 3-18,* A. *When two tube-like structures are surgically connected within the body, the new connection is an* **anastomosis** *(see Figure 3-18,* B*). A* **colocolostomy** *is an anastomosis, a new connection between two previously unconnected portions of the colon.*

tracheostomy _____
See Figure 3-19.

-therapy	treatment	radiotherapy _____

chemotherapy _____

cryotherapy _____
Skin lesions, such as warts, are removed with cryotherapy. Liquid nitrogen or carbon dioxide snow is applied and blistering followed by necrosis results.

 Radiotherapy versus radiology

Radiotherapy is directed by a radiation oncologist, a medical doctor specializing in **treating** cancer using radiation to kill tumor cells. Radiology is the specialty of a radiologist, also a medical doctor, who primarily **diagnoses** conditions using x-ray, magnetic wave, and ultrasound techniques.

3

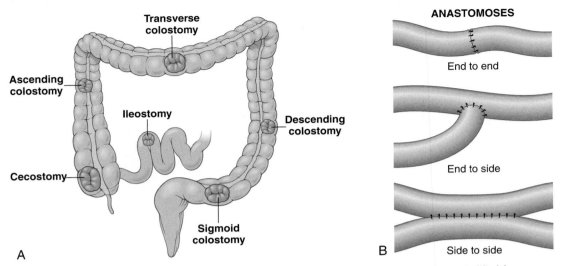

Figure 3-18 • **A,** Locations of **stomas** in the ileum and colon. **B, Anastomoses.** (**B,** *Modified from Chabner D-E: The Language of Medicine, ed 9, Philadelphia, 2011, Saunders.*)

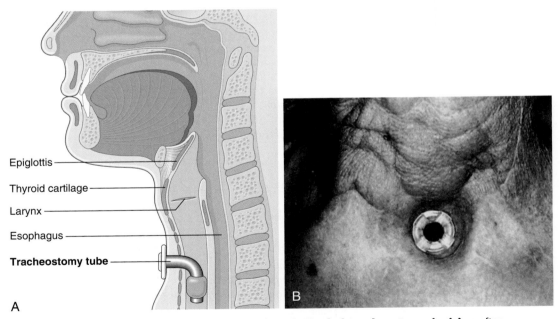

Figure 3-19 • **A, Tracheostomy** with tube in place. **B, Healed tracheostomy incision** after laryngectomy. (**B,** *From Black JM, Matassarin-Jacobs E: Medical-Surgical Nursing: Clinical Management for Continuity of Care, ed 5, Philadelphia, 1997, Saunders.*)

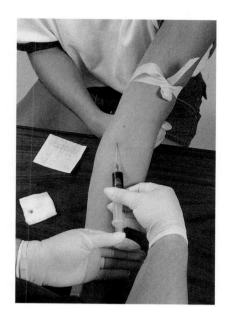

Figure 3-20 • **Phlebotomy.** After a vein is entered with a needle inserted through the skin, the plunger of the syringe is slowly pulled out to withdraw blood. *(From Bonewit-West K: Clinical Procedures for Medical Assistants, ed 6, Philadelphia, 2004, Saunders.)*

3

-tomy   incision, cutting into   cranio<u>tomy</u> _____

laparo<u>tomy</u> _____

phlebo<u>tomy</u> _____
See Figure 3-20.

 -TOMY versus -STOMY

-TOMY indicates a temporary incision, as opposed to -STOMY, which is a permanent or semipermanent opening.

IN PERSON

This first-person narrative describes the symptoms and treatment of a 42-year-old woman with gallbladder stones.

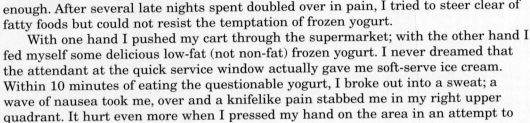

Everyone enjoys a little dessert after dinner, but when the ice cream or a creamy tart leads to pain, most would avoid it. I loved sweets, and despite the revenge they took on my waistline, I still would not pass up an ice cream cone—until my gallbladder decided it had had enough. After several late nights spent doubled over in pain, I tried to steer clear of fatty foods but could not resist the temptation of frozen yogurt.

With one hand I pushed my cart through the supermarket; with the other hand I fed myself some delicious low-fat (not non-fat) frozen yogurt. I never dreamed that the attendant at the quick service window actually gave me soft-serve ice cream. Within 10 minutes of eating the questionable yogurt, I broke out into a sweat; a wave of nausea took me, over and a knifelike pain stabbed me in my right upper quadrant. It hurt even more when I pressed my hand on the area in an attempt to brace the pain.

Several months earlier, after a similar painful episode, I had undergone an ultrasound of my gallbladder, and the surgeon then recommended cholecystectomy. The U/S showed multiple stones in my gallbladder. Most of the stones were just the right size to lodge in the common bile duct and cause blockage of the outflow of bile that occurs after a fatty meal. When I heard the ultrasound results, I swore off all fatty foods.

I just did not imagine that ice cream masquerading as "low-fat yogurt"would be the straw that broke the camel's back! Soon enough, I abandoned my shopping cart and apologized to the manager of the store for vomiting all over aisle 4. The unrelenting pain did not cease when I vomited—it only intensified. I have no idea how I made it home and into bed, but my husband found me several hours later in a deep sweat. I managed to call my surgeon and arrange for "semiemergent" surgery the next morning.

Dr. Fernandez and his team performed a laparoscopic cholecystectomy and relayed to me as I came out of anesthesia that I no longer had a "bag of marbles" for a gallbladder. I had a gassy, distended feeling in my abdomen over the two weeks after surgery (carbon dioxide gas is injected into the abdomen before surgery to allow space between abdominal organs). I felt "tight as a drum" for the first few days and then day by day it went away. My four tiny incisions healed just fine, and in about 2 weeks I was feeling back to "normal." Now I can eat ice cream to my heart's content, only suffering the padding on my waistline, not the stabbing pain just above. Without missing a beat, my liver now delivers the bile into my small intestine right after I eat a fatty meal. The bile emulsifies (breaks down) the fat. I just don't have a storage bag to hold bile in reserve.

I've had an appendectomy, my wisdom teeth removed, and now I gave up my gallbladder! How many more "useless" body parts are there to go?

Elizabeth Chabner Thompson is a physician, teacher, ultra-marathoner, and the mother of four children, ages 8 to 13.

? EXERCISES AND ANSWERS

Complete these exercises and check your answers. An important part of your success in learning medical terminology is checking your answers carefully with the Answers to Exercises beginning on page 112. Visit the Evolve website (http://evolve.elsevier.com/Chabner/medtermshort) for additional interactive activities and information.

A **Give meanings for the following suffixes.**

1. -megaly _____

2. -pathy _____

3. -rrhea _____

4. -rrhagia _____

5. -osis _____

6. -ia _____

B **Give suffixes for the following meanings.**

1. inflammation _____

2. condition of pain _____

3. blood condition _____

4. tumor, mass _____

5. hardening _____

6. condition of urine _____

3

C Match the following medical terms with their meanings below. Write each term next to its meaning.

adenocarcinoma   hepatomegaly   myeloma
cardiomyopathy   ischemia   otalgia
esophagitis   leukocytosis   pneumonia
hematoma

1. Enlargement of the liver _____

2. Pain in the ear _____

3. Holding back blood from an organ (depriving it of blood supply) _____

4. Abnormal condition of white blood cells (slight increase in normal cells to fight infection) _____

5. Abnormal condition of the lung (inflammation and accumulation of material often caused by bacterial infection) _____

6. Tumor (malignant) of bone marrow _____

7. Inflammation of the tube leading from the throat to the stomach _____

8. Disease of heart muscle _____

9. Collection or mass of blood _____

10. Tumor (cancerous) of glandular tissue _____

3

D Underline the suffix meaning <u>pertaining to</u> in the following terms and give the area or part of the body referred to.

1. esophageal _____

2. inguinal _____

3. renal _____

4. vascular _____

5. pelvic _____

6. pulmonary _____

7. axillary _____

8. peritoneal _____

9. mammary _____

10. myocardial _____

E Give meanings for the following suffixes related to procedures.

1. -ectomy _____

2. -gram _____

3. -centesis _____

4. -graphy _____

5. -plasty _____

6. -lysis _____

7. -stomy _____

8. -scopy _____

9. -tomy _____

10. -therapy _____

3

F Select from the following terms to complete the sentences below.

angiography
angioplasty
bronchoscopy
chemotherapy

colocolostomy
colostomy
hysterectomy
laryngoscopy

mammogram
oophorectomy
phlebotomy
thoracentesis

1. Surgical repair of a blood vessel using a catheter (tube), balloon, and stent is

   _____.

2. Treatment using chemicals to destroy malignant cells is _____.

3. X-ray record of the breast is a/an _____.

4. Surgical puncture to remove fluid from the chest is _____.

5. A new opening of the large intestine to the outside of the body is a/an _____.

6. A new internal connection (anastomosis) between two parts of the large bowel

   (intestine) is a/an _____.

7. Removal of the uterus is a/an _____.

8. Process of recording x-ray images of blood vessels after injection of contrast is

   _____.

9. Visual examination of the voice box is _____.

10. Incision of a vein to withdraw blood is _____.

G Write the medical term for the following definitions.

1. Excessive bleeding (discharge of blood) _____.

2. Hardening of fatty plaque (in the lining of the arteries) _____.

3. Pertaining to time (occurring over a long period of time) _____.

4. X-ray record of the spinal cord _____.

5. Sharp, sudden, brief _____

6. Treatment using cold temperatures _____

7. Record of electricity in the brain _____

8. Surgical puncture to remove fluid from the membrane surrounding the fetus

_____

9. Muscle pain _____

10. Malignant tumor of bone marrow _____

11. Enlargement of the heart _____

12. Abnormal condition of the death of cells _____

13. Disease condition of the kidney _____

14. Incision of the skull _____

H **What part of the body is inflamed?**   **3**

1. neuritis _____   11. meningitis _____

2. arthritis _____   12. bronchitis _____

3. salpingitis _____   13. rhinitis _____

4. otitis _____   14. peritonitis _____

5. hepatitis _____   15. vasculitis _____

6. nephritis _____   16. mastitis _____

7. esophagitis _____   17. tonsillitis _____

8. laryngitis _____   18. colitis _____

9. encephalitis _____   19. pharyngitis _____

10. osteitis _____   20. phlebitis _____

I Provide the terms for the following procedures.

1. Excision of the gallbladder _____

2. Excision of the appendix _____

3. Excision of a breast _____

4. Excision of the uterus _____

5. Excision of an ovary _____

6. Excision of the voice box _____

7. Excision of a kidney _____

8. Excision of a gland _____

9. Excision of the large intestine _____

10. Excision of a fallopian tube _____

11. Excision of tonsils _____

12. Incision of the skull _____

13. Incision of the abdomen _____

14. Incision of the chest _____

15. Opening of the windpipe to the outside of the body _____

16. Opening of the colon to the outside of the body _____

17. Surgical puncture to remove fluid from the chest _____

18. Surgical puncture to remove fluid from a joint _____

19. Incision of a vein (needle or catheter is inserted) _____

20. Visual examination of the voice box _____

J Supply the correct medical term for the following:

1. A stroke is a **cerebro**_____ _____ [two words].

2. A heart attack is a **myo**_____ _____ [two words].

3. Use of a machine that filters wastes from the blood is **hemo** _____.

4. Injection of fluid into the abdominal cavity and then withdrawal of that fluid

    (containing waste material) is **peri**_____ _____

    [two words].

5. A noncancerous tumor of muscle is a **my**_____.

6. A cancerous tumor of muscle is a **myo**_____.

7. High levels of wastes (urea) in the blood is **ur**_____.

8. Blood in the urine is **hemat**_____.

9. High numbers of malignant (cancerous) white blood cells is **leuk**_____.

10. Slightly elevated numbers of white blood cells due to an infection in the body is

    leuko_____.

11. Normal discharge of blood during menstruation is **men**_____.

12. Excessive bleeding during menstruation is **men**_____.

13. Hardening of arteries is called **arterio**_____.

14. Use of high-energy rays to treat cancerous tumors is **radio**_____.

K Circle the term that best completes the meaning of the sentences in the following medical vignettes.

1. After routine breast self-examination, Nora felt a small lump in her breast. She consulted her doctor, who scheduled a diagnostic **(mammoplasty, mastectomy, mammogram).** The examination showed a stellate (star-shaped) mass, and a **(biopsy, necropsy, laparoscopy)** revealed an infiltrating ductal carcinoma. Nora decided to have her breast removed **(hysterectomy, mastectomy, salpingectomy),** although her physician gave her the option of having lumpectomy followed by **(cryotherapy, thoracotomy, radiotherapy).**

2. In addition to her surgery, Nora had a sentinel node biopsy of a/an **(inguinal, thoracic, axillary)** lymph node to determine whether the cancer had spread. Injection of contrast revealed the primary (sentinel) lymph node, which was removed and microscopically examined.

3

3. Sylvia had irregular bleeding in between her periods. She was 50 years old and beginning menopause. On pelvic exam, Dr. Hawk felt a large, lobulated uterus. Biopsy revealed a large fibroid, which is a benign (noncancerous) tumor of muscle tissue (**myeloma, myoma, hematoma**). The doctor discussed three surgical options: removal of the fibroid, blockage of blood flow to the fibroid (embolization), or a total abdominal (**gastrectomy, hysterectomy, cholecystectomy**).

4. Victoria had never been comfortable with the bump on her nose. She saw a plastic surgeon, who performed (**mammoplasty, rhinoplasty, angioplasty**).

5. Sam was experiencing cramps, diarrhea, and a low-grade fever. He was diagnosed with ulcerative (**colitis, meningitis, laryngitis**) and had several bouts of (**uremia, menorrhagia, septicemia**) caused by inflammation and rupture of the bowel wall.

6. Bill felt chest pain every time he climbed a flight of stairs. He went to his doctor, who did a coronary (**myelogram, angiogram, dialysis**), which revealed (**adenocarcinoma, nephrosis, atherosclerosis**) in one of his coronary arteries. The doctor recommended (**angioplasty, thoracentesis, amniocentesis**). This would prevent further (**myosarcoma, ischemia, leukocytosis**) and help Bill avoid a (**peritoneal, vascular, myocardial**) infarction, or heart attack, in the future.

3 ANSWERS TO EXERCISES

A
1. enlargement
2. disease condition
3. flow, discharge
4. excessive discharge
5. condition, abnormal condition
6. condition of blood

B
1. -itis
2. -algia
3. -emia
4. -oma
5. -sclerosis
6. -uria

C
1. hepatomegaly
2. otalgia
3. ischemia
4. leukocytosis
5. pneumonia
6. myeloma (also called multiple myeloma)
7. esophagitis
8. cardiomyopathy
9. hematoma
10. adenocarcinoma

D
1. esophag**eal**—esophagus (tube leading from the throat to the stomach)
2. inguin**al**—groin (area where the thigh meets the trunk of the body)
3. ren**al**—kidney
4. vascul**ar**—blood vessels
5. pelv**ic**—hip area
6. pulmon**ary**—lungs
7. axill**ary**—armpit (underarm area)
8. periton**eal**—peritoneum (membrane surrounding the abdominal cavity)
9. mamm**ary**—breast
10. myocard**ial**—heart muscle

E
1. removal, excision, resection
2. record
3. surgical puncture to remove fluid
4. process of recording
5. surgical repair
6. separation; breakdown
7. new opening
8. process of visual examination
9. cutting into, incision, section
10. treatment

F
1. angioplasty
2. chemotherapy
3. mammogram
4. thoracentesis
5. colostomy
6. colocolostomy
7. hysterectomy
8. angiography
9. laryngoscopy
10. phlebotomy

G

1. hemorrhage
2. atherosclerosis
3. chronic
4. myelogram
5. acute
6. cryotherapy
7. electroencephalogram
8. amniocentesis
9. myalgia
10. myeloma or multiple myeloma
11. cardiomegaly
12. necrosis
13. nephropathy
14. craniotomy

H

1. nerve
2. joint
3. fallopian tubes
4. ear
5. liver
6. kidney
7. esophagus
8. larynx (voice box)
9. brain
10. bone
11. meninges (membranes surrounding the brain and spinal cord)
12. bronchial tubes
13. nose
14. peritoneum
15. blood vessels
16. breast
17. tonsils
18. colon (large intestine)
19. throat (pharynx)
20. veins

I

1. cholecystectomy
2. appendectomy
3. mastectomy
4. hysterectomy
5. oophorectomy
6. laryngectomy
7. nephrectomy
8. adenectomy
9. colectomy
10. salpingectomy
11. tonsillectomy
12. craniotomy
13. laparotomy
14. thoracotomy
15. tracheostomy
16. colostomy
17. thoracentesis
18. arthrocentesis
19. phlebotomy
20. laryngoscopy

J

1. cerebro**vascular accident**—clot or hemorrhage in an artery of the brain leads to decreased blood flow (ischemia) to brain tissue and necrosis (death of brain cells).
2. myo**cardial infarction**—ischemia of heart muscle leads to infarction (necrosis of heart muscle cells).
3. hemo**dialysis**—complete separation of waste material from the blood using a machine that receives the patient's blood and after filtration sends the blood back into the patient's body
4. peri**toneal dialysis**—fluid is introduced into the abdominal cavity and then removed after wastes have passed into the fluid from the peritoneal blood vessels.
5. my**oma**—benign muscle tumors occurring in the uterus are fibroids.
6. myo**sarcoma**—malignant tumors of connective or flesh tissue are sarcomas.
7. ur**emia**—this indicates failure of the kidneys to eliminate nitrogen-containing wastes, such as urea, creatinine, and uric acid, from the bloodstream.
8. hemat**uria**—this indicates bleeding in the urinary tract.
9. leuk**emia**—immature, cancerous white blood cells are produced in excess from the bone marrow or lymph nodes.
10. leuko**cytosis**—normal, mature white blood cells are produced to fight infection.
11. men**orrhea**—lining of the uterus breaks down as a result of changes in hormone levels.
12. men**orrhagia**—long or heavy menstrual periods; often caused by benign muscle tumors or fibroids in the uterus
13. arterio**sclerosis**—the most common type is atherosclerosis or collection of fatty plaques in arteries.
14. radio**therapy**—using high-energy x-rays, gamma rays, and protons to destroy cancerous cells

K

1. mammogram, biopsy, mastectomy, radiotherapy
2. axillary
3. myoma, hysterectomy
4. rhinoplasty
5. colitis, septicemia
6. angiogram, atherosclerosis, angioplasty, ischemia, myocardial

3

PRONUNCIATION OF TERMS

*The terms that you have learned in this chapter are presented here with their pronunciations. The capitalized letters in **BOLDFACE** represent the accented syllable. Pronounce each word out loud; then write the meaning in the space provided. Meanings of all terms can be checked with the **Mini-Dictionary: Glossary of Medical Terms** beginning on page 341 and on the audio section of the Evolve website (http://evolve.elsevier.com/Chabner/medtermshort).*

TERM	PRONUNCIATION	MEANING
acute	ah-**KUT**	
adenocarcinoma	ah-deh-no-kar-sih-**NO**-mah	
adenoma	ah-deh-**NO**-mah	
amniocentesis	am-ne-o-sen-**TE**-sis	
anastomosis	ah-nah-sto-**MO**-sis	
angiography	an-je-**OG**-rah-fe	
angioplasty	**AN**-je-o-plas-te	
arteriosclerosis	ar-te-re-o-skleh-**RO**-sis	
arthralgia	ar-**THRAL**-je-ah	
arthropathy	ar-**THROP**-ah-the	
atherosclerosis	ah-theh-ro-skleh-**RO**-sis	
axillary	**AKS**-ih-lair-e	
bronchitis	brong-**KI**-tis	
bronchoscopy	bron-**KOS**-ko-pe	
carcinoma	kar-sih-**NO**-mah	
cardiomegaly	kar-de-o-**MEG**-ah-le	
cardiomyopathy	kar-de-o-mi-**OP**-ah-the	
chemotherapy	ke-mo-**THER**-ah-pe	

cholecystectomy   ko-le-sis-**TEK**-to-me _____

chronic   **KRON**-ik _____

colitis   ko-**LI**-tis _____

colostomy   ko-**LOS**-to-me _____

colocolostomy   ko-lo-ko-**LOS**-to-me _____

craniotomy   kra-ne-**OT**-o-me _____

cystitis   sis-**TI**-tis _____

dialysis   di-**AL**-ih-sis _____

electroencephalography   e-lek-tro-en-sef-ah-**LOG**-rah-fe _____

encephalopathy   en-sef-ah-**LOP**-ah-the _____

erythrocytosis   eh-rith-ro-si-**TO**-sis _____

esophageal   e-sof-ah-**JE**-al _____

esophagitis   e-sof-ah-**JI**-tis _____

hematuria   he-mah-**TUR**-e-ah _____

hemorrhage   **HEM**-o-rij _____

hysterectomy   his-teh-**REK**-to-me _____

infarction   in-**FARK**-shun _____

inguinal   **ING**-gwih-nal _____

ischemia   is-**KE**-me-ah _____

laparoscopy   lap-ah-**ROS**-ko-pe _____

laparotomy   lap-ah-**ROT**-o-me _____

laryngitis   lah-rin-**JI**-tis _____

laryngoscopy   lah-rin-**GOS**-ko-pe _____

leukemia   loo-**KE**-me-ah _____

3

leukocytosis	loo-ko-si-**TO**-sis _____
mammogram	**MAM**-o-gram _____
mammography	mah-**MOG**-rah-fe _____
mammoplasty	**MAM**-o-plas-te _____
mastectomy	mas-**TEK**-to-me _____
meningitis	men-in-**JI**-tis _____
menorrhagia	men-or-**RA**-jah _____
menorrhea	men-o-**RE**-ah _____
myalgia	mi-**AL**-jah _____
myelogram	**MI**-eh-lo-gram _____
myeloma	mi-eh-**LO**-mah _____
myocardial	mi-o-**KAR**-de-al _____
myoma	mi-**O**-mah _____
myosarcoma	mi-o-sar-**KO**-mah _____
necrosis	neh-**KRO**-sis _____
nephrosis	neh-**FRO**-sis _____
neuralgia	nu-**RAL**-jah _____
oophorectomy	o-of-o-**REK**-to-me _or_ oo-for-**EK**-to-me _____
otalgia	o-**TAL**-jah _____
pelvic	**PEL**-vik _____
peritoneal	per-ih-to-**NE**-al _____
phlebitis	fleh-**BI**-tis _____
phlebotomy	fleh-**BOT**-o-me _____

3

pneumonia	noo-**MO**-ne-ah _____
pulmonary	**PUL**-mo-nair-re _____
radiotherapy	ra-de-o-**THAIR**-ah-pe _____
renal	**RE**-nal _____
rhinoplasty	**RI**-no-plas-te _____
rhinorrhea	ri-no-**RE**-ah _____
salpingectomy	sal-pin-**JEK**-to-me _____
septicemia	sep-tih-**SE**-me-ah _____
thoracentesis	tho-rah-sen-**TE**-sis _____
tonsillectomy	ton-sih-**LEK**-to-me _____
tracheostomy	tra-ke-**OS**-to-me _____
uremia	u-**RE**-me-ah _____
vascular	**VAS**-ku-lar _____

3

PRACTICAL APPLICATIONS

Answers are found on page 119.

MATCHING

A Match the procedure in Column I with an abnormal condition (diagnosis) it is associated with in Column II.

COLUMN I		COLUMN II
PROCEDURE		ABNORMAL CONDITION (DIAGNOSIS)
1. angioplasty	_____	A. uterine adenocarcinoma
2. mammoplasty	_____	B. ligament tear of the patella (kneecap)
3. cholecystectomy	_____	C. ovarian cyst
4. tonsillectomy	_____	D. blockage of the windpipe
5. dialysis	_____	E. renal failure
6. hysterectomy	_____	F. absence of a breast (postmastectomy)
7. thoracentesis	_____	G. pleural effusion (collection of fluid)
8. oophorectomy	_____	H. coronary atherosclerosis
9. tracheostomy	_____	I. gallbladder calculi (stones)
10. arthroscopy	_____	J. pharyngeal lymph node enlargement

B Match the sign/symptom (abnormal condition) in Column I with an organ or tissue in Column II.

COLUMN I		COLUMN II
SIGN/SYMPTOM (ABNORMAL CONDITION)		ORGAN OR TISSUE
1. colitis	_____	A. uterus
2. phlebitis	_____	B. ear
3. menorrhagia	_____	C. bone marrow
4. myocardial ischemia	_____	D. coronary arteries
5. otalgia	_____	E. large bowel
6. uremia	_____	F. membrane surrounding spinal cord or brain
7. meningitis	_____	G. vein
8. leukemia	_____	H. kidney

PRINCIPAL DIAGNOSIS

*The **principal diagnosis** is the cause, after evaluation, of the patient's admission to the hospital. Physician notes, which document clinical investigations and findings, are important for medical billing and coding. A careful reading of physician notes will identify the principal diagnosis, as in the following example.*

Physician Notes

A 45-year-old obese woman presents complaining of menorrhagia [heavy periods] with cramping pelvic pain, dizziness when standing, and rapid heart rate. Manual physical examination demonstrates multiple enlarged masses in her uterus. Blood workup reveals low RBCs [red blood cells] and hematocrit [percentage of red blood cells in a volume of blood], normal WBCs and platelets, and slightly elevated blood sugar level. U/S [ultrasound] of the abdomen and pelvis show multiple fibroids [leiomyomas] of the uterine wall. Patient is admitted to the hospital with recommendation for hysterectomy. During the course of admission she speaks to the resident dietitian about a compulsive eating disorder and agrees to undergo therapy at the hospital's weight loss clinic.

Using the information presented in the physician notes, select the principal diagnosis from the following:

    A. Pelvic pain—female (625.9)

    B. Obesity (278.00)

    C. Anemia (285.9)

    D. Menorrhagia (626.2)

    E. Fibroid uterus (218.9)

(The numbers in parentheses are medical codes as given in the *International Classification of Diseases, Ninth Revision [ICD-9] Coding Handbook 2011*.)

3

ANSWERS TO THE PRACTICAL APPLICATIONS

Matching

A	1. H	3. I	5. E	7. G	9. D
	2. F	4. J	6. A	8. C	10. B

B	1. E	3. A	5. B	7. F
	2. G	4. D	6. H	8. C

Principal Diagnosis

Answer: E. Fibroid uterus
A. Pelvic pain is a **POA (present on admission) diagnosis.***
B. Obesity is a **POA diagnosis.**
C. Anemia is an **admitting diagnosis.**†
D. Menorrhagia is a **POA diagnosis.**

*A **POA (present on admission) diagnosis** reflects incidental conditions that are noted and treated if necessary but are not a cause for hospital admission. Such conditions are not life-threatening (at the time of admission) but may require treatment and monitoring during the patient's stay.
†An **admitting diagnosis** is a cause, before further evaluation, for admission to the hospital. Such conditions may not resolve in the ED and can become life-threatening without proper treatment.

PICTURE SHOW

Answer the questions that follow each image. Correct answers are found on page 122.

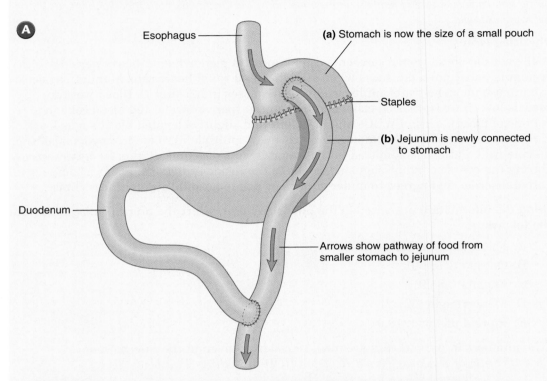

A

Esophagus

(a) Stomach is now the size of a small pouch

Staples

(b) Jejunum is newly connected to stomach

Duodenum

Arrows show pathway of food from smaller stomach to jejunum

3

1. The figure shows a surgical procedure **(bariatric surgery)** used to treat extreme obesity. First, the stomach **(a)** is stapled so that it is reduced to the size of a small pouch. Next, the jejunum **(b),** which is the second part of the small intestine, is brought up to connect with the smaller stomach. This diverts food so that it has a shorter travel time through the intestine with less time for absorption into the bloodstream. What is the name of this surgical procedure?
   a. esophageal bypass
   b. total gastric resection
   c. gastric bypass
   d. duodenal resection

2. The new connection, or anastomosis, between the stomach and the second part of the small intestine is a:
   a. gastrostomy
   b. jejunostomy
   c. gastroduodenostomy
   d. gastrojejunostomy

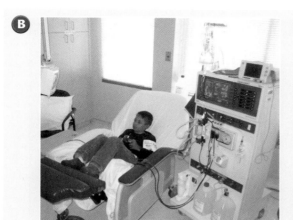

(From Lewis SM, Heitkemper MM, Dirksen SR: Medical-Surgical Nursing: Assessment and Management of Clinical Problems, ed 5, St Louis, 2000, Mosby.)

1. In the image shown, blood leaves the patient's body to enter a machine that filters out impurities. The filtered blood then circulates back to the patient's body. This procedure is:
   a. pericardiocentesis
   b. peritoneal dialysis
   c. hemodialysis
   d. amniocentesis

2. The procedure is a treatment for patients with failure of the:
   a. kidneys
   b. pancreas
   c. liver
   d. all three organs listed

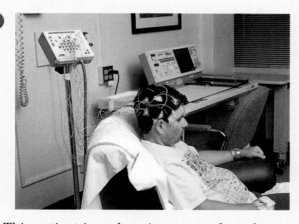

(From Chipps EM, Clanin NJ, Campbell VG: Neurologic Disorders, St Louis, 1992, Mosby.)

1. This patient is undergoing a procedure that records brain wave activity. It is called:
   a. electrocardiography
   b. electroencephalography
   c. electromyography
   d. electrocraniography

2. It may be used to diagnose:
   a. seizure disorders (epilepsy)
   b. dyspnea
   c. paraplegia
   d. quadriplegia
   e. all four disorders listed

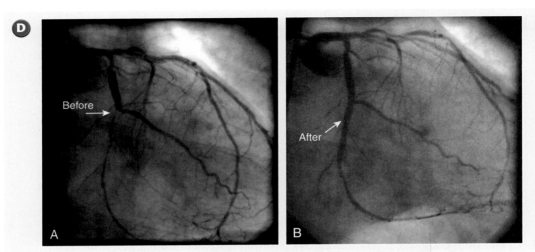

(Courtesy Dr. Daniel Simon and Mr. Paul Zampino.)

1. The *arrow* in **A** shows a narrowing of a coronary artery, preventing blood flow to the heart muscle. A condition caused by decreased blood flow is called:
   a. nephrosis
   b. uremia
   c. cardiomegaly
   d. ischemia

2. **B** shows the coronary artery after stenting. The imaging procedure that is shown is:
   a. electrocardiography
   b. angiography
   c. radiotherapy
   d. mammography

3. The treatment procedure in which coronary arteries are opened using a balloon catheter and stenting is:
   a. rhinoplasty
   b. phlebotomy
   c. angioplasty
   d. thoracentesis

ANSWERS TO PICTURE SHOW

A	1. c	2. d	
B	1. c	2. a	
C	1. b	2. a	
D	1. d	2. b	3. c

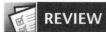 **REVIEW**

Write the meanings for the following word parts. Remember to check your answers with the Answers to Review section on page 125.

SUFFIXES

SUFFIX	MEANING	SUFFIX	MEANING
1. -al		15. -megaly	
2. -algia		16. -oma	
3. -ar		17. -osis	
4. -ary		18. -pathy	
5. -centesis		19. -plasty	
6. -eal		20. -rrhage	
7. -ectomy		21. -rrhagia	
8. -emia		22. -rrhea	
9. -gram		23. -sclerosis	
10. -graphy		24. -scopy	
11. -ia		25. -stomy	
12. -ic		26. -therapy	
13. -itis		27. -tomy	
14. -lysis		28. -uria	

3

COMBINING FORMS

COMBINING FORM	MEANING	COMBINING FORM	MEANING
1. aden/o		4. arteri/o	
2. amni/o		5. arthr/o	
3. angi/o		6. ather/o	

7. axill/o _____

8. bronch/o _____

9. carcin/o _____

10. cardi/o _____

11. chem/o _____

12. cholecyst/o _____

13. chron/o _____

14. col/o _____

15. crani/o _____

16. cry/o _____

17. cyst/o _____

18. encephal/o _____

19. erythr/o _____

20. esophag/o _____

21. hemat/o _____

22. hepat/o _____

23. hyster/o _____

24. inguin/o _____

25. isch/o _____

26. lapar/o _____

27. laryng/o _____

28. leuk/o _____

29. mamm/o _____

30. mast/o _____

31. men/o _____

32. mening/o _____

33. my/o _____

34. myel/o _____

35. necr/o _____

36. nephr/o _____

37. neur/o _____

38. oophor/o _____

39. oste/o _____

40. ot/o _____

41. pelv/o _____

42. peritone/o _____

43. phleb/o _____

44. pneumon/o _____

45. pulmon/o _____

46. radi/o _____

47. ren/o _____

48. rhin/o _____

49. salping/o _____

50. sarc/o _____

51. septic/o _____

52. thorac/o _____

53. tonsill/o _____

54. trache/o _____

55. ur/o _____

56. vascul/o _____

3

ANSWERS TO REVIEW

SUFFIXES

1. pertaining to
2. condition of pain, pain
3. pertaining to
4. pertaining to
5. surgical puncture to remove fluid
6. pertaining to
7. removal, resection, excision
8. blood condition
9. record
10. process of recording
11. condition
12. pertaining to
13. inflammation
14. separation, breakdown, destruction
15. enlargement
16. tumor, mass
17. abnormal condition
18. disease condition
19. surgical repair
20. excessive discharge of blood
21. excessive discharge of blood
22. flow, discharge
23. hardening
24. visual examination
25. opening
26. treatment
27. incision; cutting into
28. urine condition

COMBINING FORMS

1. gland
2. amnion
3. vessel
4. artery
5. joint
6. plaque, collection of fatty material
7. armpit
8. bronchial tubes
9. cancerous
10. heart
11. drug, chemical
12. gallbladder
13. time
14. colon (large intestine)
15. skull
16. cold
17. urinary bladder
18. brain
19. red
20. esophagus
21. blood
22. liver
23. uterus
24. groin
25. to hold back
26. abdomen
27. larynx (voice box)
28. white
29. breast
30. breast
31. menstruation
32. meninges
33. muscle
34. spinal cord or bone marrow
35. death
36. kidney
37. nerve
38. ovary
39. bone
40. ear
41. hip area
42. peritoneum
43. vein
44. lung
45. lung
46. x-rays
47. kidney
48. nose
49. fallopian tube
50. flesh
51. pertaining to infection
52. chest
53. tonsil
54. trachea (windpipe)
55. urine, urinary tract
56. blood vessel

3

TERMINOLOGY CHECKUP

Before you leave this chapter, here are important concepts that you should thoroughly understand. Check the box next to each item when you know you've "got" it!

☐ 1. **Ischemia:** Ischemia is a deficiency of blood flow to any area of the body. Depriving cells of blood supply containing oxygen and nutrients leads to necrosis (death of cells). If ischemia and necrosis occur in the heart muscle, a myocardial infarction (heart attack) results. If ischemia and necrosis occur in the brain, a cerebrovascular accident (stroke) results.

☐ 2. **-Tomy, -ectomy, and -stomy:** These are three important surgical suffixes! A procedure ending in **-tomy** is an incision or section. A procedure ending in **-ectomy** is an excision or resection. A procedure ending in **-stomy** is the creation of a new opening in an organ to the outside of the body. If two different structures or two parts of the same organ are newly connected or opened to each other within the body, it is an anastomosis (colocolostomy).

☐ 3. **Uremia and dialysis: Uremia** occurs when the kidneys fail to function. Waste products (urea, creatinine, and uric acid) accumulate in the bloodstream. One common option for treating uremia is **dialysis.** There are two types of dialysis. In **hemodialysis,** the patient's own blood flows through a machine, and waste materials are filtered out before the blood is returned. In **peritoneal dialysis,** a special fluid is inserted via a catheter into the peritoneal cavity. Waste materials seep into that fluid, which is then drained from the body.

☐ 4. **My/o and myel/o:** Be careful about spelling these combining forms. They have different meanings! **My/o** is always muscle, as in myoma. **Myel/o,** however, means both bone marrow AND spinal cord. **Myeloma** is a malignant tumor of bone marrow and a **myelogram** is an x-ray record of the spinal cord.

☐ 5. **Cholecystectomy, splenectomy, and oophorectomy:** These procedures are resections of the gallbladder, spleen, and ovaries, respectively. What happens when these organs are removed? After **cholecystectomy**, without a gallbladder to store bile, the liver secretes bile as needed. After **splenectomy,** without a spleen to produce white blood cells and process worn-out red blood cells, lymph nodes and the liver take over these functions. After **bilateral oophorectomy,** without ovaries to produce eggs and female hormones, adrenal glands produce small amounts of estrogen and progesterone.

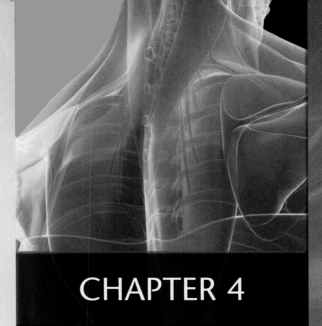

Prefixes

CHAPTER 4

CHAPTER OBJECTIVES
- To identify and define common prefixes used in medical terms
- To analyze, spell, and pronounce medical terms that contain prefixes
- To apply medical terms in real-life situations

Introduction

This chapter reviews the prefixes you studied in Chapter 1 and introduces new prefixes. The list of Combining Forms and Suffixes that follows will help you understand the terminology presented beginning on page 130. Remember to complete all exercises and check your answers. The Pronunciation of Terms and Review are opportunities to test your understanding of all terminology in this chapter.

COMBINING FORMS AND SUFFIXES

COMBINING FORM	MEANING
abdomin/o	abdomen
an/o	anus (opening of the digestive tract to the outside of the body)
bi/o	life
cardi/o	heart
carp/o	carpals (wrist bones)
cis/o	to cut
cost/o	ribs
crani/o	skull
cutane/o	skin
dur/o	dura mater (outermost meningeal membrane surrounding the brain and spinal cord)
gen/o	to produce, to begin
glyc/o	sugar
hemat/o	blood
later/o	side
men/o	menses (monthly discharge of blood from the lining of the uterus)
nat/i	birth
neur/o	nerve
norm/o	rule, order
oste/o	bone
peritone/o	peritoneum (membrane surrounding the organs in the abdomen)
plas/o	formation, growth, development
ren/o	kidney
scapul/o	scapula (shoulder blade)
son/o	sound
thyroid/o	thyroid gland
top/o	to put, place, position
troph/o	development, nourishment
urethr/o	urethra (tube leading from the bladder to the outside of the body)
uter/o	uterus
ven/o	vein
vertebr/o	vertebra (backbone)

4

SUFFIX	MEANING
-al	pertaining to
-ation	process, condition
-cision	process of cutting
-crine	secretion
-dipsia	thirst
-emia	blood condition
-gen	to produce
-graphy	process of recording
-ia	condition
-ic	pertaining to
-ine	pertaining to
-ism	condition, process
-lapse	to fall, slide
-lysis	loosening, breakdown, separation, destruction
-meter	to measure
-mission	to send
-mortem	death
-oma	tumor, mass
-ous	pertaining to
-partum	birth
-pathy	disease condition
-phagia	eating
-phasia	speech
-plasia	formation (condition)
-plasm	formation (tissue)
-plegia	paralysis
-pnea	breathing
-rrhea	flow, discharge
-scopy	process of visual examination
-section	to cut
-stasis	to stand, place, stop, control
-tension	pressure
-thesis	to put, place (state of putting or placing)
-tic	pertaining to
-trophy	nourishment; development
-um	structure
-uria	urine condition
-y	process, condition

4

Prefixes and Terminology

PREFIX	MEANING	TERMINOLOGY	MEANING
a-, an-	no, not, without	apnea _____	

In this term, the root (PNE, meaning breathing) is embedded in the suffix (-PNEA). Sleep apnea occurs when breathing stops suddenly during sleep.

aphasia _____

A stroke affecting the language area of the brain can produce this condition.

atrophy _____

Disuse of a muscle can result in muscular atrophy. Muscles shrink as cells decrease in size.

anemia _____

Anemia is a condition in which there is a lower-than-normal number of red blood cells or a decrease in hemoglobin within the cells. Table 4-1 lists different forms of anemia.

amenorrhea _____

PREFIX	MEANING	TERMINOLOGY	MEANING
ab-	away from	abnormal _____	
ad-	toward, near	adrenal glands _____	

See Figure 4-1.

Table 4-1 ANEMIAS	
aplastic anemia	Bone marrow fails to produce red blood cells (erythrocytes), white blood cells (leukocytes), and clotting cells (platelets).
hemolytic anemia	Red blood cells are destroyed (-LYTIC), and bone marrow cannot compensate for their loss. This condition can be hereditary or acquired (after infection or chemotherapy) or can occur when the immune system acts against normal red blood cells (autoimmune condition).
iron deficiency anemia	Low iron levels lead to low hemoglobin concentration or deficiency of red blood cells.
pernicious anemia	The mucous membrane of the stomach fails to produce a substance (intrinsic factor) that is necessary for the absorption of vitamin B_{12} and the proper formation of red blood cells.
sickle cell anemia	Erythrocytes assume an abnormal crescent or sickle shape; this "sickling" is due to the inheritance of an abnormal type of hemoglobin. The sickle-shaped cells clump together, causing clots that block blood vessels.

4

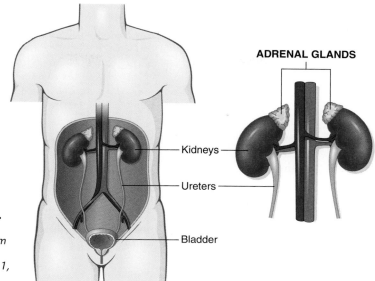

ADRENAL GLANDS

Kidneys

Ureters

Bladder

Figure 4-1 • Adrenal glands. These two endocrine glands are above each kidney. *(Modified from Chabner D-E:* The Language of Medicine, *ed 9, Philadelphia, 2011, Saunders.)*

4

ana-	up, apart	analysis _____
ante-	before, forward	antepartum _____
anti-	against	antibody _____

An antibody is a protein made by white blood cells— literally, a "body" working "against" foreign substances.

antigen _____

Antigens are foreign substances, such as bacteria and viruses. When antigens enter the body, they stimulate white blood cells to produce antibodies that act against the antigens.

Analysis of urine

A **urinalysis** (urine + analysis) is the separation of urine to determine its components. The following chart shows typical urinalysis findings:

Test	Normal	Abnormal
1. Color	light yellow	red (hematuria)
2. Clarity	clear	cloudy (infection)
3. pH (chemical nature)	slightly acidic	alkaline (infection)
4. Protein	very slight	proteinuria (renal disease)
5. Sugar	none	glycosuria (diabetes mellitus)

antibiotic _____

Antibiotics differ from antibodies. They are produced ***outside*** *the body by microorganisms and primitive plants called molds. Examples are penicillin and erythromycin. As disease-fighting medications, they are taken by mouth or through intravenous injection or applied topically to be absorbed through the skin.*

bi-	two, both	bilateral _____
brady-	slow	bradycardia _____
con-	with, together	congenital _____

A congenital anomaly is an irregularity (anomaly) present at birth. Examples are webbed fingers and toes and heart defects.

dia-	complete, through	diarrhea _____

Feces (stools) are loose and watery. Normal water reabsorption through the walls of the colon is impaired.

dys-	bad, painful, difficult, abnormal	dyspnea _____
		dysphagia _____
		dysplasia _____
		dysmenorrhea _____
		dysuria _____

Dysuria is often a symptom of a urinary tract infection (UTI).

ec-	out, outside	ectopic pregnancy _____

Figure 4-2 shows possible sites of ectopic pregnancies. Figure 4-3 indicates uterine levels in a normal pregnancy.

 -Plasia, -phagia, and -phasia

Don't confuse these very different suffixes. **-Plasia** means formation, **-phagia** means eating or swallowing, and **-phasia** means speech.

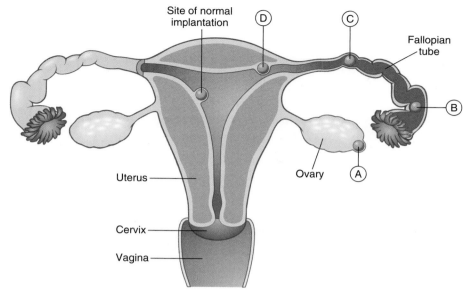

Figure 4-2 • **Ectopic pregnancy.** A, B, C, and D are ectopic sites for implantation of the fertilized egg. The fallopian tube is the most common site for ectopic pregnancies (95%), but they can also occur on the ovary or on the surface of the peritoneum. Normal implantation takes place on the inner lining (endometrium) of the uterus.

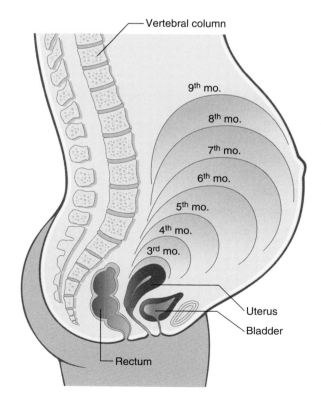

Figure 4-3 • **Uterine levels in pregnancy.**

4

Table 4-2 TYPES OF ENDOSCOPY PROCEDURES*

arthroscopy	Visual examination of a joint
bronchoscopy	Visual examination of the bronchial tubes
colonoscopy	Visual examination of the colon (large intestine)
cystoscopy	Visual examination of the urinary bladder
esophagogastroscopy	Visual examination of the esophagus and stomach
hysteroscopy	Visual examination of the uterus
laparoscopy	Visual examination of the abdomen
laryngoscopy	Visual examination of the larynx (voice box)
mediastinoscopy	Visual examination of the mediastinum
sigmoidoscopy	Visual examination of the sigmoid colon (the lower, S-shaped part of the large intestine)

*For images of these procedures, visit the Evolve companion website.

endo-   within, in, inner   endoscopy _____

Table 4-2 lists types of endoscopy procedures.

endocrine glands _____

The adrenal glands are endocrine glands. Table 4-3 lists the major endocrine glands and the hormones that they secrete.

Table 4-3 MAJOR ENDOCRINE GLANDS AND SELECTED HORMONES

Gland	Hormones
adrenal glands	Adrenaline (epinephrine)
ovaries	Estrogen Progesterone
pancreas	Insulin
parathyroid glands	Parathyroid hormone (PTH)
pituitary gland	Adrenocorticotropic hormone (ACTH) Follicle-stimulating hormone (FSH) Growth hormone (GH) Thyroid-stimulating hormone (TSH)
testes	Testosterone
thyroid gland	Thyroxine (T$_4$)

4

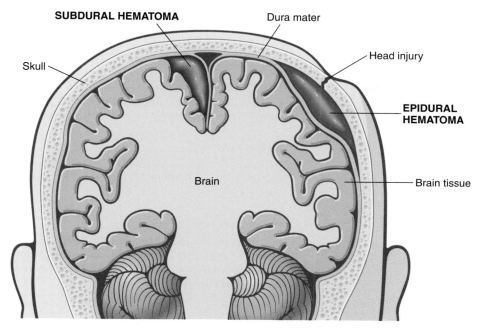

SUBDURAL HEMATOMA

Dura mater

Skull

Head injury

EPIDURAL HEMATOMA

Brain

Brain tissue

Figure 4-4 • Epidural and subdural hematomas. The dura mater is the outermost of the three meninges (membranes) around the brain and spinal cord.

4

epi-	above, upon	epidural hematoma _____
		Figure 4-4 illustrates epidural and subdural hematomas.
		epidermis _____
		The three layers of the skin, from outermost to innermost, are the epidermis, dermis, and subcutaneous layer. Check Appendix I.
ex-	out	excision _____
extra-	outside of	extrahepatic _____
hemi-	half	hemigastrectomy _____
		hemiplegia _____
		One side of the body is paralyzed; usually caused by a cerebrovascular accident or brain lesion, such as a tumor. The resulting paralysis occurs on the side opposite the brain disorder.

hyper-   excessive, too much, above

hyperthyroidism _____

Figure 4-5 shows the position of the thyroid gland in the neck.

hypertrophy _____

*Cells increase in size, not in number. The opposite of hypertrophy is **atrophy** (cells shrink in size).*

hypertension _____

Risk factors that contribute to high blood pressure are increasing age, smoking, obesity, heredity, and a stressful lifestyle.

hyperglycemia _____

*May also be a sign of **diabetes mellitus.** Insulin either is not secreted or is improperly utilized so that sugar accumulates in the bloodstream and spills over into the urine (glycosuria).*

hypo-   deficient, too little, below

hypoglycemia _____

Overproduction of insulin or an overdose (from outside the body—exogenously) of insulin can lead to hypoglycemia, as glucose is removed from the blood at an increased rate.

4

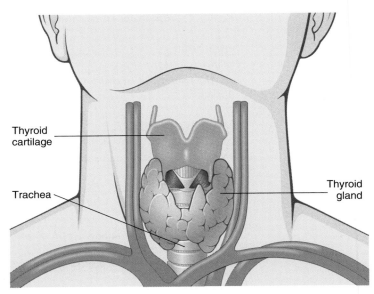

Thyroid cartilage

Trachea

Thyroid gland

Figure 4-5 • **Thyroid gland,** located in the front of the trachea in the neck. The thyroid gland produces too much hormone in hyperthyroidism.

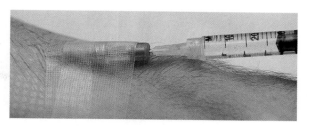

Figure 4-6 • **Administration of medication by intravenous bolus.** A bolus, in the context of an intravenous injection, is a dose of a substance. *(From Potter PA, Perry AG: Fundamentals of Nursing, ed 6, St Louis, 2005, Mosby.)*

in-	in, into	incision _____
inter-	between	intervertebral _____
		An intervertebral disk lies between any two vertebrae.
intra-	within	intrauterine _____
		intravenous _____
		The abbreviation for intravenous is IV. See Figure 4-6.
mal-	bad	malignant _____
meta-	change, beyond	metastasis _____
		This term literally means a "change of place" (-STASIS). It is the spread of a cancerous tumor from its original place to a secondary location in the body.
		metacarpals _____
		The carpal bones are the wrist bones, and the metacarpals are the hand bones, which are beyond the wrist. See the x-ray image of the hand in Figure 4-7.

4

Malignant versus benign

The root IGN comes from the Latin *ignis,* meaning "fire." A malignant tumor is a cancerous growth that spreads like a "wild fire" from its original location to other organs. A benign tumor (BEN- means "good") is a noncancerous growth that does not spread.

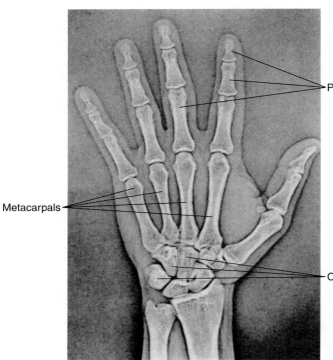

Phalanges

Metacarpals

Carpals

Figure 4-7 • **Metacarpals.** This x-ray image of a hand shows metacarpals, carpals (wrist bones), and phalanges (finger bones).

4

neo-	new	neoplasm _____
		neoplastic _____
		neonatal _____

Neonates who are born prematurely are often cared for in the neonatal intensive care unit (NICU) . *See Figure 4-8.*

para-	beside, near, along the side of	parathyroid glands _____

Figure 4-9 shows the position of the parathyroid glands on the back side of the thyroid gland. The parathyroid glands are endocrine glands that regulate the amount of calcium in bones and in the blood.

Intensive care units

Note the pronunciations and meanings of other hospital intensive care units:

MICU (**MIK**-u)   medical intensive care unit
MSICU (**M-SIK**-u)   medical/surgical intensive care unit
PICU (**PIK**-u)   pediatric or psychiatric intensive care unit
SICU (**SIK**-u)   surgical intensive care unit

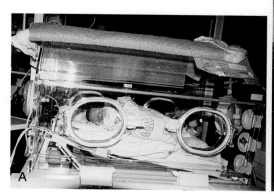 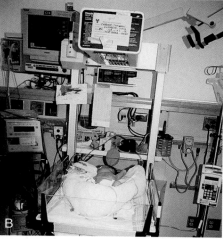

Figure 4-8 • **Neonates in the neonatal intensive care unit (NICU). A,** Benjamin Oliver Chabner, born May 22, 2001, at 32 weeks (8 weeks premature). **B,** Samuel August "Gus" Thompson, born August 13, 2001, at 36 weeks. Gus needed an endotracheal tube through which he received surfactant, a substance necessary to inflate his lungs. Both children are healthy and a delight to their grandmother.

paralysis _____

This term came from the Greek paralytikos, *meaning "one whose side was loose or weak," as after a stroke. Now it means a loss of movement in any part of the body caused by a break in the connection between nerve and muscle.*

4

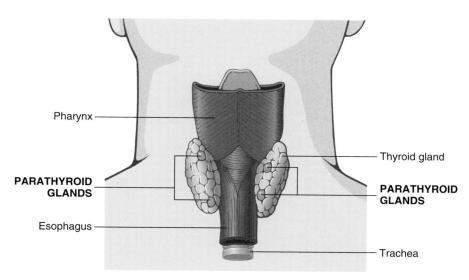

Figure 4-9 • **Parathyroid glands.** These are four endocrine glands on the posterior (back side) of the thyroid gland.

paraplegia _____

-PLEGIA means paralysis, and this term originally meant paralysis of any limb or side of the body. Since the nineteenth century, however, it has indicated paralysis of the lower half of the body.

peri-	surrounding	periosteum _____
		perianal _____
poly-	many, much	polyuria _____
		polyneuropathy _____
		polydipsia _____

Symptoms of diabetes mellitus are polyuria and polydipsia.

post-	after, behind	postpartum _____
		postmortem _____
pre-	before	precancerous _____

*An example of a precancerous lesion is **polyps** (benign growths), commonly found in the colon. These neoplasms are often removed via colonoscopy, because they may eventually become malignant.*

prenatal _____

Polyuria and diuretics

Diuretics (DI- from DIA-, meaning "complete") are drugs that promote an abnormally large quantity of urine (polyuria). They are used in the treatment of hypertension to lower blood pressure by removing excess fluid from the body.

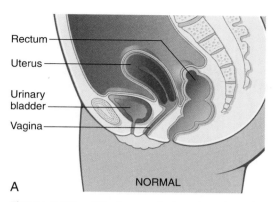
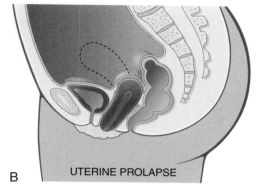

Rectum

Uterus

Urinary
bladder

Vagina

A   NORMAL

B   UTERINE PROLAPSE

Figure 4-10 • **Uterine prolapse.** A prolapsed uterus is shown in **B.** Normally, the uterus is tilted forward above the urinary bladder **(A).**

pro-	before, forward	prolapse _____

-LAPSE *means to slide. Figure 4-10 shows both the normal position of the uterus and its position when prolapsed.*

pros-	before, forward	prosthesis _____

An artificial limb is a prosthesis (literally meaning "placed" or "put"). Figure 4-11 shows Amy Palmiero-Winters running with a prosthetic leg. Figure 4-12 shows a total hip replacement and a total knee joint replacement.

4

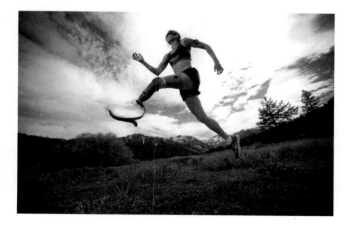

Figure 4-11 • Amy Palmiero-Winters is the first female with a prosthetic leg to finish the Badwater 135, a 135-mile race from Badwater in Death Valley to Mount Whitney, California.

4

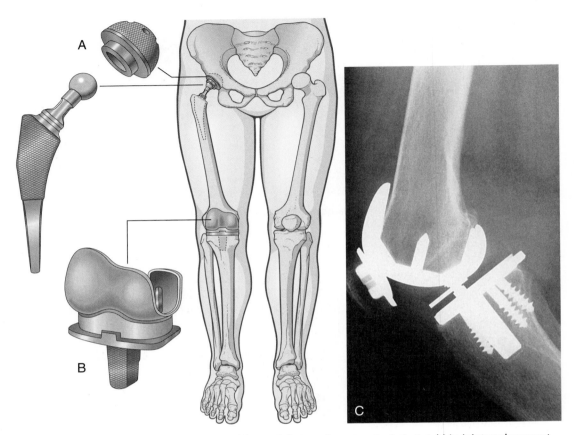

A

B

C

Figure 4-12 • **Total hip joint and total knee joint replacement. A,** In total hip joint replacement, a cementless prosthesis allows porous ingrowth of bone. **B,** In total knee joint replacement, the prosthesis includes a tibial metal retainer and a femoral component. The femoral component is chosen individually for each patient according to the amount of healthy bone present. **C,** X-ray image of knee replacement. (**C** *From Mettler FA:* Essentials of Radiology, *ed 2, Philadelphia, 2005, Saunders.*)

quadri-	four	quadriplegia _____ *Paralysis of all four limbs.*
re-	back, behind	relapse _____ *Symptoms of disease return when a patient has a relapse.* ***Exacerbation*** *is an increase in the severity of a disease or any of its symptoms.*
		remission _____ *Symptoms of disease lessen when the disease goes into remission.*
		resection _____

retro-   back, behind   retroperitoneal _____

The kidneys and adrenal glands are retroperitoneal organs. (See Figure 2-4 on page 52.)

sub-   under, less than   subcostal _____

subcutaneous _____

subtotal _____

A subtotal gastrectomy is a partial resection of the stomach.

subscapular _____

The scapula is the shoulder bone. Figure 4-13 shows its location.

syn-   with, together   syndrome _____

-DROME means running or occurring. Syndromes are groups of symptoms or signs of illness that occur together. Table 4-4 gives examples of syndromes.

tachy-   fast   tachycardia _____

tachypnea _____

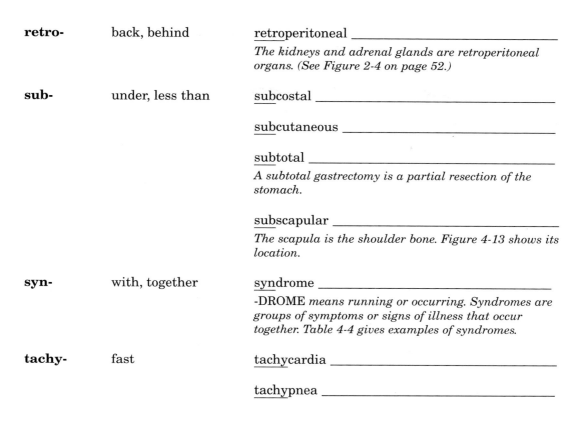
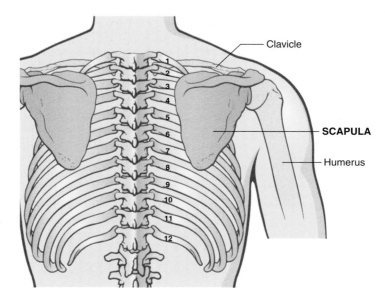

Figure 4-13 • Scapula (shoulder bone), posterior view. The clavicle is the collarbone, and the humerus is the upper arm bone. *(Modified from Chabner D-E: The Language of Medicine, ed 9, Philadelphia, 2011, Saunders.)*

Table 4-4 SYNDROMES*

Syndrome	Signs and Symptoms
acquired immunodeficiency syndrome (AIDS)	Severe infections, malignancy (Kaposi sarcoma and lymphoma), fever, malaise (discomfort), and gastrointestinal disturbances. It is caused by a virus that damages lymphocytes (white blood cells).
carpal tunnel syndrome	Pain, tingling, burning, and numbness of the hand and wrist. A nerve leading to the hand is compressed by connective tissue fibers in the wrist.
Down syndrome	Mental retardation, flat face with a short nose, slanted eyes, broad hands and feet, stubby fingers, and protruding lower lip. The syndrome occurs when an extra chromosome is present in each cell of the body.
mitral valve prolapse syndrome	Abnormal sounds (murmurs) heard through a stethoscope placed on the chest. These murmurs indicate that the mitral valve is not closing properly. Chest pain, dyspnea (difficult breathing), and fatigue are other symptoms.
toxic shock syndrome	High fever, vomiting, diarrhea, rash, hypotension (low blood pressure), and shock. It typically is caused by a bacterial infection in the vagina of menstruating women using superabsorbent tampons.

*See the Evolve website for additional information about syndromes (http://evolve.elsevier.com/Chabner/medtermshort).

4

trans-   across, through   transabdominal _____

transurethral _____

A ***transurethral resection*** *of the prostate gland is a* TURP. *Pieces of the prostate gland are removed through the urethra to relieve symptoms of **benign prostatic hypertrophy (BPH)**.*

tri-   three   tricuspid valve _____

-CUSPID *means "pointed end," as of a spear. The tricuspid valve is on the right side of the heart, while the mitral (bicuspid) valve is on the left side of the heart. Figure 4-14 shows the location of both valves and indicates the pathway of blood through the heart.*

ultra-   beyond   ultrasonography _____

Figure 4-15 shows an ultrasonogram (sonogram) of a fetus.

uni-   one   unilateral _____

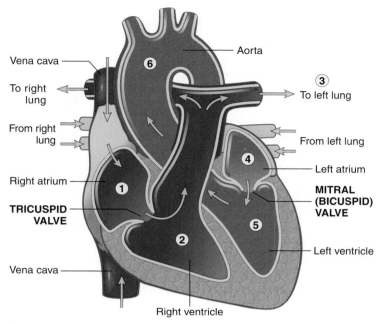

Figure 4-14 • **Tricuspid and mitral valves of the heart.** Blood enters the *right atrium* of the heart (1) from the big veins (venae cavae) and passes through the *tricuspid valve* to the *right ventricle* (2). Blood then travels to the *lungs* (3), where it loses carbon dioxide (a gaseous waste) and picks up oxygen. Blood returns to the heart into the *left atrium* (4) and passes through the *mitral (bicuspid) valve* to the *left ventricle* (5). It is then pumped from the left ventricle out of the heart into the largest artery, the *aorta* (6), which carries the blood to all parts of the body.

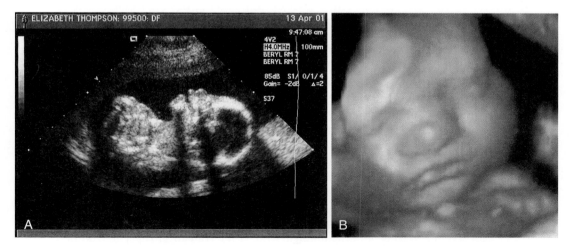

Figure 4-15 • **A, Ultrasonogram** showing my grandson Samuel August "Gus" Thompson as a 19-week-old fetus. **B,** Three-dimensional sonogram. (**A,** *courtesy Dr. Elizabeth Chabner Thompson.* **B,** *From Hagen-Ansert SL:* Textbook of Diagnostic Ultrasonography, *ed 6, St Louis, 2006, Mosby.*)

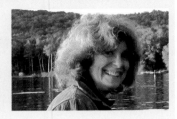

IN PERSON

The following is a first-person narrative describing the experience of a woman of a "certain age" (in her words) who had a knee replacement procedure.

Writing about my TKR [total knee replacement] more than two years after the operation is a singular experience. The main advantage of the passage of time is that—unlike psychic trauma, which seems to make inroads in the very structure of our brains—the release of the body from physical pain leaves amnesia in its wake. If that were not the case, no woman would ever have a second child—and no biped a second knee replacement. I know, even if my body doesn't remember, that I endured much pain in the aftermath of the surgery and for many weeks thereafter. In fact, unlike most other physical ailments, joint replacement necessitates working through the pain in order to regain mobility. It's when you feel you simply cannot bend it any more that you "start" working. . . So the pain is actually functional, and rather relentless. And yet I know—and accept—that sometime in the not-too-distant future, my left knee will follow my right in seeking a replacement. And that is because the osteoarthritis that depleted the first is depleting the second, and all my glucosamine-chondroitin pills, my quad exercises, my frequent massages, and even my nightshade-free diet are at best only putting off by several months or a year the inevitable.

I had endured many years of diminishing mobility in my right leg, alleviated somewhat by occasional cortisone shots and two arthroscopic surgeries (while stitching the second arthroscopic wound, my Israeli orthopedist said, "Nothing more to be done with this one. . . next stop: total knee replacement!') With all the research that I did in preparation for the Big Surgery, I became convinced—and still hold some version of this conviction—that TKR entails sawing the leg in two, like Houdini's blonde assistant in the box, and then screwing it back together with better screws. It didn't change that image much when my orthopedic surgeon at MGH [Massachusetts General Hospital], Dr. Dennis Burke, surely the best in his field in the universe, assured me that he is, in his spare time, a master carpenter . . ..

Okay—as this narrative demonstrates, the truth is a bit more complex and less grotesque. Still the procedure is very radical and involves major trauma to all the supporting muscles, tendons, nerves, and blood vessels. Hence a long period of recuperation is involved. I took advantage of the extra day that was offered to me at MGH (bless Medicare!) for a total hospitalization of five days, during which I had to learn how to perform the most basic functions in new ways. I found, after many trials, that a walker is preferable to crutches. Both are hard on the hands but the walker is more stable, and the attachable basket is a boon.

For those of a "certain age" who are contemplating TKR, the question of where to do the rehab is crucial. If, as I did, you have the conditions to recover at home, that is preferable. The necessary conditions are, first, a partner or caregiver who is available 24/7 for the first few days and who doesn't decide to take a prolonged vacation after that . . . The second relates to the physical conditions at home. Preferably the living area should all be on one level; although climbing stairs becomes one of the protocols of physical therapy, it takes a while to get to that point, and one is not very steady until that time. Easy access to bathrooms and to other living areas is crucial. The third necessary condition is the availability of the physical therapist. Living in the summer and fall months in rural New Hampshire, I was fortunate to qualify for the services of the local VNA [Visiting Nurse Association], and a marvelous physical therapist visited me three times a week for about six weeks. In between visits, I worked hard to win her approval and, although it seemed at first like tackling Everest to lift my leg even one inch off the floor, let alone walk, within about six weeks I could drive, even if I was getting around outside with crutches; within two months I had regained good mobility, and six months later I was as good as new, and ever so grateful . . . .

Although I consider this procedure to be nothing short of miraculous, like any major elective surgery, one should not undertake it unless the pain of daily life outweighs its joys . . . . when the doctors ask you about the pain, on a scale of 1 to 10, take them seriously. Don't undergo this surgery until it hovers around 8 or 9 . . . And then—well, enjoy the results!

Sidra DeKoven Ezrahi is a professor of Comparative Literature at the Hebrew University and is a Guggenheim Fellow. She divides her time between Jerusalem, Israel and Wilmot, New Hampshire.

? EXERCISES AND ANSWERS

Complete these exercises and check your answers. An important part of your success in learning medical terminology is checking your answers carefully with the Answers to Exercises beginning on page 155. Don't forget to wRite, Review, and Repeat!

A Give meanings for the following prefixes.

1. anti- _____
2. ana- _____
3. ad- _____
4. bi- _____
5. brady- _____
6. ab- _____
7. a-, an- _____
8. ante- _____
9. con- _____
10. dia- _____

B Complete the following sentences with the medical terms below.

analysis   antigen   bradycardia
anemia   apnea   diarrhea
antibiotic   atrophy
antibody   bilateral

1. A patient with hearing loss in both ears has a/an _____ condition.

2. When airways collapse or are blocked during sleep, a condition called sleep

   _____ may occur.

3. A protein produced by white blood cells in response to a foreign substance, such as

   a bacterium or virus, is a/an _____.

4. A foreign substance, such as a bacterium or virus, is a/an _____.

5. Decrease in hemoglobin in the blood to below the normal range produces a

   condition known as _____.

6. A condition of frequent loose, watery stools that seem to "flow through" the body is

   called _____.

7. The separation of substances into their component parts is known as _____.

8. A medication produced from molds or synthesized in a laboratory to destroy

   microorganisms is a/an _____.

9. A condition in which the heart rate is less than 60 beats per minute is

   _____.

10. Having an arm in a cast and not using it can cause _____.

C Give medical terms for the following meanings.

1. Without speech: _____

2. Lack of menstrual flow: _____

3. Before birth: _____

4. Glands located near the kidneys: _____ glands

5. An irregularity appearing with birth: _____ anomaly

6. Separation of waste materials from the blood when the kidneys fail:

_____

D **Give meanings for the following prefixes.**

1. ec- _____   6. dys- _____

2. epi- _____   7. endo- _____

3. hemi- _____   8. ex- _____

4. hyper- _____   9. extra- _____

5. hypo- _____   10. in- _____

E **Complete the following sentences using the medical terms listed below.**

dysmenorrhea   dysuria   extrahepatic
dysphagia   endoscopy   incision
dysplasia   epidermis
dyspnea   excision

1. Pain associated with menstrual flow is _____.

2. Cutting into a part of the body is a/an _____.

3. Any abnormal development in tissues or organs is _____.

4. Cutting out of a part of the body is a/an _____.

5. Painful burning sensation upon urination is _____.

6. Painful breathing that may be caused by anxiety, strenuous exercise, or certain

   heart conditions is _____.

7. The outer layer of skin is the _____.

8. Pertaining to outside the liver is _____.

9. Difficulty in swallowing is called _____.

10. Visual examination (via an endoscope) of what is within an organ is

_____.

F Complete the following medical terms using the meanings provided.

1. High blood pressure is _____tension.

2. A mass of blood above the membrane surrounding the brain is a/an

   _____dural hemat_____.

3. A pregnancy that is out of place and usually located in a fallopian tube is a/an

   _____topic pregnancy.

4. A condition of excessive (too much) blood sugar is _____emia.

5. A condition of deficient (too little) blood sugar is _____emia.

6. Glands that secrete hormones within the body are _____crine glands.

7. Increase in development (individual cells increase in size) often caused by overuse

   of a muscle or organ is hyper_____.

8. Paralysis of half of the body related to a stroke is _____plegia.

9. Excessive secretion of hormone from a gland in front of the trachea in the neck is

   hyper_____.

G Give meanings for the following prefixes.

1. intra- _____   6. inter- _____

2. mal-_____   7. meta- _____

3. para- _____   8. neo- _____

4. peri- _____   9. post- _____

5. poly- _____   10. pre- _____

H Give meanings for the following medical terms.

1. intervertebral _____

2. metastasis _____

3. metacarpals _____

4. intravenous _____

5. postmortem _____

6. periosteum _____

7. precancerous _____

8. neonatal _____

9. paraplegia _____

10. malignant _____

Ⓘ Complete each of the sentences below by selecting from the following list of terms. The bold words in each sentence should help you choose the correct term.

adrenal glands	neoplasm	polyneuropathy
dyspnea	parathyroid glands	polyuria
extracranial	perianal	postpartum
intrauterine	polydipsia	

1. An injury to the **outside** of the skull is a/an _____ lesion.

2. Four small glands in the neck region **near** (posterior to) another endocrine gland

   are the _____.

3. Common symptoms of diabetes are **much** urination, or _____,

   and **much** thirst, or _____.

4. People suffering from asthma often have **difficult** breathing, which is called

   _____.

5. Bleeding can occur from cracks or sores **surrounding** the opening to the rectum.

   These are _____ fissures.

6. Two glands each located **near** (above) a kidney are _____.

7. A **new** growth, which can be malignant or benign, is a/an _____.

8. Disease of **many** nerves is known as a/an _____.

9. Any problem that affects the fetus **within** the womb is a/an _____

   condition.

10. Women may experience moodiness and sad feelings **after** birth, a condition known

    as _____ depression.

J Give meanings for the following prefixes.

1. pro- _____

2. quadri- _____

3. sub- _____

4. tachy- _____

5. trans- _____

6. uni- _____

7. re- _____

8. pros- _____

9. retro- _____

10. syn- _____

11. ultra- _____

12. tri- _____

K Select from the following terms to complete each of the sentences below.

prolapse
prosthesis
quadriplegia
relapse

remission
resection
subtotal
syndrome

tachypnea
tricuspid
ultrasonography
unilateral

1. Removal or cutting out of an organ is a/an _____.

2. Test that shows the structure of organs using sound waves beyond the normal range of hearing is _____.

3. An artificial part of the body is a/an _____.

4. Recurrence of symptoms of an illness is a/an _____.

5. Recovery and disappearance of symptoms is a/an _____.

6. Rapid breathing is _____.

7. If the spinal cord is severed in the cervical region, paralysis of all four limbs, known as _____ , occurs.

8. The _____ valve has three parts and is on the right side of the heart, between the upper and lower chambers.

9. If a patient has a/an _____ gastrectomy, less than the complete stomach is removed.

10. Pain, tingling, burning, and numbness of the hand are symptoms of carpal tunnel _____.

L Define the following terms that describe parts of the body.

1. subscapular _____

2. transabdominal _____

3. retroperitoneal _____

4. subcutaneous _____

5. intervertebral _____

M Select from the following terms to complete the sentences below.

anemia   prolapse   tachycardia
aphasia   relapse   transurethral
paralysis   remission

1. After her ninth child, muscles in Ms. Smith's uterine wall weakened, causing her

   uterus to fall and _____ through her vagina.

2. After Mr. Jones' heart attack, his cardiologist noticed a rapid heart rhythm, or

   _____.

3. A cerebrovascular accident (CVA) on the left side of the brain can cause a loss of

   speech, or _____.

4. Menorrhagia and lack of iron in Sharon's diet led to a condition of low hemoglobin

   and iron deficiency _____.

5. The operation to remove part of Bill's enlarged prostate gland involved placing a

   catheter through his urethra and removing pieces of the gland. The surgery, called

   a TURP, or _____ resection of the prostate gland,

   improved his ability to urinate. The prostate gland is at the base of the urinary

   bladder in males (see Figure 4-16).

4

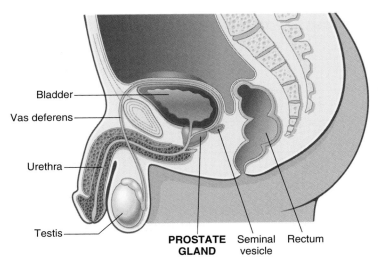

Bladder

Vas deferens

Urethra

Testis

PROSTATE GLAND

Seminal vesicle

Rectum

Figure 4-16 • **Prostate gland.**

4

N Circle the correct meaning in each of the following.

1. Dys- and mal- both mean **(outside, good, bad)**.

2. Hypo- and sub- both mean **(under, above, outside)**.

3. Epi- and hyper- both mean **(inside, beneath, above)**.

4. Con- and syn- both mean **(apart, near, with)**.

5. Ultra- and meta- both mean **(new, beyond, without)**.

6. Ante-, pre-, and pro- all mean **(before, surrounding, between)**.

7. Ec- and extra- both mean **(within, many, outside)**.

8. Endo-, intra-, and in- all mean **(painful, within, through)**.

9. Post-, re-, and retro- all mean **(behind, slow, together)**.

10. Uni- mean**s** **(one, two, three)**.

11. Tri- means **(one, two, three)**.

12. Bi- means **(one, two, three)**.

O Circle the term that best completes the meaning of the sentences in the following medical vignettes.

1. As part of her **(intravenous, postpartum, prenatal)** care, Beatrix underwent **(ultrasonography, endoscopy, urinalysis)** to determine the age, size, and development of her fetus.

2. Ellen's pregnancy test was positive, but she had excruciating pelvic pain. After a careful pelvic exam and ultrasound scan, the doctors diagnosed a/an **(epidural, ectopic, subscapular)** pregnancy. She then underwent emergency surgery to remove the implanted tissue from the fallopian tube.

3. After noticing a suspicious-looking mole on her upper arm, Carole was diagnosed with **(malignant, benign, subtotal)** melanoma. This type of skin cancer is a/an **(intrauterine, extrahepatic, neoplastic)** process and has a high likelihood of **(paralysis, dysplasia, metastasis)** to other areas of the body.

4. Carole's daughter, Annabelle, found a mole on her back and quickly had it checked by her physician. Fortunately, after a biopsy, the pathology revealed a **(transabdominal, precancerous, perianal)** nevus (mole) that was considered **(chronic, unilateral, benign)**. In the future, Annabelle will need close follow-up for other suspicious lesions.

5. Milton's blood pressure was 160/110 mm Hg. Normal blood pressure is 120/80 mm Hg. To reduce Milton's risk of stroke, his physician prescribed medication to treat his **(bradycardia, hypertension, dyspnea)**.

4

ANSWERS TO EXERCISES

A
1. against
2. up, apart
3. toward, near
4. two, both
5. slow
6. away from
7. no, not, without
8. before, forward
9. with, together
10. through, complete

B
1. bilateral
2. apnea
3. antibody
4. antigen
5. anemia
6. diarrhea
7. analysis
8. antibiotic
9. bradycardia
10. atrophy

C
1. aphasia
2. amenorrhea
3. antepartum, or prenatal
4. adrenal
5. congenital
6. dialysis

D
1. out, outside
2. above, upon
3. half
4. excessive, too much, above
5. deficient, too little, below
6. bad, painful, difficult, abnormal
7. within, in, inner
8. out
9. outside of
10. in, into

E
1. dysmenorrhea
2. incision
3. dysplasia
4. excision
5. dysuria
6. dyspnea
7. epidermis
8. extrahepatic
9. dysphagia
10. endoscopy

F
1. **hyper**tension
2. **epi**dural hemat**oma**
3. **ec**topic
4. **hyperglyc**emia
5. **hypoglyc**emia
6. **endo**crine
7. hyper**trophy**
8. **hemi**plegia
9. hyper**thyroidism**

G
1. within
2. bad
3. beside, near, along the side of
4. surrounding
5. many, much
6. between
7. change, beyond
8. new
9. after, behind
10. before

H
1. pertaining to between the vertebrae (backbones)
2. change of place or beyond control (spread of a cancerous tumor to a secondary location)
3. beyond the wrist bones (carpals); hand bones
4. pertaining to within a vein
5. after death
6. membrane surrounding a bone
7. pertaining to a condition that comes before a malignancy—for example, dysplastic nevi (moles) that precede malignant melanoma
8. pertaining to new birth (a neonate is a newborn)
9. condition of paralysis of the lower half of the body
10. cancerous; not benign

I
1. extracranial
2. parathyroid glands
3. polyuria; polydipsia
4. dyspnea
5. perianal
6. adrenal glands
7. neoplasm
8. polyneuropathy
9. intrauterine
10. postpartum

J
1. before, forward
2. four
3. under, less than
4. fast
5. across, through
6. one
7. back, behind
8. before, forward
9. back, behind
10. with, together
11. beyond
12. three

K
1. resection
2. ultrasonography
3. prosthesis; literally, "to put forward"
4. relapse
5. remission
6. tachypnea
7. quadriplegia
8. tricuspid
9. subtotal
10. syndrome

L
1. pertaining to under the scapula (shoulder bone)
2. pertaining to across or through the abdomen
3. pertaining to behind the peritoneum
4. pertaining to under the skin
5. pertaining to between the vertebrae (backbones)

M
1. prolapse
2. tachycardia
3. aphasia
4. anemia
5. transurethral

N
1. bad
2. under
3. above
4. with
5. beyond
6. before
7. outside
8. within
9. behind
10. one
11. three
12. two

O
1. prenatal, ultrasonography
2. ectopic
3. malignant, neoplastic, metastasis
4. precancerous, benign
5. hypertension

4

PRONUNCIATION OF TERMS

The terms that you have learned in this chapter are presented here with their pronunciations. The capitalized letters in **BOLDFACE** *represent the accented syllable. Pronounce each word out loud; then write its meaning in the space provided. All terms are defined in the* **Mini-Dictionary: Glossary of Medical Terms,** *beginning on page 341 and on the audio section of the Evolve website (http://evolve.elsevier.com/medtermshort).*

TERM	PRONUNCIATION	MEANING
abnormal	ab-**NOR**-mal	_____
adrenal glands	ah-**DRE**-nal glanz	_____
analysis	ah-**NAL**-ih-sis	_____
anemia	ah-**NE**-me-ah	_____
antepartum	**AN**-te **PAR**-tum	_____
antibiotic	an-tih-bi-**OT**-ik	_____
antibody	**AN**-tih-bod-e	_____
antigen	**AN**-tih-jen	_____
aphasia	a-**FA**-ze-ah	_____
apnea	**AP**-ne-ah	_____
atrophy	**AT**-ro-fe	_____
benign	be-**NIN**	_____
bilateral	bi-**LAT**-er-al	_____
bradycardia	bra-de-**KAR**-de-ah	_____
congenital anomaly	kon-**JEN**-ih-tal ah-**NOM**-ah-le	_____
dialysis	di-**AL**-ih-sis	_____
diarrhea	di-ah-**RE**-ah	_____
dysphagia	dis-**FA**-jah	_____
dysplasia	dis-**PLA**-zhah	_____

4

dyspnea	**DISP**-ne-ah *or* disp-**NE**-ah _____
dysuria	dis-**U**-re-ah _____
ectopic pregnancy	ek-**TOP**-ik **PREG**-nan-se _____
endocrine glands	**EN**-do-krin glanz _____
endoscopy	en-**DOS**-ko-pe _____
epidural hematoma	ep-ih-**DUR**-al he-mah-**TO**-mah _____
excision	ek-**SIZH**-un _____
extrahepatic	eks-tra-heh-**PAT**-ik _____
hemigastrectomy	heh-me-gast-**REK**-to-me _____
hemiplegia	heh-me-**PLE**-jah _____
hyperglycemia	hi-per-gli-**SE**-me-ah _____
hypertension	hi-per-**TEN**-shun _____
hyperthyroidism	hi-per-**THI**-royd-izm _____
hypertrophy	hi-**PER**-tro-fe _____
hypoglycemia	hi-po-gli-**SE**-me-ah _____
incision	in-**SIZH**-un _____
intervertebral	in-ter-**VER**-teh-bral _____
intrauterine	in-trah-**U**-ter-in _____
intravenous	in-trah-**VE**-nus _____
malignant	mah-**LIG**-nant _____
metacarpal	met-ah-**KAR**-pal _____
metastasis	meh-**TAS**-tah-sis _____
neonatal	ne-o-**NA**-tal _____
neoplastic	ne-o-**PLAS**-tik _____

4

paralysis	pah-**RAL**-ih-sis _____
paraplegia	par-ah-**PLE**-jah _____
parathyroid glands	par-ah-**THI**-royd glanz _____
perianal	per-e-**A**-nal _____
periosteum	per-e-**OS**-te-um _____
polydipsia	pol-e-**DIP**-se-ah _____
polyneuropathy	pol-e-nu-**ROP**-ah-the _____
polyuria	pol-e-**UR**-e-ah _____
postmortem	post-**MOR**-tem _____
postpartum	post-**PAR**-tum _____
precancerous	pre-**KAN**-ser-us _____
prolapse	pro-**LAPS** _____
prosthesis	pros-**THE**-sis _____
quadriplegia	quah-drah-**PLE**-jah _____
relapse	re-**LAPS** _____
remission	re-**MISH**-un _____
resection	re-**SEK**-shun _____
retroperitoneal	reh-tro-peri-ih-to-**NE**-al _____
subcostal	sub-**KOS**-tal _____
subcutaneous	sub-ku-**TA**-ne-us _____
subdural hematoma	sub-**DUR**-al he-mah-**TO**-mah _____
subscapular	sub-**SKAP**-u-lar _____
subtotal	sub-**TO**-tal _____

4

syndrome	**SIN**-drom _____
tachycardia	tak-eh-**KAR**-de-ah _____
tachypnea	tak-ip-**NE**-ah _____
transabdominal	trans-ab-**DOM**-ih-nal _____
transurethral	trans-u-**RE**-thral _____
tricuspid valve	tri-**KUS**-pid valv _____
ultrasonography	ul-trah-son-**OG**-rah-fe _____
unilateral	u-nih-**LAT**-er-al _____
urinalysis	u-rih-**NAL**-ih-sis _____

PRACTICAL APPLICATIONS

MATCHING

Match the abnormal condition in Column I with the organ, lesion, or body part in Column II that may be involved in or cause the condition. Answers are found on page 162.

COLUMN I	COLUMN II
1. aphasia	_____ A. urinary bladder
2. dysphagia	_____ B. colon
3. diarrhea	_____ C. uterine cervix
4. quadriplegia	_____ D. left-sided brain lesion
5. hyperglycemia	_____ E. pancreas
6. dysuria	_____ F. lungs
7. paraplegia	_____ G. heart
8. bradycardia	_____ H. cervical spinal cord lesion
9. dyspnea	_____ I. esophagus
10. dysplasia	_____ J. lumbar spinal cord lesion

4

PRINCIPAL DIAGNOSIS

The **principal diagnosis** *is the cause, after evaluation, of the patient's admission to the hospital. Physician notes, which document clinical investigations and findings, are important for medical billing and coding. A careful reading of physician notes will identify the principal diagnosis, as in the following example.*

Physician Notes

A 22-year-old sexually active female presents to the ED [emergency department] with history of temperature of 104° F for 2 days, vomiting, diarrhea, and a red spotty rash over her chest and abdomen. She reports that she remembered not removing a tampon from her last menstrual cycle until a week after she had stopped menstruating. Other complaints include dysmenorrhea and dysuria.

Physical examination does not reveal an acute abdomen [sudden, severe abdominal pain] or any RLQ tenderness. Blood test is negative for HCG [human chorionic gonadotropin or pregnancy test]; CBC [complete blood count] reveals elevated white blood cell count; blood cultures are positive for staphylococci.

The patient's fever and dehydration do not subside with initial emergency care, and she is subsequently admitted to the hospital. She is seen by a physician from ID [infectious disease], who confirms that the retained tampon has resulted in the above conditions. Her condition improves with IV fluids and antibiotics.

Using the information presented in the physician notes, select the principal diagnosis from the following. Answers are found on page 162.

A. Dehydration (276.51)

B. Fever (280.60)

C. Toxic shock syndrome (TSS) (040.82) with *Staphylococcus aureus* (041.10)

D. Rash (782.1)

E. Nausea/vomiting (787.01)

(The numbers in parentheses are medical codes as given in the *International Classification of Diseases, Ninth Revision [ICD-9] Coding Handbook 2011.*)

DISEASE DESCRIPTION: HYPERTHYROIDISM

From the following list, select terms to complete the sentences in the paragraphs below.

antibiotics	exophthalmos	hypoplastic
antibodies	goiter	hyposecretion
bradycardia	hyperplastic	neoplastic
dyspnea	hypersecretion	tachycardia

1. Hyperthyroidism, also known as thyrotoxicosis or Graves disease, is marked by an excess of thyroid hormones. There is much evidence for a hereditary factor in the development of this condition, and some researchers consider it to be an autoimmune disorder caused by _____ that bind to the surface of thyroid gland cells and stimulate _____ of hormones (T_3 and T_4—triiodothyronine and thyroxine). On histologic examination, the enlarged gland is composed of _____ follicles lined with hyperactive cells.

2. Signs and symptoms of hyperthyroidism include restlessness, insomnia, weight loss, sweating, and rapid heartbeat, or _____. Abnormal protrusion of the eyes, known as _____, is another clinical sign. The patient typically also has an enlarged thyroid gland, called a/an _____.

ANSWERS TO PRACTICAL APPLICATIONS

Matching

1. D	3. B	5. E	7. J	9. F
2. I	4. H	6. A	8. G	10. C

Principal Diagnosis

Answer: C. Toxic shock syndrome (TSS) with *Staphylococcus aureus*
  A. Dehydration is an **admitting diagnosis.***
  B. Fever is an **admitting diagnosis.***
  D. Rash is a **POA (present on admission) diagnosis.**†
  E. Nausea/vomiting is a **POA diagnosis.**†

Disease Description: Hyperthyroidism

1. antibodies, hypersecretion, hyperplastic   2. tachycardia, exophthalmos, goiter

*An **admitting diagnosis** is a cause, before further evaluation, for admission to the hospital. Such conditions may not resolve in the ED and can become life-threatening without proper treatment.

†A **POA (present on admission) diagnosis** reflects incidental conditions that are noted and treated if necessary but are not a cause for hospital admission. Such conditions are not life-threatening (at the time of admission) but may require treatment and monitoring during the patient's stay.

PICTURE SHOW

Answer the questions that follow each image. Correct answers are found on page 165.

A

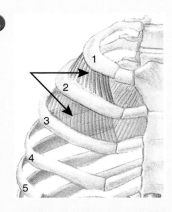

(Modified from Thibodeau GA, Patton KT: Anatomy and Physiology, *ed 5, St Louis, 2003, Mosby.)*

1. The *arrows* are pointing to muscles that lie between the ribs. They are the:
   a. intracostal muscles
   b. intercostal muscles
   c. perianal muscles
   d. intrauterine muscles

B

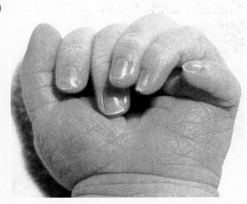

(From Zitelli BJ, Davis HW: Atlas of Pediatric Physical Diagnosis, *ed 4, St Louis, 2002, Mosby.)*

1. This image shows the hand of an infant with (HINT: the combining form for fingers is DACTYL/O):
   a. syndactyly
   b. condactyly
   c. transdactyly
   d. polydactyly

2. This condition occurs as a/an:
   a. neoplastic anomaly
   b. congenital anomaly
   c. hypertensive anomaly
   d. ectopic pregnancy

4

C

Bag

Drip chamber

Tube

Clamp

(Modified from Sorrentino SA: Mosby's Textbook for Nursing Assistants, *ed 5, St Louis, 2000, Mosby.)*

1. This equipment permits nutrients to enter the bloodstream and is used for:
   a. hemodialysis
   b. intrauterine feeding
   c. intravenous feeding
   d. peritoneal dialysis

2. Which term describes a condition or procedure that would be likely to make this equipment necessary?
   a. metacarpalgia
   b. hemigastrectomy
   c. polyneuropathy
   d. epidural hematoma
   e. ultrasonography

D

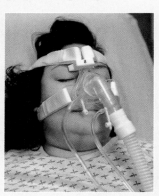

(From Elkin MK, Perry AG, Potter PA: Nursing Interventions and Clinical Skills, *ed 2, St Louis, 2000, Mosby.)*

1. The image shows a woman using a device that helps her maintain adequate blood oxygen levels while sleeping. This method is called:
   a. airway prosthesis
   b. nasogastric intubation
   c. bronchoscopy
   d. continuous positive airway pressure (CPAP)

2. The condition that may require use of such a device during sleep is:
   a. bradycardia
   b. aphasia
   c. apnea
   d. dysphagia

E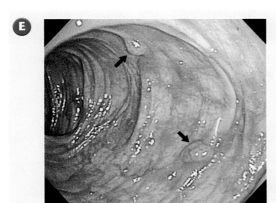

(From Weinstein WM, Hawkey CJ, Bosch J: Clinical Gastroenterology and Hepatology, *St Louis, 2005, Mosby.)*

1. The *arrows* in this image show abnormal, precancerous, neoplastic lesions in the colon. They are:
   a. polyps
   b. fibroids
   c. prolapsed mitral valves
   d. metastases

2. This image was taken via:
   a. intrauterine ultrasonography
   b. electrocardiography
   c. transabdominal ultrasonography
   d. endoscopy

4

ANSWERS TO PICTURE SHOW

A	1. b	
B	1. d	2. b
C	1. c	2. b
D	1. d	2. c
E	1. a	2. d

REVIEW

Write the meaning of each of the following word parts, and remember to check your answers with the Answers to Review on page 169.

PREFIXES

PREFIX	MEANING	PREFIX	MEANING
1. a-, an- _____		20. inter- _____	
2. ab- _____		21. intra- _____	
3. ad- _____		22. mal- _____	
4. ana- _____		23. meta- _____	
5. ante- _____		24. neo- _____	
6. anti- _____		25. para- _____	
7. bi- _____		26. peri- _____	
8. brady- _____		27. post- _____	
9. con- _____		28. pre- _____	
10. dia- _____		29. pro-, pros- _____	
11. dys- _____		30. quadri- _____	
12. ec- _____		31. re-, retro- _____	
13. endo- _____		32. sub- _____	
14. epi- _____		33. syn- _____	
15. ex-, extra- _____		34. tachy- _____	
16. hemi- _____		35. trans- _____	
17. hyper- _____		36. tri- _____	
18. hypo- _____		37. ultra- _____	
19. in- _____		38. uni- _____	

4

COMBINING FORMS

COMBINING FORM	MEANING	COMBINING FORM	MEANING
1. abdomin/o	_____	16. neur/o	_____
2. an/o	_____	17. norm/o	_____
3. bi/o	_____	18. oste/o	_____
4. cardi/o	_____	19. peritone/o	_____
5. carp/o	_____	20. plas/o	_____
6. cis/o	_____	21. ren/o	_____
7. cost/o	_____	22. scapul/o	_____
8. crani/o	_____	23. son/o	_____
9. cutane/o	_____	24. thyroid/o	_____
10. dur/o	_____	25. top/o	_____
11. gen/o	_____	26. troph/o	_____
12. glyc/o	_____	27. urethr/o	_____
13. hemat/o	_____	28. uter/o	_____
14. later/o	_____	29. ven/o	_____
15. nat/i	_____	30. vertebr/o	_____

4

SUFFIXES

SUFFIX	MEANING	SUFFIX	MEANING
1. -al		20. -partum	
2. -ation		21. -pathy	
3. -cision		22. -phagia	
4. -crine		23. -phasia	
5. -dipsia		24. -plasia	
6. -emia		25. -plasm	
7. -gen		26. -plegia	
8. -graphy		27. -pnea	
9. -ia		28. -rrhea	
10. -ic		29. -scopy	
11. -ine		30. -section	
12. -ism		31. -stasis	
13. -lapse		32. -tension	
14. -lysis		33. -thesis	
15. -meter		34. -tic	
16. -mission		35. -trophy	
17. -mortem		36. -um	
18. -oma		37. -uria	
19. -ous		38. -y	

4

ANSWERS TO REVIEW

PREFIXES

1. no, not, without
2. away from
3. toward
4. up, apart
5. before, forward
6. against
7. two
8. slow
9. with, together
10. through, complete
11. bad, painful, difficult, abnormal
12. out, outside
13. within, in, inner
14. above, upon
15. out, outside
16. half
17. excessive, above
18. below, under
19. in, into
20. between
21. within
22. bad
23. change, beyond
24. new
25. beside, near, along the side of
26. surrounding
27. after, behind
28. before
29. before, forward
30. four
31. back, behind
32. under, less than
33. with, together
34. fast
35. across, through
36. three
37. beyond
38. one

COMBINING FORMS

1. abdomen
2. anus
3. life
4. heart
5. wrist bones
6. to cut
7. ribs
8. skull
9. skin
10. dura mater
11. to produce
12. sugar
13. blood
14. side
15. birth
16. nerve
17. rule, order
18. bone
19. peritoneum
20. formation, growth
21. kidney
22. shoulder blade (bone)
23. sound
24. thyroid gland
25. to put, place
26. development, nourishment
27. urethra
28. uterus
29. vein
30. vertebra (backbone)

SUFFIXES

1. pertaining to
2. process, condition
3. process of cutting
4. secretion
5. condition of thirst
6. blood condition
7. to produce
8. process of recording
9. condition
10. pertaining to
11. pertaining to
12. condition, process
13. to fall, slide
14. loosening, breakdown, separation, destruction
15. to measure
16. to send
17. death
18. tumor
19. pertaining to
20. birth
21. disease condition
22. to eat, swallow
23. to speak
24. formation
25. formation
26. paralysis
27. breathing
28. flow, discharge
29. process of visual examination
30. incision
31. to stand, place, stop, control
32. pressure
33. to put, place
34. pertaining to
35. nourishment; development
36. structure
37. urine condition
38. process, condition

4

✓ TERMINOLOGY CHECKUP

Before you leave this chapter, here are important terminology concepts and information that you should thoroughly understand. Check the box next to each item when you know you've "got" it!

☐ 1. **Antigens, antibodies, and antibiotics: Antigens** are foreign substances (bacteria, viruses, fungi) that stimulate white blood cells to make **antibodies**, which destroy the antigens. **Antibiotics**, however, are medications produced *outside* the body to kill or inhibit the growth of antigens such as bacteria and other microorganisms.

☐ 2. **Primary malignant tumor and metastasis**: A **primary malignant tumor** originates and grows in a tissue or specific organ, such as the lung, breast, or liver. A **metastasis,** however, is a malignant tumor that has traveled from a primary location to a secondary site, such as a lymph node or a vital organ. For example, a tumor located in the lung may be a primary adenocarcinoma of the lung or a metastasis that has spread to the lung from another organ. Analysis of the biopsy sample will reveal this distinction.

☐ 3. **Remission and relapse:** A **remission** is the *lessening or absence of disease symptoms* during an illness. Patients who have no signs or symptoms of illness are described as being "in remission." A **relapse** is the *return of disease symptoms* (-LAPSE meaning to fall or slide), after a period of time.

☐ 4. **Paralysis and -plegia: Paralysis** is the *loss of muscle function.* It can be caused by a cerebrovascular accident (stroke) or nerve damage in any part of the body. The suffix **-plegia** means *paralysis.* For example, *hemiplegia* is paralysis of one half or one side of the body, as occurs with a stroke. *Quadriplegia* is paralysis of all four (QUADRI- means four) limbs of the body when spinal nerves in the neck are damaged.

☐ 5. **Syndrome and disease:** A **syndrome** is a group of signs and symptoms that occur together indicating a particular condition, the cause of which is not always known. An example is chronic fatigue syndrome. A **disease** is a specific medical condition often marked by an identifiable cause. Synonyms for disease are illness, sickness, and morbidity.

4

Medical Specialists and Case Reports

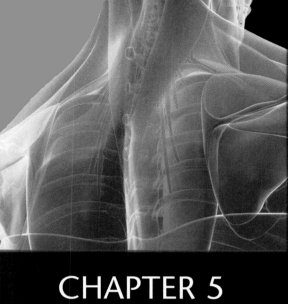

CHAPTER 5

CHAPTER OBJECTIVES

- To describe the training process of physicians
- To identify medical specialists and describe their specialties
- To identify combining forms used in terms that describe specialists
- To decipher medical terminology as written in case reports

171

Introduction

This chapter reviews many of the terms you have learned in previous chapters and adds others related to medical specialists. In the following section, the training of physicians is described and specialists are listed with their specialties. Next, on page 175, useful combining forms are presented with terminology to increase your medical vocabulary. Finally, short case reports beginning on page 180 illustrate the use of the medical language in context. As you read these reports, I guarantee that you will be impressed with your ability to understand medical terminology!

Medical Specialists

Doctors complete 4 years of medical school and then pass national medical board examinations to receive an MD degree (MD stands for Latin *Medicinae Doctor,* "teacher [doctor] of medicine"). They may then begin postgraduate training, which lasts at least 3 years and in some cases longer. This postgraduate training is known as *residency training.* Examples of residency programs are

Anesthesiology	Administration of agents capable of bringing about a loss of sensation
Dermatology	Diagnosis and treatment of skin disorders
Emergency medicine	Care of patients that requires sudden and immediate action
Family practice	Primary care of all members of the family on a continuing basis
Internal medicine	Diagnosis and treatment of usually complex, nonsurgical disorders in adults
Ophthalmology	Diagnosis and treatment of eye disorders
Pathology	Diagnosis of the cause and nature of disease
Pediatrics	Diagnosis and treatment of children's disorders
Psychiatry	Diagnosis and treatment of disorders of the mind
Radiology	Diagnosis using x-ray studies including ultrasound and magnetic resonance imaging (MRI)
Surgery	Treatment by manual (SURG- means hand) or operative methods

Examinations are administered after the completion of each residency program to certify the doctor's competency in that specialty area.

A physician may then choose to specialize further by doing *fellowship training.* Fellowship programs (lasting 2 to 5 years) train doctors in *clinical* (patient care) and *research* (laboratory) skills. For example, an *internist* (specialist in internal medicine) may choose fellowship training in internal medicine specialties such as neurology, nephrology, endocrinology, and oncology. A surgeon interested in further specialization may do fellowship training in thoracic surgery, neurosurgery, or plastic surgery. On completion of training and examinations, the doctor is then recognized as a specialist in that area of medical practice.

Medical specialists and an explanation of their specialties are listed below:

MEDICAL SPECIALIST	AREA OF PRACTICE
allergist	Treatment of hypersensitivity reactions
anesthesiologist	Administration of agents to prevent pain and unpleasant awareness during surgical and other procedures
cardiologist	Treatment of heart disease
cardiovascular surgeon	Surgery on the heart and blood vessels
colorectal surgeon	Surgery on the colon and rectum
dermatologist	Treatment of skin disorders
emergency practitioner	Immediate evaluation and treatment of acute injury and illness in a hospital setting
endocrinologist	Treatment of endocrine gland disorders
family practitioner	Primary care and treatment for families on a continuing basis
gastroenterologist	Treatment of stomach and intestinal disorders
geriatrician	Treatment of diseases of old age
gynecologist	Surgery and treatment for diseases of the female reproductive system
hematologist	Treatment of blood disorders
hospitalist	General medical care of hospitalized patients
infectious disease specialist	Treatment of diseases caused by microorganisms (bacteria, viruses, fungi, others)
internist	Comprehensive care for adults in an office or a hospital setting
nephrologist	Treatment of kidney diseases
neurologist	Treatment of nerve disorders
neurosurgeon	Surgery on the brain, spinal cord, and nerves
obstetrician	Treatment of pregnant women; delivery of babies
oncologist	Diagnosis and medical treatment of malignant and benign tumors
ophthalmologist	Surgical and medical treatment of eye disorders
orthopedist	Surgical treatment of bone, muscle, and joint conditions
otolaryngologist	Surgical treatment of ear, nose, and throat disorders
pathologist	Diagnosis of disease by analysis of cells
pediatrician	Treatment of diseases of children
physiatrist	Treatment to restore function after illness; physical medicine and rehabilitation specialist
psychiatrist	Treatment of mental disorders
pulmonologist	Treatment of lung diseases
radiologist	Examination of x-ray images to determine a diagnosis; interpretation of ultrasound, MRI, and nuclear medicine studies
radiation oncologist	Treatment of disease with high-energy radiation
rheumatologist	Treatment of systemic diseases affecting joints and muscles
thoracic surgeon	Surgery on chest organs
urologist	Surgery on the urinary tract and for treatment of male reproductive disorders

5

To help you identify medical specialists and what they do, select from the list of medical specialists to match the test or procedure described. Answers are found on page 201.

A Match the medical specialists with the procedures and tests that they perform. Write the name of the specialist on the line provided.

allergist   cardiovascular surgeon   gynecologist
anesthesiologist   endocrinologist   hematologist
cardiologist   gastroenterologist   ophthalmologist

PROCEDURE/TEST	MEDICAL SPECIALIST
1. Esophagoscopy and colonoscopy	_____
2. Blood cell counts; bone marrow biopsy	_____
3. Ultrasound examination of the heart; angioplasty	_____
4. Skin testing to determine sensitivity to antigens	_____
5. Serum (blood) level of hormones	_____
6. Vision tests; retinoscopy	_____
7. Coronary artery bypass grafting (CABG)	_____
8. Catheter and IV line insertion for sedation during surgery	_____
9. Pap smear (microscopic examination of cells from the cervix and organs); hysterectomy	_____

B Select from the list of medical specialists to match the test or procedure described.

neurologist   pathologist   radiologist
nephrologist   psychiatrist   radiation oncologist
orthopedist   pulmonologist   urologist

PROCEDURE/TEST	MEDICAL SPECIALIST
1. Nephrectomy; cystectomy; prostatectomy	_____
2. Personality and mental function tests	_____

5

3. Use of high-energy beams (photon and proton) to kill tumor cells   _____

4. Fixation of bone fracture; arthroscopic surgery   _____

5. Breathing function (spirometry) tests   _____

6. Microscopic examination of biopsy samples; autopsies   _____

7. CT scan; MRI; ultrasound examination   _____

8. Kidney function tests; dialysis   _____

9. Spinal and cranial nerve reflex tests   _____

COMBINING FORMS AND VOCABULARY

The combining forms listed below should be familiar because they are found in the list of terms describing medical specialists. A medical term is included to illustrate the use of the combining form. Write the meaning of the medical term in the space provided. You can always check your answers with the ***Mini-Dictionary: Glossary of Medical Terms*** beginning on page 341.

COMBINING FORM	MEANING	MEDICAL TERM	MEANING
cardi/o	heart	cardiomegaly	_____
col/o	colon (large intestine)	colitis	_____
dermat/o	skin	dermatitis	_____
endocrin/o	endocrine glands	endocrinology	_____

Ulcerative colitis and Crohn disease

Both of these conditions are types of **inflammatory bowel disease (IBD),** with similar signs and symptoms, such as abdominal pain, diarrhea, and bleeding from the rectum. While ulcerative colitis is confined to the colon, Crohn's commonly affects the last part of the small intestine and may involve other areas of the gastrointestinal tract. Lesions can be identified, but causes of both types of IBD are unknown. See the In Person feature on page **192**.

enter/o	intestines	enteritis _____
esthesi/o	sensation	anesthesiology _____
gastr/o	stomach	gastroscopy _____
ger/o	old age	geriatrics _____
gynec/o	woman, female	gynecology _____
hemat/o	blood	hematoma _____
iatr/o	treatment	iatrogenic _____

IATR/O *means treatment by a physician or with medicines. An iatrogenic illness is produced (-GENIC) adversely and unexpectedly by a treatment.*

laryng/o	voice box	laryngeal _____
lymph/o	lymph	lymphadenopathy _____

Lymph "glands" are actually lymph nodes, located all over the body but especially in **axillary** *(armpit),* **inguinal** *(groin),* **cervical** *(neck), and* **mediastinal** *(area between the lungs) regions. Lymphadenopathy often refers to the presence of malignant cells in lymph nodes.*

nephr/o	kidney	nephrostomy _____

A catheter (tube) is inserted into the kidney for drainage of fluid.

neur/o	nerve	neuralgia _____
nos/o	disease	nosocomial _____

A nosocomial infection is acquired during hospitalization (COMI/O means to care for).

obstetr/o	midwife	obstetric _____

odont/o	tooth	orthodontist _____
		ORTH/O *means straight.*
onc/o	tumor	oncogenic _____
		Oncogenic viruses give rise to tumors.
ophthalm/o	eye	ophthalmologist _____
opt/o	eye	optometrist _____
		An optometrist examines (METR/O means to measure) eyes and prescribes corrective lenses but cannot treat eye diseases.
optic/o	eye	optician _____
		Opticians grind lenses and fit glasses, and may treat eye diseases.
orth/o	straight	orthopedist _____
		PED/O comes from paidos, *the Greek word for "child." In the past, orthopedists were concerned with straightening bone deformities in children. Today, they treat bone, muscle, and joint disorders in adults as well.*
ot/o	ear	otitis _____
path/o	disease	pathology _____
ped/o	child	pediatrics _____
psych/o	mind	psychosis _____
pulmon/o	lung	pulmonary _____

Dental specialists

The following are other specialists in dental medicine:

Dental Specialist	**Area of Expertise**
periodontist	Gums (PERI- means surrounding)
endodontist	Root canal therapy (the root canal is the inner part of a tooth containing blood vessels and nerves)
pedodontist	Children (PED/O means child)
prosthodontist	Replacement of missing teeth with artificial appliances (PROSTH/O = artificial replacement)

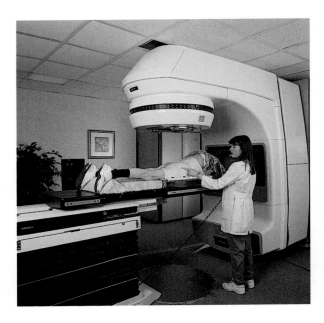

Figure 5-1 • **Radiation therapy.** The patient is positioned under a radiation therapy machine (containing a linear accelerator) to receive treatment for a lesion in the posterior portion of his hip. *(Courtesy Dr. Arthur Brimberg, Riverhill 21st Century Radiation Oncology, Yonkers, New York.)*

5

radi/o	x-rays	radiotherapy _____

Radiotherapy is also called radiation therapy. See Figure 5-1.

rect/o	rectum	rectocele _____

-CELE means a hernia or protrusion. The walls of the rectum weaken and bulge forward toward the vagina. See Figure 5-2.

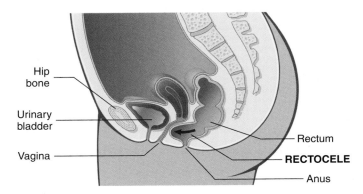

Hip bone

Urinary bladder

Vagina

Rectum

RECTOCELE

Anus

Figure 5-2 • **Rectocele.** *(Modified from Chabner D-E: The Language of Medicine, ed 9, Philadelphia, 2011, Saunders.)*

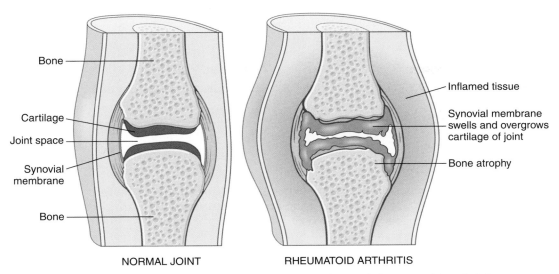

Figure 5-3 • **Differences between a normal joint and rheumatoid arthritis.**

rheumat/o   flow, fluid

rheumatology _____

Joints can fill with fluid when diseased—hence,
RHEUMAT/O *indicates a problem with a swollen joint.*
 Rheumatoid arthritis is a chronic inflammatory
disease of joints and connective tissues that leads to
deformation of joints. See Figures 5-3 and 5-4.

5

Rheumatoid arthritis and osteoarthritis

Rheumatoid arthritis first appears when patients (often women) are young, and it has an autoimmune component (antibodies are found that destroy joint tissue). Osteoarthritis most often appears in older patients (both men and women) and is marked by degenerative changes that cause destruction of the joint space. Knee and hip replacements may be helpful treatments for patients with osteoarthritis.

Figure 5-4 • **Advanced rheumatoid arthritis of the hands.** Notice the soft tissue swelling and deformed joints—fingers, knuckles, and wrist. Atrophy of muscles and tendons (connecting muscles to bones) allows one joint surface to slip past the other (subluxation). *(From Lewis SM, Heitkemper MM, Dirksen SR:* Medical-Surgical Nursing: Assessment and Management of Clinical Problems, *ed 6, St Louis, Mosby, 2004.)*

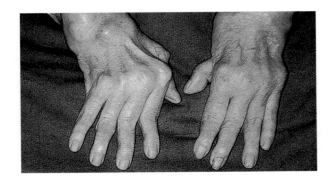

rhin/o	nose	rhinorrhea	_____
thorac/o	chest	thoracotomy	_____
ur/o	urinary tract	urology	_____
vascul/o	blood vessels	vasculitis	_____

Case Reports

Here are short case reports related to medical specialties. Many of the terms will be familiar to you; others are explained in the **_Mini-Dictionary: Glossary of Medical Terms_** (beginning on page 341). For every case report, write the meaning of the **boldface** terms in the spaces provided.

CASE 1 **_Cardiology_**

Mr. Rose was admitted to the cardiac care unit (CCU) with **angina** and a history of **hypertension.**

A **coronary angiogram** (Figure 5-5, _A_) showed **spasm** of the right coronary artery _(closed arrow)_, causing **acute myocardial ischemia.** The electrocardiogram (ECG) showed **ventricular arrhythmias** as well.

Nitroglycerin was administered, and within minutes, the angiogram showed reversal of the spasm (Figure 5-5, _B_). The ECG recorded reversal of the life-threatening arrhythmias as well. To prevent further ischemia and **myocardial infarction,** Mr. Rose's treatment will include **antiarrhythmic, diuretic,** and **anticoagulant** drugs. In the future, he may need an additional procedure to place a **stent** in his coronary artery to keep it open.

Continued on following page

CASE 1 *Cardiology* (Continued)

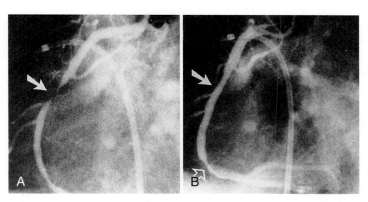

Figure 5-5 • **A, Coronary angiogram** showing spasm of the right coronary artery *(arrow).*
B, Angiogram showing reversal of the spasm *(arrow).* (**A** *and* **B,** *From Zipes DP, et al:* Braunwald's Heart Disease: A Textbook of Cardiovascular Medicine, *ed 7, Philadelphia, 2005, Saunders.)*

acute myocardial ischemia _____

angina _____

antiarrhythmic _____

anticoagulant _____

coronary angiogram _____

diuretic _____

hypertension _____

myocardial infarction _____

nitroglycerin _____

spasm _____

stent _____

ventricular arrhythmias _____

5

CASE 2 *Gynecology*

Ms. Sessions has had **dysmenorrhea** and **menorrhagia** for several months. She is also **anemic.** Because of the presence of a large **fibroid,** as seen on a pelvic **ultrasound** image (**sonogram**) (see Figure 5-6, *A*), a **hysterectomy** was recommended. After it was removed, the uterus was opened to reveal multiple fibroids (**leiomyomas**) bulging into the uterine cavity and displaying a firm, white appearance. See Figure 5-6, *B.*

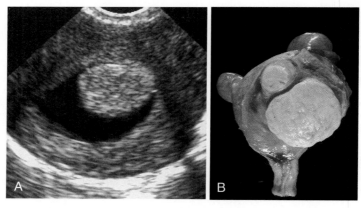

Figure 5-6 • **A, Pelvic sonogram. B, Fibroids (leiomyomas).** These are benign tumors of the uterus. *(A, From Salem S: The uterus and adnexa. In Rumack CM, Wilson SR, Charboneau JW, editors:* Diagnostic Ultrasound, *ed 2, St Louis, 1998, Mosby;* **B,** *from Cotran RS, Kumar V, Collins T:* Robbins' Pathologic Basis of Disease, *ed 6, Philadelphia, 1999, Saunders.)*

anemic _____

dysmenorrhea _____

fibroids _____

hysterectomy _____

leiomyomas _____

menorrhagia _____

sonogram _____

ultrasound _____

CASE 3 *Oncology*

John Smith, a 26-year-old law student, was admitted to the hospital after experiencing several months of fatigue, low-grade fevers, chest pain, and night sweats. A chest **MRI** scan (see Figure 5-7) revealed large **mediastinal** masses, as shown by *arrows*. **Needle biopsy** confirmed a **diagnosis** of **Hodgkin disease.** There was no evidence of **lymphadenopathy** or **hepatic** involvement. Treatment included **chemotherapy** followed by **radiotherapy** to the chest. Mr. Smith's **prognosis** is good.

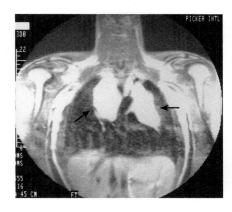

Figure 5-7 • **Magnetic resonance imaging of the upper body.** *(From Chabner D-E:* The Language of Medicine, *ed 9, Philadelphia, 2011, Saunders.)*

chemotherapy _____

diagnosis _____

fatigue _____

hepatic _____

Hodgkin disease _____

lymphadenopathy _____

mediastinal _____

MRI _____

needle biopsy _____

prognosis _____

radiotherapy _____

CASE 4 *Urology*

Scott Jones has a history of lower back pain, associated with **hematuria** and **dysuria.** An abdominal x-ray film (Figure 5-8, *A*) shows a **renal calculus** *(black arrow)* in the right upper quadrant. His doctor tells him that renal calculi should be suspected any time a calcification is seen within the renal outline or along the expected course of the **ureter** *(dotted lines).*

Treatment with shock wave **lithotripsy** (Figure 5-8, *B*) is expected to crush the stone and relieve his **symptoms.**

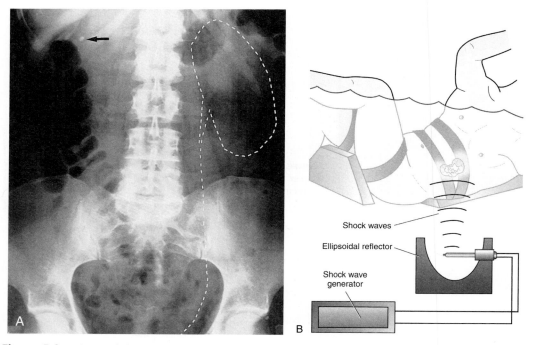

Figure 5-8 • **A,** An abdominal x-ray image showing a **renal calculus** *(arrow).* **B, Lithotripsy.** (**A,** *From Mettler FA:* Essentials of Radiology, *ed 2, Philadelphia, 2005, Saunders;* **B,** *from Rakel D:* Integrative Medicine, *ed 2, Philadelphia, 2007, Saunders.)*

dysuria _____

hematuria _____

lithotripsy _____

renal calculus _____

symptoms _____

ureter _____

CASE 5 *Gastroenterology*

Mr. Pepper suffers from **dyspepsia,** acid reflux, and sharp **abdominal** pain. A recent episode of **hematemesis** has left him very weak and **anemic. Gastroscopy** and an **upper GI series** with **barium** revealed the presence of a large **ulcer.** Figure 5-9 shows a photograph of a peptic ulcer located in the stomach. Mr. Pepper will be admitted to the hospital, treated with medication to reduce gastric acid output and with antibiotics to control a bacterium (*Helicobacter* or *H. pylori*) known to cause ulcers. He will also be scheduled for a partial **gastrectomy.**

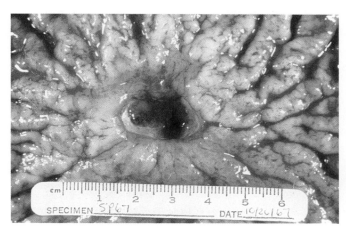

Figure 5-9 • **Peptic (gastric) ulcer.** *(From Lewis SM, Heitkemper MM, Dirksen SR:* Medical-Surgical Nursing: Assessment and Management of Clinical Problems, *ed 5, St Louis, 2004, Mosby.)*

abdominal _____

anemic _____

barium _____

dyspepsia _____

gastrectomy _____

gastroscopy _____

hematemesis _____

ulcer _____

upper GI series _____

CASE 6 *Radiology*

Evaluation of David Green's **posteroanterior** chest x-ray film (Figure 5-10, *A, arrows*) shows an ill-defined mass near the right **hilum.** The **lateral** view (Figure 5-10, *B, arrows*) also shows the mass, and its shaggy outline is very suggestive of **carcinoma.** Further evaluation by **CT scan** (Figure 5-10, *C*) clearly shows the mass in relation to the **mediastinal** structures such as the **pulmonary artery** (PA) and **aorta** (Ao).

Impression: Lung cancer

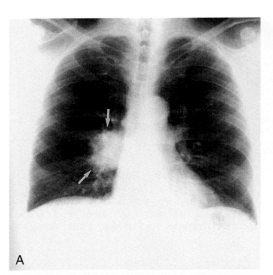

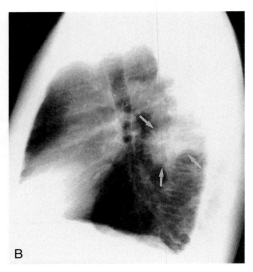

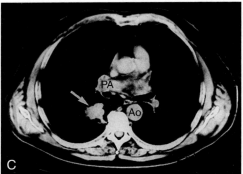

Figure 5-10 • **A, Posteroanterior chest x-ray** shows an ill-defined mass *(arrows).* **B, Lateral chest x-ray** view clearly shows the mass to be posterior to the hilum. **C, Computed tomography** image clearly shows the mass *(arrow)* in relation to the mediastinal structures. (**A-C,** *From Mettler FA:* Essentials of radiology, *ed 2, Philadelphia, 2005, Saunders.)*

Continued on following page

CASE 6 ***Radiology*** (Continued)

aorta _____

carcinoma _____

CT scan _____

hilum _____

lateral _____

mediastinal _____

posteroanterior _____

pulmonary artery _____

5

CASE 7 *Orthopedics*

A 20-year-old male patient was admitted to the hospital after a motorcycle accident. He was found to have **fractures** of the right **fibula** (see Figure 5-11, *A*), right **femur,** and **pelvis** and **intra-abdominal** injuries. He was taken to surgery, and internal **fixation** of the right femur was performed. A cast was applied to the femur for immobilization, and the fibula healed on its own with **callus** formation (Figure 5-11, *B*).

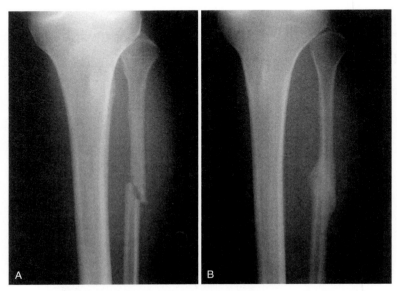

Figure 5-11 • A, Fracture of the fibula. B, Callus formation, 6 weeks later. *(Courtesy Dr. Barbara Weissman, Brigham and Women's Hospital, Boston, Massachusetts. **A** and **B,** From Cotran RS, Kumar V, Collins T: Robbins' Pathologic Basis of Disease, ed 6, Philadelphia, 1999, Saunders.)*

callus _____

femur _____

fibula _____

fixation _____

fracture _____

intra-abdominal _____

pelvis _____

CASE 8 *Nephrology*

A 52-year-old woman with **chronic renal failure** secondary to long-standing **hypertension** has been maintained on **hemodialysis** for the past 18 months. An **arteriovenous fistula** (Figure 5-12) was created surgically to provide long-term vascular access for hemodialysis. For the past 3 weeks, during the dialysis sessions, she has become moderately **hypotensive,** with symptoms of dizziness. Consequently, we have decided to withhold her **antihypertensive** medications before dialysis.

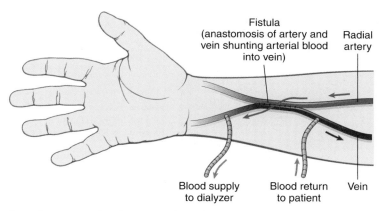

Figure 5-12 • Arteriovenous fistula created for hemodialysis. *(From Chabner D-E:* The Language of medicine, *ed 9, Philadelphia, 2011, Saunders.)*

antihypertensive _____

arteriovenous fistula _____

chronic _____

hemodialysis _____

hypertension _____

hypotensive _____

renal failure _____

5

CASE 9 *Endocrinology*

A 36-year-old woman known to have **type 1 diabetes mellitus** was brought to the emergency department after being found collapsed at home. She had experienced 3 days of extreme weakness, **polyuria,** and **polydipsia.** It was discovered that a few days before her admission, she had discontinued use of her external **insulin pump** (see Figure 5-13) in a suicide attempt.

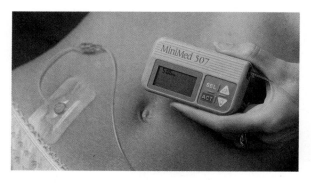

Figure 5-13 • **External insulin pump.** *(From* Mosby's Dictionary of Medicine, Nursing & Health Professions, *ed 7, St Louis, 2006, Mosby.)*

insulin pump _____

polydipsia _____

polyuria _____

type 1 diabetes mellitus _____

CASE 10 *Neurology*

Ms. Kindrick is admitted with severe, throbbing **unilateral frontal cephalgia** that has lasted for 2 days. Light makes her cringe, and she has **nausea.** Before the onset of these symptoms, she saw zigzag lines for about 20 minutes and a **scotoma** (see Figure 5-14). Diagnosis is **acute migraine** with **aura.** A **vasoconstrictor** is prescribed, and Ms. Kindrick's condition is improving. [Migraine headaches are thought to be caused by sudden **dilation** of blood vessels.]

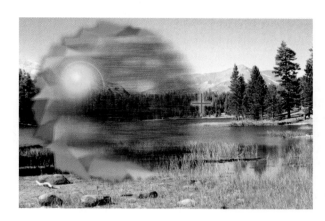

Figure 5-14 • **Scotoma.** This abnormal area of the visual field is both "positive" (consisting of bright flickering imagery) and "negative" (displaying a relatively dark area that obscures the visual field). It is called a scintillating scotoma. *(From Yanoff M, Duker JS:* Ophthalmology, *ed 2, St Louis, 2004, Mosby.)*

5

acute _____

aura _____

cephalgia _____

dilation _____

frontal _____

migraine _____

nausea _____

scotoma _____

unilateral _____

vasoconstrictor _____

IN PERSON

This first-person narrative was written by a woman living with Crohn disease ("Crohn's").

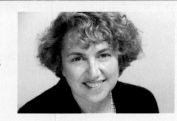

When a friend told me she was felled by the flu yesterday, I was jealous. To someone with a chronic illness, like me, having something acute always seems luxurious. Lie in bed, read glossy magazines, take over-the-counter meds, sleep it off, and in a matter of days you're okay. I have Crohn disease, a chronic inflammation of the small intestine, which is characterized by flare-ups and remission. During flare-ups, I've experienced fever, diarrhea, vomiting, pain, and intestinal obstruction. Even in remission I am never "okay."

Right now I have been in remission two years after a third surgery to remove yet another portion of my small bowel. This time internal bleeding, a rather rare symptom of Crohn's, necessitated the surgery. I was enduring weekly iron infusions, which turned into bimonthly blood transfusions, as my hemoglobin plummeted to 6 (12 is normal). It was no way to live. After the surgery, the bleeding stopped, but I had bouts of urgent, watery diarrhea for a year. That was no way to live either, and unfortunately, as wonderful as my doctor is, I've found that few GIs want to address after-effects of small bowel surgery. After visiting several doctors and trial-and-error, I finally got these symptoms under control with codeine, Lomotil, and Metamucil, but I will never be able to absorb vitamin B_{12}, so I must inject it monthly for the rest of my life. In addition to taking medicine to cope with having less and less small bowel, I take medicine in the hopes of preventing the next flare-up. Every few weeks, I inject myself with a biologic medicine, Humira, but I must eventually be weaned off this drug because it has possible long-term side effects, the scariest of which is lymphoma. At 52 and with two school-age children, however, I have learned to think of valuing my present quality of life the most, over possible unknown dangers lurking in the future.

I do often think about the past. What would my life be like if our family doctor hadn't told my parents that my constant episodes of diarrhea—which occurred since I was a child—were caused by "nerves?" By the time I was 21, my weight had dropped below 100 pounds, and I was twisted in pain after every meal. My dad arranged for me to visit his own doctor, who gave me a small bowel series that showed I had Crohn's and that a portion of my small intestine was "as narrow as a pencil." By then it was too late for even prednisone (then the drug of choice despite side effects ranging from puffy face to psychosis) to open up the inflamed passage, and I had my first surgery just months after I was diagnosed. Thinking of those times—as well as all the other flare-up times—makes me flinch. While you can never relive pain, you can remember what it felt like. In my case, it was as if a large metal bike lock chain was being forced through my tender gut.

Before that first surgery, I was just out of college and longing to make my mark on the world, but I spent most of my evenings curled up in my small bedroom, listening to the soothing strains of "Make Believe Ballroom Hour" on the radio. Or, because vomiting and diarrhea usually accompanied the pain, I lay with my back pressed against the cold tiles of the bathroom floor. Later on, as a mom with two young children, I would lie on the couch watching life swirl around me, feeling guilty that I could not take part.

There was a silver lining to those flare-ups, and that is the tender affection of those around me: husband, family, and friends. When you have Crohn's, no one knows you have it until things get unbearable. It's not the kind of illness you discuss, but when you have pain and fever, you can kind of approximate those times of being felled by the flu. Yet you know that it will take more than a dose of Nyquil or a night's sleep to get "better." You know you'll face another course of medications—often untried ones—or that you will likely end up in the hospital undergoing yet another surgery.

Nancy J. Brandwein is a writer, editor, and food columnist.

? EXERCISES AND ANSWERS

Complete these exercises and check your answers. An important part of your success in learning medical terminology is checking your answers carefully with the Answers to Exercises beginning on page 200.

A **Match each of the following residency programs to its description below.**

anesthesiology	internal medicine	psychiatry
dermatology	ophthalmology	radiology
emergency medicine	pathology	surgery
family practice	pediatrics	

1. Treatment by operation or manual (hand) methods _____

2. Diagnosis and treatment of often complex medical disorders in adult patients

   _____

3. Diagnosis and treatment of disorders of the mind _____

4. Primary care of all family members on a continuing basis _____

5. Diagnosis and treatment of skin disorders _____

6. Diagnosis and treatment of eye disorders _____

7. Diagnosis of disease using x-rays _____

8. Diagnosis and treatment of children's disorders _____

9. Care of patients with illness that requires immediate action _____

10. Administration of agents that produce loss of sensation/awareness _____

11. Diagnosis of disease by examining cells and tissues _____

5

B Name the physician who treats the following problems (first letters are given).

1. kidney diseases: n_____

2. tumors: o_____

3. broken bones: o_____

4. female diseases: g_____

5. eye disorders: o_____

6. heart disorders: c_____

7. nerve disorders: n_____

8. lung disorders: p_____

9. mental disorders: p_____

10. stomach and intestinal disorders: g_____

C Match the medical specialists in Column I to their specialties in Column II.

COLUMN I		COLUMN II
1. urologist	_____	A. operates on the large intestine
2. thoracic surgeon	_____	B. treats blood disorders
3. radiation oncologist	_____	C. treats thyroid and pituitary gland disorders
4. colorectal surgeon	_____	D. rehabilitates after spinal injuries
5. endocrinologist	_____	E. treats disorders of childhood
6. obstetrician	_____	F. operates on the urinary tract
7. radiologist	_____	G. treats disorders of the skin
8. pediatrician	_____	H. delivers babies
9. hematologist	_____	I. operates on the chest
10. dermatologist	_____	J. examines x-ray images to diagnose disease
11. physiatrist	_____	K. treats tumors using high-energy radiation

5

D **Complete each of the sentences below using a term from the following list.**

clinical   oncologist   pathologist
geriatrician   ophthalmologist research
hospitalist   optician   surgeon
infectious disease specialist optometrist   orthopedist

1. A doctor who diagnoses and treats diseases that are caused by microorganisms is

   a/an _____.

2. A doctor who performs bone surgery is a/an _____.

3. A doctor who takes care of patients practices _____ medicine.

4. A medical professional who grinds lenses and fills prescriptions for eye glasses is

   a/an _____.

5. A doctor who reads biopsy samples and performs autopsies is a/an _____.

6. A doctor who treats cancerous tumors is a/an _____.

7. A medical professional (non-physician) who examines eyes, prescribes eyeglasses,

   and treats eye disorders is a/an _____.

8. A doctor who operates on patients is a/an _____.

9. A doctor who does experiments with test tubes and laboratory equipment is

   interested in _____ medicine.

10. A doctor who specializes in surgery and medical treatment of disorders of the eye is

    a/an _____.

11. A doctor who specializes in the treatment of older people is a/an

    _____ .

12. A physician who cares for hospitalized patients is a/an _____.

E Which medical specialist would you consult for the following medical conditions? The first letter of the specialist is given.

1. Arthritis: r_____

2. Otitis media: o_____

3. Anemia: h_____

4. Urinary bladder displacement: u_____

5. Chronic bronchitis: p_____ _

6. Cerebrovascular accident: n_____

7. Breast cancer: o _____

8. Coronary artery blockages (bypass surgery):   c_____

9. Dislocated shoulder bone: o _____

10. Thyroid gland enlargement: e_____

11. Kidney disease: n_____

12. Acne (skin disorder):   d_____

13. Hay fever (hypersensitivity reaction):   a_____

14. Viral and bacterial diseases: i _____

15. Rehabilitation after herniated disk: p_____

5

F **Give the meaning for each of the following medical terms.**

1. neuralgia _____

2. pathology _____

3. cardiomegaly _____

4. nephrostomy _____

5. thoracotomy _____

6. laryngeal _____

7. otitis _____

8. colitis _____

9. pulmonary _____

10. iatrogenic _____

11. gastroscopy _____

12. radiotherapy _____

13. anesthesiology _____

14. enteritis _____

15. nosocomial _____

5

G Use the following combining forms and suffixes to make the medical terms called for.

COMBINING FORMS		SUFFIXES	
aden/o	onc/o	-algia	-pathy
col/o	ophthalm/o	-ectomy	-scopy
laryng/o	ot/o	-genic	-stomy
lymph/o	path/o	-itis	-therapy
nephr/o	psych/o	-logy	-tomy
neur/o	thorac/o	-osis	

1. Inflammation of the ear _____

2. Removal of a nerve _____

3. Incision of the chest _____

4. Study of tumors _____

5. Pertaining to producing disease _____

6. Inflammation of the voice box _____

7. Opening of the large intestine to the outside of the body _____

8. Visual examination of the eye _____

9. Abnormal condition of the mind _____

10. Inflammation of the kidney _____

11. Removal of the large intestine _____

12. Pain in the ear _____

13. Treatment of the mind _____

14. Pertaining to producing tumors _____

15. Disease of lymph glands (nodes) _____

H Circle the **bold** term that best completes the meaning of the sentences in the following medical vignettes.

1. Dr. Butler is a physician who operates on hearts. He trained as a **(neurologic, cardiovascular, pulmonary)** surgeon. Often, his procedures require that Dr. Smith, a/an **(gynecologic, ophthalmic, thoracic)** surgeon, assist him when the surgical problem involves the chest and lungs.

2. Pauline noticed a rash over most of her body. First she saw Dr. Cole, her **(family practitioner, oncologist, radiologist),** who performs her yearly physicals. Dr. Cole, who is not a/an **(endocrinologist, orthopedist, dermatologist)** by training, referred her to a skin specialist to make the proper diagnosis and treat the rash.

3. Dr. Liu is a/an **(internist, obstetrician, pediatrician)** as well as a/an **(nephrologist, urologist, gynecologist)** and can take care of her female patients before, during, and after their pregnancies.

4. After her sixth pregnancy, Sally developed an abnormal condition at the lower end of her colon. She went to a/an **(gastroenterologist, hematologist, optometrist),** who made the diagnosis of protrusion of the rectum into the vagina. She then consulted colorectal and gynecologic surgeons to make an appropriate treatment plan for her condition, known as a **(vasculitis, rectocele, colostomy).**

5. In the cancer clinic, patients often see a medical **(oncologist, orthopedist, rheumatologist),** who prescribes and monitors chemotherapy, and a/an **(psychiatrist, radiation oncologist, radiologist),** who prescribes and supervises **(drugs, surgery, radiation therapy)** to treat tumors with high-energy beams.

6. During a lengthy hospitalization, Janet developed a cough and fever (unrelated to any treatment or procedure she received). Her surgeon ordered a chest x-ray, which showed a/an **(oncogenic, nosocomial, iatrogenic)** pneumonia. A/an **(anesthesiologist, neurologist, infectious disease specialist)** was called in to diagnose and treat the hospital-acquired disease condition.

7. Sam had noticed bright red rectal bleeding for several days when he finally saw his family practitioner. This physician referred him to a/an **(endocrinologist, urologist, gastroenterologist).** A **(laparoscopy, colonoscopy, bronchoscopy)** was scheduled, which revealed a large pedunculated (on a stalk) polyp (benign growth) in the descending colon. See Figure 5-15. The polyp was resected and sent to the **(pathology, hematology, infectious disease)** department for evaluation. Fortunately, it was a noncancerous or **(malignant, metastatic, benign)** lesion. Sam will need follow-up **(laparotomy, endoscopy, laparoscopy)** in a year.

5

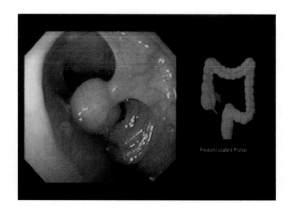

Figure 5-15 • Pedunculated polyp in the descending colon. It arises from the mucosal surface of the colon and is projecting into the lumen of the colon. *(From Lewis SM, Heitkemper MM, Dirksen SR: Medical-Surgical Nursing: Assessment and Management of Clinical Problems, ed 5, St Louis, 2004, Mosby.)*

ANSWERS TO EXERCISES

A
1. surgery
2. internal medicine
3. psychiatry
4. family practice
5. dermatology
6. ophthalmology
7. radiology
8. pediatrics
9. emergency medicine
10. anesthesiology
11. pathology

B
1. nephrologist
2. oncologist
3. orthopedist
4. gynecologist
5. ophthalmologist
6. cardiologist (internist) or cardiovascular surgeon (surgeon)
7. neurologist
8. pulmonary specialist
9. psychiatrist
10. gastroenterologist

C
1. F
2. I
3. K
4. A
5. C
6. H
7. J
8. E
9. B
10. G
11. D

D
1. infectious disease specialist
2. orthopedist
3. clinical
4. optician
5. pathologist
6. oncologist
7. optometrist
8. surgeon
9. research
10. ophthalmologist
11. geriatrician
12. hospitalist

E
1. rheumatologist
2. otolaryngologist
3. hematologist
4. urologist
5. pulmonary specialist
6. neurologist
7. oncologist
8. cardiovascular surgeon
9. orthopedist
10. endocrinologist
11. nephrologist
12. dermatologist
13. allergist
14. infectious disease specialist
15. physiatrist

F
1. nerve pain
2. study of disease
3. enlargement of the heart
4. opening from the kidney to the outside of the body
5. incision of the chest
6. pertaining to the voice box
7. inflammation of the ear
8. inflammation of the colon
9. pertaining to the lungs
10. pertaining to an abnormal condition that is produced by treatment
11. process of visual examination of the stomach (using an endoscope)
12. treatment of disease using high-energy radiation
13. study of loss of sensation or feeling
14. inflammation of the intestines (usually small intestine)
15. pertaining to a disease acquired in the hospital

G
1. otitis
2. neurectomy
3. thoracotomy
4. oncology
5. pathogenic
6. laryngitis
7. colostomy
8. ophthalmoscopy
9. psychosis
10. nephritis
11. colectomy
12. otalgia
13. psychotherapy
14. oncogenic
15. lymphadenopathy

H
1. cardiovascular, thoracic
2. family practitioner, dermatologist
3. obstetrician, gynecologist
4. gastroenterologist, rectocele
5. oncologist, radiation oncologist, radiation therapy
6. nosocomial, infectious disease specialist
7. gastroenterologist, colonoscopy, pathology, benign, endoscopy

5

Medical Specialists Matching Exercises (on pages 174-175)

A
1. gastroenterologist
2. hematologist
3. cardiologist

4. allergist
5. endocrinologist
6. ophthalmologist

7. cardiovascular surgeon
8. anesthesiologist
9. gynecologist

B
1. urologist
2. psychiatrist
3. radiation oncologist

4. orthopedist
5. pulmonologist
6. pathologist

7. radiologist
8. nephrologist
9. neurologist

 PRONUNCIATION OF TERMS

The terms that you have learned in this chapter are presented here with their pronunciations. The capitalized letters in **BOLDFACE** *represent the accented syllable. Pronounce each word out loud; then write the meaning in the space provided. Meanings of all terms can be checked with the* **Mini-Dictionary: Glossary of Medical Terms** *beginning on page 341 and on the audio section of the Evolve website (http://evolve.elsevier.com/Chabner/medtermshort).*

TERM	PRONUNCIATION	MEANING
anesthesiology	an-es-the-ze-**OL**-o-je	
cardiologist	kar-de-**OL**-o-jist	
cardiovascular surgeon	kar-de-o-**VAS**-ku-lar **SUR**-jun	
clinical	**KLIN**-ih-kal	
colitis	ko-**LI**-tis	
colorectal surgeon	ko-lo-**REK**-tal **SUR**-jun	
dermatologist	der-mah-**TOL**-o-jist	
dermatology	der-mah-**TOL**-o-je	
emergency medicine	e-**MER**-jen-se **MED**-ih-sin	
endocrinologist	en-do-krih-**NOL**-o-jist	
enteritis	en-teh-**RI**-tis	
family practitioner	**FAM**-ih-le prak-**TIH**-shun-er	
gastroenterologist	gas-tro-en-ter-**OL**-o-jist	
gastroscopy	gas-**TROS**-ko-pe	

5

geriatric	jer-e-**AH**-trik
geriatrician	jer-e-ah-**TRISH**-un
gynecologist	gi-neh-**KOL**-o-jist
gynecology	gi-neh-**KOL**-o-je
hematologist	he-mah-**TOL**-o-jist
hematoma	he-mah-**TO**-mah
hospitalist	**HOS**-pih-tah-list
iatrogenic	i-ah-tro-**JEN**-ik
infectious disease	in-**FEK**-shus dih-**ZEZ**
internal medicine	in-**TER**-nal **MED**-ih-sin
laryngitis	lah-rin-**JI**-tis
lymphadenopathy	limf-ah-deh-**NOP**-ah-the
nephrologist	neh-**FROL**-o-jist
nephrostomy	neh-**FROS**-to-me
neuralgia	nu-**RAL**-jah
neurologist	nu-**ROL**-o-jist
neurosurgeon	nu-ro-**SUR**-jun
nosocomial	nos-o-**KO**-me-al
obstetrician	ob-steh-**TRISH**-an
obstetrics	ob-**STET**-riks
oncogenic	ong-ko-**JEN**-ik
oncologist	ong-**KOL**-o-jist
ophthalmologist	of-thal-**MOL**-o-jist
ophthalmology	of-thal-**MOL**-o-je

5

optician	op-**TISH**-an _____
optometrist	op-**TOM**-eh-trist _____
orthopedist	or-tho-**PE**-dist _____
otitis	o-**TI**-tis _____
otolaryngologist	o-to-lah-rin-**GOL**-o-jist _____
pathologist	pah-**THOL**-o-jist _____
pathology	pah-**THOL**-o-je _____
pediatric	pe-de-**AT**-rik _____
pediatrician	pe-de-ah-**TRISH**-un _____
physiatrist	fih-**ZI**-ah-trist _____
psychiatrist	si-**KI**-ah-trist _____
psychosis	si-**KO**-sis _____
pulmonary specialist	**PUL**-mo-nair-e **SPESH**-ah-list _____
radiation oncologist	ra-de-**A**-shun ong-**KOL**-o-jist _____
radiologist	ra-de-**OL**-o-jist _____
radiotherapy	ra-de-o-**THER**-ah-pe _____
rectocele	**REK**-to-sel _____
research	**RE**-surch _____
rheumatologist	roo-mah-**TOL**-o-jist _____
rheumatology	roo-mah-**TOL**-o-je _____
rhinorrhea	ri-no-**RE**-ah _____
surgery	**SUR**-jer-e _____
thoracic surgeon	tho-**RAS**-ik **SUR**-jun _____
thoracotomy	tho-rah-**KOT**-o-me _____

5

urologist   u-**ROL**-o-jist _____

vasculitis   vas-ku-**LI**-tis _____

 ## PRACTICAL APPLICATIONS

This section provides three groups of exercises on allied health specialists and their job descriptions. Answers are on page 207. **Appendix 4** *on page 331 lists health professions with education requirements, national association information, and certificate and licensing requirements.*

A Match each allied health specialist to the appropriate job description: Write your answer on the blank line.

- audiologist
- blood bank technologist
- chiropractor
- clinical laboratory technician
- dental assistant
- dental hygienist
- diagnostic medical sonographer
- dietitian/nutritionist
- nurse anesthetist
- nurse practitioner

1. Treats health problems associated with the muscular, nervous, and skeletal

   systems, especially the spine _____

2. Examines, diagnoses, and treats patients under the direct supervision of a physician

   _____

3. Works with people who have hearing problems by using testing devices to measure

   hearing loss _____

4. Provides preventive dental care and teaches the practice of good oral hygiene

   _____

5. Collects, types, and prepares blood and its components for transfusions

   _____

6. Aids in the delivery of anesthesia during surgery _____

7. Assists a dentist with dental procedures _____

8. Performs diagnostic ultrasound procedures _____

9. Plans nutrition programs and supervises the preparation and serving of meals

   _____

10. Performs tests to examine and analyze body fluids, tissues, and cells

   _____

B Select from the list of specialists to match the job description.

- ECG technician
- emergency medical technician/paramedic
- health information management professional
- home health aide
- licensed practical nurse
- medical assistant
- medical laboratory technician
- nuclear medicine technologist
- nursing aide
- occupational therapist

1. Cares for elderly, disabled, and ill persons in their own homes, helping them live there instead of in an institution _____

2. Performs routine tests and laboratory procedures _____

3. Designs, manages, and administers the use of heath care data and information

   _____

4. Operates an electrocardiograph to record ECGs and for Holter monitoring and stress tests _____

5. Performs radioactive tests and procedures under the supervision of a nuclear medicine physician, who interprets the results _____

6. Gives immediate care to acutely ill or injured persons and transports them to medical facilities _____

7. Helps physicians examine and treat patients and performs tasks to keep offices running smoothly _____

8. Cares for the sick, injured, convalescing, and handicapped, under the direct supervision of physicians and registered nurses; provides basic bedside care

   _____

9. Helps individuals with mentally, physically, developmentally, or emotionally disabling conditions to develop, recover, or maintain daily living and working skills _____

10. Helps care for physically or mentally ill, injured, or disabled patients confined to nursing, hospital, or residential care facilities; also known as nursing assistants or hospital attendants _____

5

C Match the specialist to the appropriate job description.

- ophthalmic medical technician
- phlebotomist
- physical therapist
- physician assistant
- radiation therapist
- radiographer/radiologic technologist
- registered nurse
- respiratory therapist
- speech-language pathologist
- surgical technologist

1. Evaluates, treats, and cares for patients with breathing disorders

   _____

2. Draws and tests blood under the supervision of a medical technologist or laboratory

   manager _____

3. Cares for sick and injured people by assessing and recording symptoms, assisting

   physicians during treatments and examinations, and administering medications

   _____

4. Prepares cancer patients for treatment and administers prescribed doses of ionizing

   radiation to specific areas of the body _____

5. Helps ophthalmologists provide medical eye care _____

6. Examines, diagnoses, and treats patients under the direct supervision of a physician

   _____

7. Assists in operations under the supervision of surgeons or registered nurses

   _____

8. Improves mobility, relieves pain, and prevents or limits permanent physical

   disabilities in patients suffering from injuries or disease _____

9. Produces x-ray images of parts of the body for use in diagnosing medical problems

   _____

10. Assesses and treats persons with speech, language, voice, and fluency disorders

    _____

5

ANSWERS TO PRACTICAL APPLICATIONS

A
1. chiropractor
2. nurse practitioner
3. audiologist
4. dental hygienist
5. blood bank technologist
6. nurse anesthetist
7. dental assistant
8. diagnostic medical sonographer
9. dietitian/nutritionist
10. clinical laboratory technician

B
1. home health aide
2. medical laboratory technician
3. health information management professional
4. ECG technician
5. nuclear medicine technologist
6. emergency medical technician/paramedic
7. medical assistant
8. licensed practical nurse
9. occupational therapist
10. nursing aide

C
1. respiratory therapist
2. phlebotomist
3. registered nurse
4. radiation therapist
5. ophthalmic medical technician
6. physician assistant
7. surgical technologist
8. physical therapist
9. radiographer/radiologic technologist
10. speech-language pathologist

5

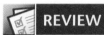

REVIEW

Test your understanding of the combining forms and suffixes used in this chapter by completing this review. Remember to check your responses with the Answers to Review on page 209.

COMBINING FORMS

COMBINING FORM	MEANING	COMBINING FORM	MEANING
1. aden/o		18. obstetr/o	
2. cardi/o		19. onc/o	
3. col/o		20. ophthalm/o	
4. dermat/o		21. opt/o, optic/o	
5. endocrin/o		22. orth/o	
6. enter/o		23. ot/o	
7. esthesi/o		24. path/o	
8. gastr/o		25. ped/o	
9. ger/o		26. psych/o	
10. gynec/o		27. pulmon/o	
11. hemat/o		28. radi/o	
12. iatr/o		29. rect/o	
13. laryng/o		30. rheumat/o	
14. lymph/o		31. rhin/o	
15. nephr/o		32. thorac/o	
16. neur/o		33. ur/o	
17. nos/o		34. vascul/o	

SUFFIXES

SUFFIX	MEANING	SUFFIX	MEANING
1. -algia	_____	10. -oma	_____
2. -ary	_____	11. -osis	_____
3. -cele	_____	12. -pathy	_____
4. -eal	_____	13. -rrhea	_____
5. -genic	_____	14. -scopy	_____
6. -ist	_____	15. -stomy	_____
7. -itis	_____	16. -therapy	_____
8. -logy	_____	17. -tomy	_____
9. -megaly	_____		

ANSWERS TO REVIEW

5

COMBINING FORMS

1. gland
2. heart
3. colon
4. skin
5. endocrine glands
6. intestines
7. sensation
8. stomach
9. old age
10. woman
11. blood
12. treatment
13. voice box
14. lymph
15. kidney
16. nerve
17. disease
18. midwife
19. tumor
20. eye
21. eye
22. straight
23. ear
24. disease
25. child
26. mind
27. lung
28. x-rays
29. rectum
30. flow, fluid
31. nose
32. chest
33. urinary tract
34. blood vessels

SUFFIXES

1. pain
2. pertaining to
3. hernia, protrusion
4. pertaining to
5. pertaining to producing
6. specialist
7. inflammation
8. study of
9. enlargement
10. mass, tumor
11. abnormal condition
12. disease, emotion
13. flow
14. process of visual examination
15. opening
16. treatment
17. incision

5

 TERMINOLOGY CHECKUP

Before you leave this chapter, here are important concepts that you should understand. Check the box next to each item when you know you've "got" it!

☐ 1. **Medical specialists:** Note the differences between the following medical doctors:

- **orthopedist and rheumatologist.** An **orthopedist** is a surgeon who diagnoses and treats bone, muscle, and joint conditions, while a **rheumatologist** is an internal medicine specialist who primarily diagnoses and treats disorders of joints.

- **nephrologist and urologist.** A **nephrologist** is an internal medicine specialist who diagnoses and treats disorders of the kidneys, while a **urologist** is a surgeon who operates on the kidneys, urinary tract, and male reproductive organs.

- **cardiologist and cardiovascular surgeon.** A **cardiologist** is an internal medicine specialist who diagnoses and treats disorders of the heart, while a **cardiovascular surgeon** operates on the heart and blood vessels.

- **pulmonologist, otolaryngologist, and thoracic surgeon.** A **pulmonologist** is an internal medicine specialist who diagnoses and treats diseases of the lungs, while an **otolaryngologist** is a surgeon who operates on the ear, nose, throat, head, and neck. A **thoracic surgeon**, however, operates on organs in the chest, such as the heart, lungs, and esophagus.

- **neurologist and neurosurgeon.** A **neurologist** is an internal medicine specialist who diagnoses and treats disorders of the brain, spinal cord, and nerves, while a **neurosurgeon** operates on the brain, nerves, and spinal cord.

- **pathologist and oncologist.** A **pathologist** is an internal medicine specialist who examines dead bodies (performs autopsies) and specimens of living cells (biopsies) to determine the correct diagnosis. An **oncologist**, also a specialist in internal medicine, diagnoses and treats malignant tumors.

- **radiologist and radiation oncologist.** A **radiologist** is primarily a diagnostic physician who examines images from x-ray, CT, ultrasound, and MRI studies, while a **radiation oncologist** treats malignancies with high-energy radiation (photons and protons).

☐ 2. **Specialists and conditions they treat:** Carefully review Exercises A to E beginning on page 193. It is important to identify physicians and their areas of expertise to gain proper perspective on the medical community as a whole.

☐ 3. **Case reports:** Read over the cases beginning on page 180 and congratulate yourself on how much medical terminology you are able to decipher on your own.

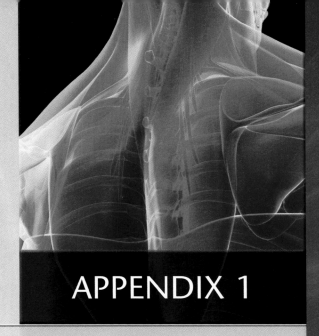

Body Systems

APPENDIX 1

This appendix contains full-color diagrams of body systems. For each system, the material presented is divided into seven sections. **Anatomy** shows major organs and structures with labels and combining forms (in parentheses) for each body part. The parts of the body are defined and explained in the ***Mini-Dictionary: Glossary of Medical Terms*** (beginning on page 341). **Terminology** reviews combining forms and their meanings and gives examples of medical terminology using each combining form. **Pathology** explains terms related to common pathological conditions. **Laboratory Tests and Diagnostic Procedures** presents common tests and procedures, which can be cross-referenced for additional information in ***Appendix 2, Diagnostic Tests and Procedures.*** **Treatment Procedures** explains procedures that treat abnormal conditions in each system. **Useful Abbreviations** lists selected abbreviations for easy reference. **Matching Exercises** review the terminology to test your understanding; answers to all exercises are provided at the end of the appendix, beginning on page 288.

Use this appendix both as a study guide for classroom work and as a reference for your work in the medical field.

Cardiovascular System

ANATOMY

Circulation of Blood

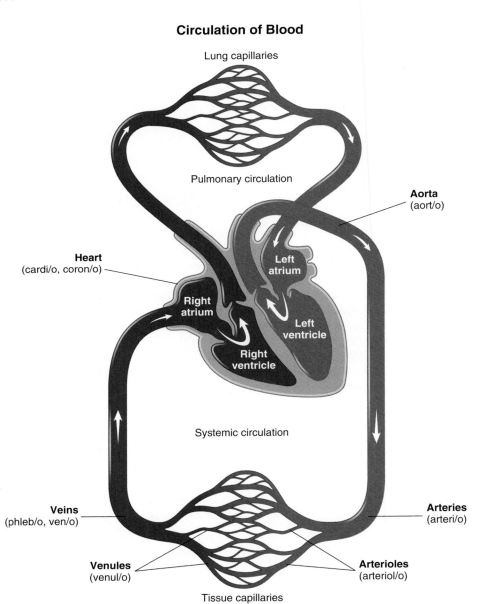

Lung capillaries

Pulmonary circulation

Aorta
(aort/o)

Left atrium

Heart
(cardi/o, coron/o)

Right atrium

Left ventricle

Right ventricle

Systemic circulation

Veins
(phleb/o, ven/o)

Arteries
(arteri/o)

Venules
(venul/o)

Arterioles
(arteriol/o)

Tissue capillaries

Red vessels contain blood that is rich in oxygen. Blue vessels contain blood that is oxygen-poor. *Arrows* show the path of blood flow from the tissue capillaries through venules and veins toward the heart, to the lung capillaries, back to the heart, out of the aorta to the arteries and arterioles, and then back to the tissue capillaries.

TERMINOLOGY

Meanings for terminology are found in the *Mini-Dictionary: Glossary of Medical Terms,* beginning on page 341.

COMBINING FORM	MEANING	TERMINOLOGY	MEANING
angi/o	vessel	angioplasty _____	
aort/o	aorta	aortic stenosis _____	
arteri/o	artery	arteriosclerosis _____	
arteriol/o	arteriole	arteriolitis _____	
cardi/o	heart	cardiomyopathy _____	
		pericardium _____	
coron/o	heart	coronary arteries _____	
phleb/o	vein	phlebotomy _____	
ven/o	vein	intravenous _____	
venul/o	venule	venulitis _____	

PATHOLOGY

Definitions for additional terms in **boldface** are found in the *Mini-Dictionary: Glossary of Medical Terms.*

Aneurysm: Local widening of an artery caused by weakness in the arterial wall or breakdown of the wall from **atherosclerosis.**

Angina: Chest pain caused by decreased blood flow to heart muscle. Also called angina pectoris (chest).

Arrhythmia: Abnormal heartbeat (rhythm); **fibrillation** and **flutter** are examples.

Atherosclerosis: Hardening of arteries with a collection of cholesterol-like plaque.

Congestive heart failure: Inability of the heart to pump its required amount of blood. Blood accumulates in the lungs, causing **pulmonary edema.**

Hypertension: High blood pressure. Essential hypertension is high blood pressure with no apparent cause. In secondary hypertension, another illness (kidney disease or an adrenal gland disorder) is the cause of the high blood pressure.

Myocardial infarction: Heart attack. An **infarct** is an area of dead (**necrotic**) tissue.

Shock: A group of signs and symptoms (paleness of skin, weak and rapid pulse, shallow breathing) indicating poor oxygen supply to tissues and insufficient return of blood to the heart.

LABORATORY TESTS AND DIAGNOSTIC PROCEDURES

Consult *Appendix 2,* beginning on page 291, for pronunciation of terms and additional information.

Angiography: Recording (via x-ray images) blood vessels after the injection of contrast into the bloodstream.

Cardiac catheterization: Introducing a catheter (a flexible, tubular instrument) into a vein or artery to measure pressure and flow patterns of blood.

Cardiac enzyme tests: Measurements of enzymes released into the bloodstream after a heart attack (myocardial infarction).

Doppler ultrasound: Measuring blood flow in vessels via sound waves.

Echocardiography: Producing images of the heart via sound waves or echoes.

Electrocardiography: Recording electricity flowing through the heart.

Holter monitoring: Detection of abnormal heart rhythms (**arrhythmias**) that involves having a patient wear a compact version of an electrocardiograph for 24 hours.

Lipid tests: Measurements of cholesterol and triglyceride levels in the blood.

Lipoprotein tests: Measurements of **high-density lipoprotein (HDL)** and **low-density lipoprotein (LDL)** in the blood.

Magnetic resonance imaging (MRI): Producing an image, by beaming magnetic waves at the heart, that gives detailed information about congenital heart disease, cardiac masses, and disease within large blood vessels.

MUGA scan: Imaging the motion of heart wall muscles and assessing the function of the heart via a *mu*ltiple-*g*ated *a*cquisition scan, which uses radioactive chemicals.

Positron emission tomography (PET) scan: Radioactive chemicals, which release radioactive particles, are injected into the bloodstream and travel to the heart. Cross-sectional images show the flow of blood and the functional activity of the heart muscle.

Stress test: An electrocardiogram plus blood pressure and heart rate measurements shows the heart's response to physical exertion (treadmill test).

Technetium Tc 99m sestamibi scan: A radioactive chemical (sestamibi "tagged" with technetium-99m) is injected intravenously and shows perfusion (flow) of blood in heart muscle. It is taken up in the area of a myocardial infarction, producing "hot spots." In an ETT-MIBI exercise tolerance test, an intravenous radioactive substance is given before the patient reaches maximal heart rate on a treadmill.

Thallium-201 scan: A radioactive test that shows where injected thallium-201 (a radioactive substance) localizes in heart muscle.

TREATMENT PROCEDURES

Cardiac catheter ablation: Flexible tube is threaded through blood vessels into the heart to destroy (ablate) abnormal tissue that causes arrhythmias.

Cardioversion: Brief discharges of electricity passing across the chest to stop a cardiac **arrhythmia.** Also called **defibrillation.**

Coronary artery bypass grafting (CABG): Vessels taken from the patient's legs or chest are connected to coronary arteries to make detours around blockages.

Endarterectomy: Surgical removal of the innermost lining of an artery to remove fatty deposits and clots.

Heart transplantation: A donor heart is transferred to a recipient.

Percutaneous coronary intervention (PCI): A balloon-tipped catheter (a flexible, tubular instrument) is threaded into a coronary artery to compress fatty deposits and open the artery. **Stents** (expandable slotted tubes) create wider openings that make the recurrence of blockages less likely. Also called **balloon angioplasty.**

Thrombolytic therapy: Drugs such as tPA (tissue plasminogen activator) and streptokinase are injected into a patient's bloodstream to dissolve clots that may cause a heart attack.

USEFUL ABBREVIATIONS

See *Appendix 3,* beginning on page 311, for a more complete list of medical abbreviations.

ACS	Acute coronary syndrome (disease changes in coronary arteries leading to plaque/clot formation and heart attack or other heart problems)
AED	Automated external defibrillator
AMI	Acute myocardial infarction (heart attack)
BP	Blood pressure
CABG	Coronary artery bypass grafting (surgical placement of vessels, either vein or artery, to detour blocked coronary arteries)
CAD	Coronary artery disease
CCU	Coronary care unit
CHF	Congestive heart failure (heart is unable to pump its required amount of blood)
CPR	Cardiopulmonary resuscitation
ECG	Electrocardiography
ECHO	Echocardiography
HDL	High-density lipoprotein
HTN	Hypertension (high blood pressure)
ICD	Implantable cardioverter-defibrillator
LDL	Low-density lipoprotein
PCI	Percutaneous coronary intervention (placement of a catheter and stent in a coronary artery to open the artery; balloon angioplasty)

MATCHING EXERCISES

The following exercises will help you review terminology related to the cardiovascular system. Answers begin on page 288.

Ⓐ Match the term in Column I with its meaning in Column II. These terms are illustrated in the diagram on page 212 and are defined in the *Mini-Dictionary: Glossary of Medical Terms,* beginning on page 341.

COLUMN I	COLUMN II
1. aorta _____	A. Blood vessels that carry blood to the heart from the body tissues
2. lung capillaries _____	B. Largest artery in the body
3. arteries _____	C. Tiny blood vessels that lie near cells and through whose walls gases, food, and wastes can pass
4. arterioles _____	
5. venules _____	D. Small veins
6. veins _____	E. Small arteries
7. pulmonary circulation _____	F. Blood vessels that carry blood away from the heart
8. systemic circulation _____	G. Passage of blood from the heart to the body tissues and back
9. tissue capillaries _____	H. Hollow muscular organ that pumps blood all over the body
10. heart _____	I. Tiny blood vessels surrounding lung tissue through which gases pass into and out of the blood
	J. Passage of blood from the heart to the lungs and back to the heart

B Match the combining form in Column I with its meaning in Column II.

COLUMN I		COLUMN II
1. phleb/o	_____	A. Artery
2. arteriol/o	_____	B. Vessel
3. angi/o	_____	C. Heart
4. venul/o	_____	D. Vein
5. arteri/o	_____	E. Small artery
6. coron/o	_____	F. Small vein

C Match the medical term in Column I with its meaning in Column II.

COLUMN I		COLUMN II
`1. intravenous	_____	A. Inflammation of small veins
2. arteriosclerosis	_____	B. Narrowing of the largest artery
3. phlebotomy	_____	C. Disease of heart muscle
4. cardiomyopathy	_____	D. Pertaining to within a vein
5. angioplasty	_____	E. Inflammation of small arteries
6. arteriolitis	_____	F. Hardening of arteries
7. venulitis	_____	G. Incision of a vein
8. aortic stenosis	_____	H. Surgical repair of blood vessels
9. pericardium	_____	I. Pertaining to the heart
10. coronary	_____	J. Membrane surrounding the heart

D Match the pathologic condition in Column I with its meaning in Column II.

COLUMN I	COLUMN II
1. hypertension _____	A. Abnormal heartbeat
2. atherosclerosis _____	B. Local widening of an artery
3. angina _____	C. Heart attack
4. shock _____	D. Chest pain
5. myocardial infarction _____	E. High blood pressure
	F. Inability of the heart to pump its required amount of blood
6. arrhythmia _____	G. Group of signs and symptoms: pale skin, weak rapid pulse, and shallow respirations
7. congestive heart failure _____	H. Hardening of arteries with cholesterol-like plaque
8. aneurysm _____	

E Match the test or procedure in Column I with its description in Column II.

COLUMN I	COLUMN II
1. lipid tests _____	A. Sound waves produce images of the heart
2. MUGA scan _____	B. X-ray images of blood vessels after contrast is injected into the bloodstream
3. lipoprotein tests _____	C. Measurement of HDL and LDL in blood
4. Holter monitoring _____	D. Recording electricity through the heart
	E. Measurement of substances in the blood that indicate a heart attack
5. angiography _____	F. Sound waves measure blood flow in vessels
6. cardiac enzyme test _____	G. Abnormal heart rhythms are detected with a compact ECG over a 24-hour period
7. electrocardiography _____	H. Radioactive test to detect blood perfusion in heart muscle
8. echocardiography _____	I. Measurement of triglyceride and cholesterol levels in the blood
9. sestamibi scan _____	J. Radioactive chemicals and a scanner produce images of the motion of the heart wall
10. Doppler ultrasound _____	

F Match the treatment procedure in Column I with its description in Column II.

COLUMN I	COLUMN II
1. cardioversion _____	A. Surgery to detour around blockages in coronary arteries
2. thrombolytic therapy _____	B. Drugs such as tPA dissolve clots that may cause a heart attack
3. heart transplantation _____	C. Balloon-tipped catheter with stent opens coronary arteries
4. endarterectomy _____	D. Flexible tube is threaded into the heart; abnormal tissue is destroyed
5. CABG _____	E. Brief discharges of electricity stop a cardiac arrhythmia
6. PCI _____	F. Removal of innermost lining of an artery to eliminate fatty deposits
7. cardiac catheter ablation _____	G. Donor heart is transferred to a recipient

Digestive System

ANATOMY

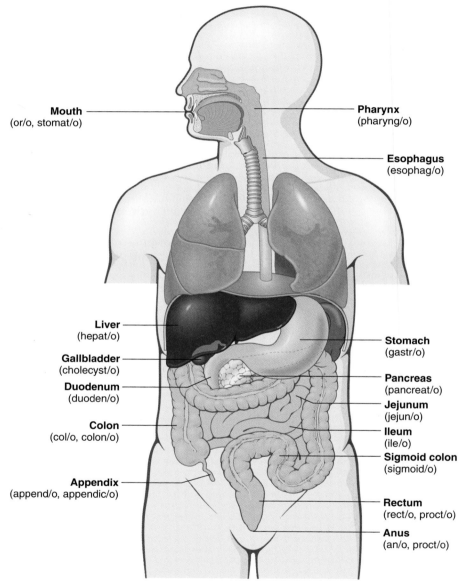

Mouth
(or/o, stomat/o)

Pharynx
(pharyng/o)

Esophagus
(esophag/o)

Liver
(hepat/o)

Gallbladder
(cholecyst/o)

Duodenum
(duoden/o)

Colon
(col/o, colon/o)

Appendix
(append/o, appendic/o)

Stomach
(gastr/o)

Pancreas
(pancreat/o)

Jejunum
(jejun/o)

Ileum
(ile/o)

Sigmoid colon
(sigmoid/o)

Rectum
(rect/o, proct/o)

Anus
(an/o, proct/o)

Food enters the body via the mouth and travels through the pharynx, esophagus, and stomach to the small intestine (duodenum). The liver, gallbladder, and pancreas make and store chemicals that aid in the digestion of foods. Digested (broken-down) food is absorbed into the bloodstream through the walls of the small intestine (jejunum and ileum). Any substance that cannot be absorbed continues into the colon (large intestine) and leaves the body through the rectum and anus. *(Modified from Chabner D-E: The Language of Medicine, ed 9, Philadelphia, 2011, Saunders.)*

TERMINOLOGY

Meanings for terminology are found in the **_Mini-Dictionary: Glossary of Medical Terms._**

COMBINING FORM	MEANING	TERMINOLOGY	MEANING
an/o	anus	anal _____	
append/o	appendix	appendectomy _____	
appendic/o	appendix	appendicitis _____	
cholecyst/o	gallbladder	cholecystectomy _____	
col/o	colon	colostomy _____	
colon/o	colon	colonoscopy _____	
duoden/o	duodenum	duodenal _____	
esophag/o	esophagus	esophageal _____	
gastr/o	stomach	gastralgia _____	
hepat/o	liver	hepatomegaly _____	
ile/o	ileum	ileostomy _____	
jejun/o	jejunum	gastrojejunostomy _____	
or/o	mouth	oral _____	
pancreat/o	pancreas	pancreatitis _____	
pharyng/o	pharynx	pharyngeal _____	
proct/o	anus and rectum	proctoscopy _____	
rect/o	rectum	rectocele _____	
sigmoid/o	sigmoid colon	sigmoidoscopy _____	
stomat/o	mouth	stomatitis _____	

PATHOLOGY

Definitions for additional terms in **boldface** are found in the *Mini-Dictionary: Glossary of Medical Terms.*

Cholelithiasis: Abnormal condition of gallstones.

Cirrhosis: Chronic disease of the liver with degeneration of liver cells.

Colonic polyposis: Condition in which **polyps** protrude from the mucous membrane lining the colon.

Diverticulosis: Abnormal condition of small pouches or sacs (**diverticula**) in the wall of the intestine (often the colon). **Diverticulitis** is inflammation and infection within diverticula.

Gastroesophageal reflux disease (GERD): A condition in which contents of the stomach flow back into the esophagus.

Hepatitis: Inflammation of the liver.

Inflammatory bowel disease (IBD): Inflammation of the terminal (last) portion of the ileum (**Crohn disease**) or inflammation of the colon (**ulcerative colitis**).

Irritable bowel syndrome (IBS): Signs and symptoms are cramping, abdominal bloating, constipation, and diarrhea. Although IBS causes distressing symptoms, it does not permanently harm the intestine. Its cause is unknown.

Hepatocellular carcinoma: Cancer (primary) of the liver.

Jaundice: Yellow-orange coloration of the skin and other tissues, from high levels of **bilirubin** in the bloodstream (**hyperbilirubinemia**).

LABORATORY TESTS AND DIAGNOSTIC PROCEDURES

Consult *Appendix 2* for pronunciation of terms and additional information.

Abdominal computed tomography (CT) scan: A series of cross-sectional x-ray images that show abdominal organs.

Abdominal magnetic resonance imaging (MRI): Magnetic and radio waves create images of abdominal organs and tissues in all three planes of the body.

Abdominal ultrasonography: Process of beaming sound waves into the abdomen to produce images of organs such as the gallbladder. **Endoscopic ultrasonography** is useful to detect enlarged lymph nodes and tumors in the upper abdomen.

Barium tests: X-ray examinations using a liquid barium mixture to locate disorders of the gastrointestinal tract. In a **barium enema (lower GI series),** barium is injected into the anus and rectum and x-ray images are taken of the colon. In an **upper GI series (barium swallow),** barium is taken in through the mouth and x-ray images reveal the esophagus, stomach, and small intestine.

Cholangiography: X-ray examination of the bile ducts (CHOLANGI/O-) after the injection of contrast material through the liver (**percutaneous transhepatic cholangiography**) or through a catheter (a flexible, tubular instrument) from the mouth, esophagus, and stomach into the bile ducts (**endoscopic retrograde cholangiopancreatography** or **ERCP**).

Gastrointestinal endoscopy: Visual examination of the gastrointestinal tract with an endoscope. Examples are **esophagoscopy, gastroscopy, colonoscopy,** and **sigmoidoscopy.**

Hemoccult test: Feces are placed on paper containing the chemical guaiac, which reacts with hidden (occult) blood. This is an important screening test for colon cancer.

Liver function tests (LFTs): Measurements of liver enzymes and other substances in the blood. Enzyme levels increase when the liver is damaged (as in hepatitis). Examples of liver enzymes are **ALT, AST,** and **alkaline phosphatase (alk phos).** High **bilirubin** (blood pigment) levels indicate **jaundice** caused by liver disease or other problems affecting the liver.

Stool culture: Feces (stools) are placed in a growth medium (culture) to test for microorganisms (such as bacteria).

Virtual colonoscopy: CT scans, MRI, and computers are used to produce two- and three-dimensional images of the colon. Also called **CT colonography.**

TREATMENT PROCEDURES

Anastomosis: Surgical creation of an opening between two gastrointestinal organs. Examples are gastrojejunostomy, cholecystojejunostomy, and choledochoduo-denostomy (CHOLEDOCH/O means common bile duct).

Colostomy: Surgical creation of a new opening of the colon to the outside of the body.

Ileostomy: Surgical creation of a new opening of the ileum to the outside of the body.

Laparoscopic surgery: Removal of organs or tissues via a laparoscope (instrument inserted into the abdomen through a small incision). Examples are **laparoscopic cholecystectomy** and **laparoscopic appendectomy,** which are types of **minimally invasive surgery.**

USEFUL ABBREVIATIONS

ALT, AST	Alanine transaminase and aspartate transaminase (liver enzymes measured as part of LFTs)
BE	Barium enema (barium, a contrast agent, is introduced through the rectum, and x-ray pictures of the colon are taken)
ERCP	Endoscopic retrograde cholangiopancreatography
GB	Gallbladder
GERD	Gastroesophageal reflux disease
GI	Gastrointestinal
IBD	Inflammatory bowel disease (Crohn disease and ulcerative colitis)
IBS	Irritable bowel syndrome
LFTs	Liver function tests (ALT, AST, bilirubin)
NPO	Nothing by mouth (*nil per os*)
TPN	Total parenteral nutrition (intravenous solutions are given to maintain nutrition)

MATCHING EXERCISES

The following exercises will help you review terminology related to the digestive system. Answers begin on page 288.

Ⓐ Match the term in Column I with its description in Column II.

COLUMN I		COLUMN II
1. mouth	_____	A. Organ that receives food from the esophagus and sends it to the intestine
2. pharynx	_____	B. Third part of the small intestine
3. esophagus	_____	C. Throat
4. stomach	_____	D. Second part of the small intestine
5. duodenum	_____	E. Large intestine
6. jejunum	_____	F. First part of the small intestine
7. ileum	_____	G. Opening that is the beginning of the digestive system
8. colon	_____	H. Tube that carries food to the stomach

Ⓑ Match the term in Column I with its description in Column II.

COLUMN I		COLUMN II
1. sigmoid colon	_____	A. Opening of the colon to the outside of the body
2. rectum	_____	B. Sac that stores bile
3. anus	_____	C. S-shaped lower portion of the large intestine
4. appendix	_____	D. Organ that makes bile, stores sugar, and produces proteins to clot blood
5. liver	_____	E. Gland that makes both digestive juices and insulin (hormone)
6. gallbladder	_____	F. Small sac that hangs from the beginning of the large intestine
7. common bile duct	_____	G. Tube that carries bile from the liver and gallbladder to the intestine
8. pancreas	_____	H. Final section of the colon

C Match the combining form in Column I with its meaning in Column II.

COLUMN I		COLUMN II
1. gastr/o	_____	A. Mouth
2. col/o	_____	B. Endocrine and exocrine gland near the stomach
3. proct/o	_____	
4. cholecyst/o	_____	C. Third part of the small intestine
5. pharyng/o	_____	D. Stomach
6. or/o	_____	E. Liver
7. hepat/o	_____	F. First part of the small intestine
8. duoden/o	_____	G. Large intestine
9. ile/o	_____	H. Anus and rectum
10. pancreat/o	_____	I. Gallbladder
		J. Throat

D Match the term in Column I with its meaning in Column II.

COLUMN I		COLUMN II
1. hepatomegaly	_____	A. Pertaining to the tube leading from the throat to the stomach
2. cholecystectomy	_____	B. Pain of the stomach
3. proctoscopy	_____	C. Enlargement of the liver
4. ileostomy	_____	D. Inflammation of the mouth
5. stomatitis	_____	E. Pertaining to the first part of the small intestine
6. gastrojejunostomy	_____	F. Removal of the gallbladder
7. pancreatitis	_____	G. Visual examination of the anus and rectum
8. duodenal	_____	H. New opening of the third part of the small intestine to the outside of the body
9. esophageal	_____	I. New opening between the stomach and second part of the small intestine
10. gastralgia	_____	J. Inflammation of a gland adjacent to the stomach

E Match the pathologic condition in Column I with its meaning in Column II.

COLUMN I	COLUMN II
1. hepatitis _____	A. Yellow-orange coloration of the skin and other tissues
2. cirrhosis _____	B. Abnormal condition of small pouches or sacs in the wall of the intestine
3. cholelithiasis _____	C. Ulcerative colitis and Crohn disease
4. colonic polyposis _____	D. Inflammation of the liver
5. jaundice _____	E. Abnormal condition of gallstones
6. inflammatory bowel disease _____	F. Chronic disease of the liver with degeneration of liver cells
7. diverticulosis _____	G. Small growths protrude from the mucous membrane lining the intestine
8. irritable bowel syndrome _____	H. Contents of the stomach flow backwards into the esophagus
9. hepatocellular carcinoma _____	I. Signs and symptoms of GI distress, but no lesions found in the GI tract
10. gastroesophageal reflux disease _____	J. Primary cancer of the liver

F Match the test or procedure in Column I with its description in Column II.

COLUMN I		COLUMN II

1. LFTs _____

2. abdominal CT _____

3. cholangiography _____

4. stool culture _____

5. GI endoscopy _____

6. hemoccult test _____

7. barium tests _____

8. abdominal MRI _____

9. anastomosis _____

10. laparoscopic surgery _____

A. X-ray examination of bile ducts

B. Minimally invasive surgery of the abdomen

C. Visual examination of the gastrointestinal tract (colonoscopy)

D. Feces are placed in a growth medium and tested for microorganisms

E. Cholecystojejunostomy

F. Magnetic waves create images of abdominal organs in three planes of the body

G. Measurements of liver enzymes (ALT, AST, alk phos) and other substances

H. Feces are tested for blood; stool guaiac test

I. Series of cross-sectional x-ray images show abdominal organs

J. X-ray images of the GI tract obtained after introduction of a radiopaque liquid into the rectum or mouth

Endocrine System

ANATOMY

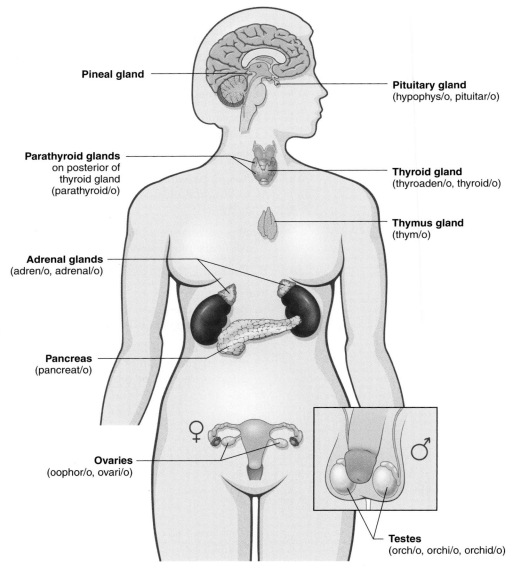

Endocrine glands secrete (form and give off) hormones into the bloodstream. The hormones travel throughout the body, affecting organs (including other endocrine glands) and controlling their actions. *(Modified from Chabner D-E:* The Language of Medicine, *ed 9, Philadelphia, 2011, Saunders.)*

TERMINOLOGY

Meanings for terminology are found in the *Mini-Dictionary: Glossary of Medical Terms.*

COMBINING FORM	MEANING	TERMINOLOGY	MEANING
adren/o	adrenal gland	adrenopathy _____	
adrenal/o	adrenal gland	adrenalectomy _____	
hypophys/o	pituitary gland	hypophyseal _____	
oophor/o	ovary	oophoritis _____	
ovari/o	ovary	ovarian cyst _____	
orch/o	testis	orchitis _____	
orchi/o	testis	orchiopexy _____	
orchid/o	testis	orchidectomy _____	
pancreat/o	pancreas	pancreatectomy _____	
parathyroid/o	parathyroid gland	hyperparathyroidism _____	
pituitar/o	pituitary gland	hypopituitarism _____	
thym/o	thymus gland	thymoma _____	
thyroaden/o	thyroid gland	thyroadenitis _____	
thyroid/o	thyroid gland	thyroidectomy _____	

PATHOLOGY

Definitions for additional terms in **boldface** are found in the *Mini-Dictionary: Glossary of Medical Terms.*

Acromegaly: Enlargement of extremities caused by hypersecretion from the anterior portion of the pituitary gland after puberty.

Cushing syndrome: A group of clinical features produced by excess secretion of **cortisol** from the adrenal cortex. These signs and symptoms include obesity, moon-like facies (fullness of the face), **hyperglycemia,** and **osteoporosis.**

Diabetes mellitus: A disorder of the pancreas that causes an increase in blood glucose levels. **Type 1 diabetes,** with the onset usually in childhood, involves complete deficiency of **insulin** in the body. **Type 2 diabetes,** with the onset usually in adulthood, involves some insulin deficiency and resistance of tissues to the action of insulin.

Goiter: Enlargement of the thyroid gland.

Hyperthyroidism: Overactivity of the thyroid gland; also called **Graves disease** or **exophthalmic** (eyeballs bulge outward) **goiter.**

LABORATORY TESTS AND DIAGNOSTIC PROCEDURES

Consult *Appendix 2* for pronunciation of terms and additional information.

Computed tomography (CT scan): Cross-sectional x-ray images of the pituitary gland and other endocrine organs.

Exophthalmometry: Measurement of eyeball protrusion (**exophthalmos**) as an indicator of **Graves disease (hyperthyroidism).**

Fasting blood sugar (glucose) test: Measurement of glucose levels in a blood sample taken from a fasting patient and in specimens taken 30 minutes, 1 hour, 2 hours, and 3 hours after the ingestion of 75 g of glucose. Delayed return of blood glucose to normal levels indicates **diabetes mellitus.**

Magnetic resonance imaging (MRI): Magnetic waves produce images of the **hypothalamus,** pituitary gland, and other endocrine organs in all three planes of the body.

Radioactive iodine uptake: The uptake of radioactive iodine, given by mouth, measured as evidence of thyroid function.

Serum and urine tests: Measurement of hormones, **electrolytes** (such as sodium and potassium), and glucose levels in blood (serum) and urine as indicators of endocrine function.

Thyroid function tests: Measurement of levels of T_4 (thyroxine), T_3 (triiodothyronine), and TSH (thyroid-stimulating hormone) in the bloodstream.

Thyroid scan: Procedure in which a radioactive compound, injected intravenously, localizes in the thyroid gland. A scanning device produces an image showing the presence of tumors or nodules in the gland.

USEFUL ABBREVIATIONS

ACTH	Adrenocorticotropic hormone (from the pituitary gland)
DM	Diabetes mellitus
GH	Growth hormone (secreted by the pituitary gland)
GTT	Glucose tolerance test (measures the ability to respond to a glucose load; test for diabetes mellitus)
K^+	Potassium (an electrolyte)
Na^+	Sodium (an electrolyte)
T_3	Triiodothyronine (hormone from the thyroid gland)
T_4	Thyroxine (hormone from the thyroid gland)
TSH	Thyroid-stimulating hormone (from the pituitary gland)

MATCHING EXERCISES

The following exercises will help you review terminology related to the endocrine system. Answers begin on page 288.

A **Match the term in Column I with its location in Column II.**

COLUMN I		COLUMN II
1. thyroid gland	_____	A. Two paired male glands located in the scrotal sac
2. ovaries	_____	B. Organ at the base of the brain in the sella turcica (round depression at the base of the skull)
3. testes	_____	
4. thymus gland	_____	C. Gland in the neck on either side of the trachea
5. parathyroid glands	_____	
6. pituitary gland	_____	D. Two glands, one above each kidney
7. pancreas	_____	E. Gland in the middle of the chest (mediastinum)
8. adrenal glands	_____	F. Gland adjacent to the stomach
		G. Four glands behind the thyroid gland
		H. Two paired organs in the female abdomen

(B) Match the combining form in Column I with the secretion or function in Column II.

COLUMN I		COLUMN II
1. hypophys/o	_____	A. Regulates calcium in the blood and bones
2. orchid/o	_____	B. Secretes epinephrine (adrenaline) and cortisone
3. thym/o	_____	
4. oophor/o	_____	C. Secretes insulin, which allows sugar to enter cells
5. thyroaden/o	_____	D. Secretes testosterone
6. pancreat/o	_____	E. Secretes thymosin and produces white blood cells
7. adren/o	_____	
8. parathyroid/o	_____	F. Secretes growth hormone and hormones that control the thyroid gland, ovaries, and testes
		G. Secretes estrogen and progesterone
		H. Secretes thyroxine (T_4), which increases metabolism of body cells

(C) Match the medical term in Column I with its meaning in Column II.

COLUMN I		COLUMN II
1. thyroadenitis	_____	A. Disease of the adrenal glands
2. oophoritis	_____	B. Tumor of the thymus gland
3. orchiopexy	_____	C. Pertaining to the pituitary gland
4. thymoma	_____	D. Inflammation of the thyroid gland
5. hyperparathyroidism	_____	E. Removal of the thyroid gland
6. thyroidectomy	_____	F. Surgical fixation of an undescended testicle
7. adrenopathy	_____	G. Increased secretion of parathyroid hormone
8. hypophyseal	_____	H. Inflammation of an ovary

D Match the pathologic condition in Column I with its description in Column II.

COLUMN I	COLUMN II
1. diabetes mellitus _____	A. Enlargement of the thyroid gland
2. acromegaly _____	B. Hypersecretion of cortisone from the adrenal glands
3. goiter _____	C. Deficiency of insulin leading to high blood sugar levels
4. Cushing syndrome _____	D. Enlargement of extremities caused by increased growth hormone from the pituitary gland
5. hyperthyroidism _____	E. Overactivity of the thyroid gland

E Match the test or procedure in Column I with its description in Column II.

COLUMN I	COLUMN II
1. thyroid scan _____	A. Measures blood glucose levels
2. exophthalmometry _____	B. Radioactive compound, injected intravenously, localizes in the thyroid gland; images are produced
3. fasting blood sugar _____	C. Measures hormones, electrolytes, and sugar in blood and urine
4. thyroid function testing _____	D. Measures localization of an element necessary for making thyroid hormone
5. CT scan _____	E. Measures eyeball protrusion
6. serum and urine testing _____	F. Cross-sectional x-ray images of endocrine organs
7. radioactive iodine uptake _____	G. Measures T_3, T_4, and TSH levels in the blood

Female Reproductive System

ANATOMY

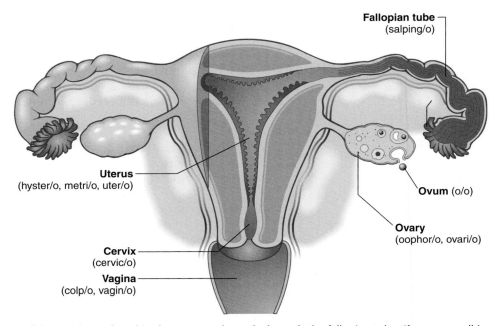

An egg cell (ovum) is produced in the ovary and travels through the fallopian tube. If a sperm cell is present and fertilization (the union of the egg and sperm cell) takes place, the resulting cell (embryo) may implant in the lining of the uterus. The embryo (later called the fetus) develops in the uterus for nine months and is delivered from the body through the cervix and vagina. *(Modified from Chabner D-E: The Language of Medicine, ed 9, Philadelphia, 2011, Saunders.)*

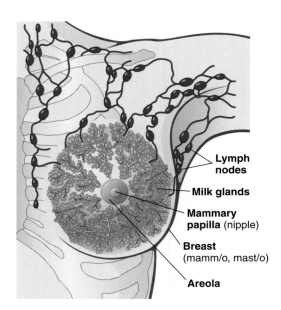

The breast contains glandular tissue that produces milk after delivery of an infant. The areola is the dark-pigmented area surrounding the mammary papilla (breast nipple). There are numerous lymph nodes around the breast and in the underarm (axilla). *(Modified from Chabner D-E: The Language of Medicine, ed 9, Philadelphia, 2011, Saunders.)*

TERMINOLOGY

Meanings for terminology are found in the ***Mini-Dictionary: Glossary of Medical Terms.***

COMBINING FORM	MEANING	TERMINOLOGY	MEANING
cervic/o	cervix	cervical _____	
colp/o	vagina	colposcopy _____	
vagin/o	vagina	vaginitis _____	
hyster/o	uterus	hysterectomy _____	
mamm/o	breast	mammogram _____	
mast/o	breast	mastectomy _____	
metri/o	uterus	endometrium _____	
uter/o	uterus	uterine _____	
o/o	egg	oocyte _____	
oophor/o	ovary	oophorectomy _____	
ovari/o	ovary	ovarian cancer _____	
salping/o	fallopian tube	salpingectomy _____	

PATHOLOGY

Definitions for additional terms in **boldface** are found in the ***Mini-Dictionary: Glossary of Medical Terms.***

Amenorrhea: Absence of menstrual flow.

Dysmenorrhea: Painful menstrual flow.

Ectopic pregnancy: Pregnancy that is not in the uterus; usually occurring in a fallopian tube.

Endometriosis: Tissue from the inner lining of the uterus (**endometrium**) occurs abnormally in other pelvic or abdominal locations (**fallopian tubes, ovaries,** or **peritoneum**).

Fibroids: Benign tumors in the uterus. Also called a **leiomyoma**; LEI/O means smooth (referring to **visceral muscle** within an internal organ).

Menorrhagia: Excessive discharge (-RRHAGIA) of blood from the uterus during menstruation.

Pelvic inflammatory disease: Inflammation (often caused by bacterial infection) in the region of the pelvis. Because the condition primarily affects the fallopian tubes, it is also called **salpingitis.**

LABORATORY TESTS AND DIAGNOSTIC PROCEDURES

Consult *Appendix 2* for pronunciation of terms and additional information.

Amniocentesis: Surgical puncture of the amniotic sac (surrounding the fetus) to withdraw fluid for chemical and chromosomal analysis.
Aspiration: Withdrawal of fluid from a cavity or sac. In breast aspiration, a needle is used to remove fluid from cystic lesions in the breast. The fluid is analyzed for the presence of malignant cells.
Colposcopy: Visual examination of the vagina and cervix with a colposcope (a small, magnifying instrument resembling a mounted pair of binoculars).
Conization: Removal of a cone-shaped section of the cervix for **biopsy.**
Hysterosalpingography: X-ray imaging of the uterus and fallopian tubes after injection of a contrast agent into the uterus.
Mammography: X-ray imaging of the breast.
Pap smear: Procedure in which a physician inserts a wooden spatula or cotton swab to take secretions from the cervix and vagina. Microscopic analysis of the smear (spread on a glass slide) indicates the presence of cervical or vaginal disease.
Pelvic ultrasonography: Procedure that produces an image of sound waves as they bounce off organs (such as the ovaries and uterus) in the pelvic (hip) region. In **transvaginal ultrasound,** a sound probe is placed in the vagina.
Pregnancy test: Measurement of human chorionic gonadotropin (HCG), a hormone in blood and urine that indicates pregnancy.

TREATMENT PROCEDURES

Cauterization: The use of heat to destroy abnormal tissue, such as can occur, for example, in the lining of the **cervix** (lower neck-like region of the uterus).
Cryosurgery: The use of cold temperatures (liquid nitrogen) to freeze and destroy tissue (such as the lining of the cervix).
Dilation and curettage (D&C): Widening (dilation or dilatation) of the opening of the cervix and scraping (curettage) of the lining of the uterus to remove tissue and stop prolonged or heavy uterine bleeding.
Hysterectomy: Excision of the uterus either through the abdominal wall (abdominal hysterectomy) or through the vagina (vaginal hysterectomy)
Myomectomy: The surgical removal of **fibroid (myoma)** tissue from the uterus. **Uterine artery embolization** may be used instead to shrink the fibroids. Tiny pellets are injected into the uterine artery. The pellets act as emboli to block blood flow to fibrous tissue.
Tubal ligation: Procedure in which both fallopian tubes are ligated (tied off) in two places with sutures and the intervening segment is burned or removed. This prevents pregnancy.

USEFUL ABBREVIATIONS

CS	Cesarean section (fetus is removed through an abdominal incision)
D&C	Dilation and curettage
DUB	Dysfunctional uterine bleeding (not associated with menstruation)
GYN	Gynecology
HRT	Hormone replacement therapy (estrogen and progesterone)
IVF	In vitro fertilization (egg and sperm are combined outside the body in a laboratory container; fertilized eggs are injected into the uterus for pregnancy)
OB	Obstetrics (labor and delivery of a fetus)
PID	Pelvic inflammatory disease (salpingitis, oophoritis, endometritis; leading causes are sexually transmitted infections)
STI	Sexually transmitted infection; also called STD (sexually transmitted disease)
TAH-BSO	Total abdominal hysterectomy with bilateral salpingo-oophorectomy (entire uterus and both fallopian tubes and ovaries are removed)

MATCHING EXERCISES

The following exercises will help you review terminology related to the female reproductive system. Answers begin on page 288.

Ⓐ Match the term in Column I with its meaning in Column II.

COLUMN I		COLUMN II
1. ovary	_____	A. Muscular passageway from the uterus to the outside of the body
2. cervix	_____	B. Neck (lower portion) of the uterus
3. fallopian tube	_____	C. One of two paired organs in the female abdomen that produce egg cells and hormones
4. vagina	_____	D. One of two paired tubes that lead from the ovaries to the uterus
5. uterus	_____	E. One of two paired glands on the front of the chest that produce milk after childbirth
6. breast	_____	F. Muscular organ that holds and provides nourishment for the developing fetus

B Match the combining form in Column I with its meaning in Column II.

COLUMN I		COLUMN II
1. oophor/o	_____	A. Uterus
2. colp/o	_____	B. Fallopian tube
3. salping/o	_____	C. Neck of the uterus
4. hyster/o	_____	D. Ovary
5. cervic/o	_____	E. Vagina
6. mast/o	_____	F. Breast

C Match the medical term in Column I with its meaning in Column II.

COLUMN I		COLUMN II
1. salpingectomy	_____	A. Visual examination of the vagina
2. mammography	_____	B. Pertaining to the lower, neck-like region of the uterus
3. vaginitis	_____	C. Inflammation of the breast
4. colposcopy	_____	D. Removal of a fallopian tube
5. hysterectomy	_____	E. Inner lining of the uterus
6. cervical	_____	F. X-ray imaging of the breast
7. endometrium	_____	G. Resection of the uterus
8. mastitis	_____	H. Inflammation of the vagina

D Match the pathologic condition in Column I with its meaning in Column II.

COLUMN I		COLUMN II
1. fibroids	_____	A. Absence of menstrual flow
2. dysmenorrhea	_____	B. Excessive discharge of blood from the uterus between menstrual periods
3. endometriosis	_____	C. Leiomyomas (benign muscle growths) in the uterus
4. ectopic pregnancy	_____	D. Uterine tissue found in sites (ovary, fallopian tubes) other than in the uterus
5. amenorrhea	_____	E. Painful menstrual flow
6. pelvic inflammatory disease	_____	F. Salpingitis
7. menorrhagia	_____	G. Embryo develops outside the uterus

E Match the test or procedure in Column I with its description in Column II.

COLUMN I		COLUMN II
1. pregnancy test	_____	A. Endoscopic visual examination of the vagina
2. pelvic ultrasonography	_____	B. Withdrawal of fluid from a cavity or sac
3. conization	_____	C. Removal of a section of the cervix for biopsy
4. colposcopy	_____	D. X-ray imaging of the breast
5. mammography	_____	E. X-ray examination of the uterus and fallopian tubes
6. Pap smear	_____	F. Sound wave image of organs in the hip region
7. hysterosalpingography	_____	G. Secretions from the vagina and cervix are examined microscopically
8. aspiration	_____	H. Measurement of HCG levels
9. amniocentesis	_____	I. Surgical puncture to remove fluid from the sac surrounding the fetus

F Match the treatment procedure in Column I with its description in Column II.

COLUMN I		COLUMN II
1. myomectomy	_____	A. Use of cold temperatures to freeze and destroy tissue
2. cryosurgery	_____	B. Fallopian tubes are tied to prevent pregnancy
3. cauterization	_____	C. Removal of fibroids from the uterus
4. tubal ligation	_____	D. Widening the cervix and scraping the lining of the uterus
5. D&C	_____	E. Use of heat to destroy abnormal tissue

Lymphatic System

ANATOMY

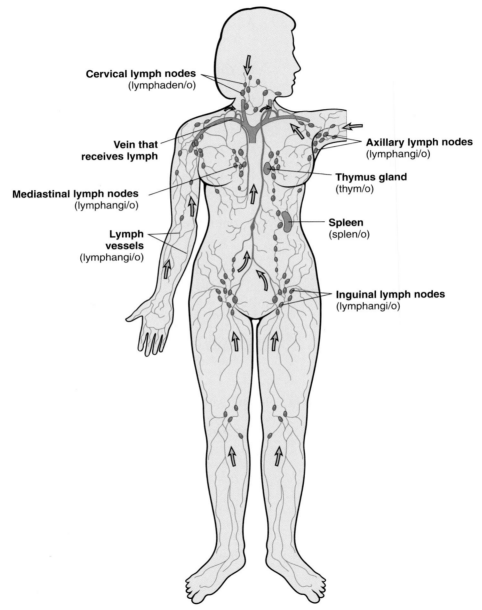

Lymph originates in the tissue spaces around cells and travels in lymph vessels and through lymph nodes to a large vein in the neck, where it enters the bloodstream. *Arrows* in the figure indicate the direction of lymph flow. Lymph contains white blood cells (lymphocytes), which help the body fight disease. The spleen produces lymphocytes and disposes of dying blood cells. The thymus gland also produces lymphocytes. *(Modified from Chabner D-E: The Language of Medicine, ed 9, Philadelphia, 2011, Saunders.)*

TERMINOLOGY

Meanings for terminology are found in the ***Mini-Dictionary: Glossary of Medical Terms.***

COMBINING FORM	MEANING	TERMINOLOGY	MEANING
lymph/o	lymph fluid	lymphoma _____	
lymphaden/o	lymph node ("gland")	lymphadenectomy _____	
		lymphadenopathy _____	
lymphangi/o	lymph vessel	lymphangiectasis _____	
splen/o	spleen	splenomegaly _____	
thym/o	thymus gland	thymoma _____	

PATHOLOGY

Definitions for additional terms in **boldface** are found in the ***Mini-Dictionary: Glossary of Medical Terms.***

Acquired immunodeficiency syndrome (AIDS): Suppression or deficiency of the immune response (destruction of **lymphocytes**) caused by exposure to **human immunodeficiency virus (HIV).**

Lymphoma: Malignant tumor of lymph nodes and lymphatic tissue. **Hodgkin disease** is an example of a lymphoma.

Mononucleosis: Acute infectious disease with enlargement of lymph nodes and increased numbers of **lymphocytes** and **monocytes** in the bloodstream.

Sarcoidosis: Inflammatory disease in which small nodules, or tubercles, form in lymph nodes and other organs. SARC/O means flesh, and -OID means resembling.

LABORATORY TESTS AND DIAGNOSTIC PROCEDURES

Consult ***Appendix 2*** for pronunciation of terms and additional information.

Computed tomography (CT) scan: X-ray views in the transverse plane for the diagnosis of abnormalities in lymphoid organs (lymph nodes, spleen, and thymus gland).

ELISA *(enzyme-linked immunosorbent assay):* A test to screen for antibodies to the **human immunodeficiency virus (HIV),** which causes **acquired immunodeficiency syndrome (AIDS).**

Western blot test: A blood test to detect the presence of antibodies to specific antigens such as the **human immunodeficiency virus.** It is regarded as a more precise test than the ELISA.

TREATMENT PROCEDURES

Chemotherapy: Treatment with powerful drugs to kill cancer cells (**Hodgkin disease, non-Hodgkin lymphoma,** and **multiple myeloma**) and viruses such as the **human immunodeficiency virus.**

Radiotherapy (radiation therapy): Treatment with high-dose radiation to destroy malignant lesions in the body.

USEFUL ABBREVIATIONS

AIDS	Acquired immunodeficiency syndrome
ELISA	Enzyme-linked immunosorbent assay (test to detect anti-HIV antibodies)
HAART	Highly active antiretroviral therapy (for AIDS)
HD	Hodgkin disease
HIV	Human immunodeficiency virus
IgA, IgD, IgE, IgG, IgM	Immunoglobulins (antibodies)
MAC	*Mycobacterium avium* complex (a group of pathogens that cause lung disease in patients with depressed immune systems)
PCP	*Pneumocystis* pneumonia (opportunistic infection seen in patients with AIDS)

MATCHING EXERCISES

The following exercises will help you review terminology related to the lymphatic system. Answers begin on page 288.

(A) Match the term in Column I with its meaning in Column II.

COLUMN I	COLUMN II
1. lymph nodes _____	A. Blood-forming organ in early life; later a storage organ for red blood cells and a source of lymphocytes
2. thymus _____	B. Gland in the mediastinum; produces lymphocytes, which play an important role in immunity
3. lymph _____	C. Stationary collections of lymph tissue throughout the body
4. spleen _____	D. Clear fluid, present in tissue spaces, that circulates in lymph vessels
5. lymph vessels _____	E. Small tubes that carry lymph fluid throughout the body

B Match the combining form in Column I with its meaning in Column II.

COLUMN I		COLUMN II
1. thym/o	_____	A. Spleen
2. lymphangi/o	_____	B. Lymph fluid
3. lymphaden/o	_____	C. Thymus gland
4. splen/o	_____	D. Lymph vessels
5. lymph/o	_____	E. Lymph nodes (glands)

C Match the medical term in Column I with its meaning in Column II.

COLUMN I		COLUMN II
1. lymphadenopathy	_____	A. Malignant tumor of lymph nodes and lymphatic tissue
2. lymphangiectasis	_____	B. Acute infectious disease with enlargement of lymph nodes and increase in lymphocytes and monocytes
3. splenomegaly	_____	
4. lymphoma	_____	C. Malignant tumor of a mediastinal lymphocyte-producing gland
5. lymphadenectomy	_____	D. Widening, dilation of lymph vessels
6. mononucleosis	_____	E. Enlargement of an abdominal organ that produces lymphocytes
7. thymoma	_____	F. Excision of lymph nodes
		G. Disease of lymph nodes

D Match the procedure or test in Column I with its description in Column II.

COLUMN I		COLUMN II
1. ELISA	_____	A. Treatment with high-dose radiation to destroy malignant tissue
2. Western blot	_____	B. X-ray images in a cross-sectional plane for diagnosis of lymph node abnormalities
3. chemotherapy	_____	
4. CT scan	_____	C. Precise blood test to detect antibodies to specific antigens as in HIV infection
5. radiotherapy	_____	D. Screening test for antibodies to the AIDS virus
		E. Treatment with powerful drugs to kill cancer cells

Male Reproductive System

ANATOMY

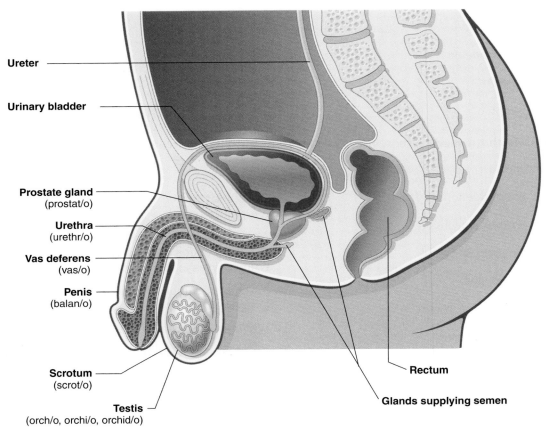

Ureter

Urinary bladder

Prostate gland
(prostat/o)

Urethra
(urethr/o)

Vas deferens
(vas/o)

Penis
(balan/o)

Scrotum
(scrot/o)

Testis
(orch/o, orchi/o, orchid/o)

Rectum

Glands supplying semen

Sperm cells are produced in the testes (*singular: testis*) and travel up into the body, through the vas deferens, and around the urinary bladder. The vas deferens unites with the urethra, which opens to the outside of the body through the penis. The prostate and the other glands near the urethra produce a fluid (semen) that leaves the body with sperm cells. *(Modified from Chabner D-E: The Language of Medicine, ed 9, Philadelphia, 2011, Saunders.)*

TERMINOLOGY

Meanings for terminology are found in the ***Mini-Dictionary: Glossary of Medical Terms.***

COMBINING FORM	MEANING	TERMINOLOGY	MEANING
balan/o	penis	balanitis _____	
orch/o	testis	orchitis _____	
orchi/o	testis	orchiectomy _____	
orchid/o	testis	orchidectomy _____	
prostat/o	prostate gland	prostatectomy _____	
scrot/o	scrotum	scrotal _____	
urethr/o	urethra	urethritis _____	
vas/o	vas deferens	vasectomy _____	

PATHOLOGY

Definitions for additional terms in **boldface** are found in the ***Mini-Dictionary: Glossary of Medical Terms.***

Benign prostatic hyperplasia: Noncancerous enlargement of the prostate gland. Also called **benign prostatic hypertrophy.**

Cryptorchism: Condition of undescended testis. The testis is not in the scrotal sac at birth. CRYPT/O means hidden.

Hydrocele: Sac of clear fluid in the scrotum. HYDR/O means water, and -CELE indicates a hernia (a bulging or swelling).

Prostatic carcinoma: Cancer of the prostate gland (prostate cancer).

Sexually transmitted infections: These affect both males and females and are spread by sexual or other genital contact. Examples are **chlamydial infection, gonorrhea, herpes genitalis,** and **syphilis.**

Testicular carcinoma: Malignant tumor of the testis. An example is a **seminoma.**

Varicocele: Enlarged, swollen veins near a testicle. VARIC/O means swollen veins.

LABORATORY TESTS AND DIAGNOSTIC PROCEDURES

Consult *Appendix 2* for pronunciation of terms and additional information.

Digital rectal examination (DRE): Examination of the prostate gland with finger palpation through the rectum.

Prostate-specific antigen (PSA): Measurement of the amount of PSA in the blood. Higher-than-normal levels are associated with prostatic enlargement and prostate cancer.

Semen analysis: Measurement of the number, shape, and motility (ability to move) of sperm cells.

TREATMENT PROCEDURES

Orchiopexy: Surgical fixation (-PEXY) of an undescended testicle in a young male infant.

Transurethral resection of the prostate gland (TURP): The removal of portions of the prostate gland with an **endoscope** inserted into the urethra. **Photoselective vaporization of the prostate** (GreenLight PVP) is a newer technique that uses a laser to treat benign prostatic hyperplasia.

Vasectomy: Procedure in which the vas deferens on each side is cut, a piece is removed, and the free ends are folded and ligated (tied) with sutures. Vasectomy produces sterilization so that sperm are not released with semen.

USEFUL ABBREVIATIONS

BPH	Benign prostatic hyperplasia
DRE	Digital rectal examination
GU	Genitourinary
PSA	Prostate-specific antigen
STI	Sexually transmitted infection; also called STD (sexually transmitted disease)
TURP	Transurethral resection of the prostate gland

MATCHING EXERCISES

The following exercises will help you review terminology related to the male reproductive system. Answers begin on page 288.

A Match the term in Column I with its meaning in Column II.

COLUMN I		COLUMN II
1. scrotum	_____	A. One of two paired male organs in the scrotum that produces sperm cells and male hormones
2. penis	_____	
3. vas deferens	_____	B. External male organ, containing the urethra, through which both urine and semen (sperm cells and fluid) leave the body
4. testis	_____	
5. prostate	_____	C. Sac on the outside of the body that contains the testes
		D. One of two tubes that carry sperm cells from the testes to the outside of the body
		E. Male organ that surrounds the base of the urinary bladder and produces fluid that leaves the body with sperm

B Match the combining form in Column I with its meaning in Column II.

COLUMN I		COLUMN II
1. prostat/o	_____	A. Tube leading from the urinary bladder to the outside of the body
2. vas/o	_____	B. Gland that produces fluid portion of semen
3. orch/o	_____	
4. scrot/o	_____	C. Penis
5. balan/o	_____	D. Testis
6. urethr/o	_____	E. Tube carrying sperm cells from the testis to the ejaculatory duct and urethra
		F. Sac containing the testes

C Match the medical term in Column I with its meaning in Column II.

COLUMN I		COLUMN II
1. urethritis	_____	A. Resection of the prostate gland
2. scrotal	_____	B. Inflammation of the penis
3. vasectomy	_____	C. Inflammation of a testis
4. orchitis	_____	D. Inflammation of the urethra
5. prostatectomy	_____	E. Pertaining to the sac containing the testes
6. orchidectomy	_____	F. Resection of a piece of each vas deferens
7. balanitis	_____	G. Excision of a testicle

D Match the pathologic condition in Column I with its meaning in Column II.

COLUMN I		COLUMN II
1. varicocele	_____	A. Undescended testicle
2. benign prostatic hyperplasia	_____	B. Malignant tumor of the prostate gland
3. hydrocele	_____	C. Hernia (collection of fluid) in the scrotal sac
4. testicular carcinoma	_____	D. Malignant tumor; one type is a seminoma
5. prostatic carcinoma	_____	E. Swollen, twisted veins near the testis
6. cryptorchism	_____	F. Nonmalignant enlargement of the prostate gland

E Match the test or procedure in Column I with its description in Column II.

COLUMN I	COLUMN II

1. orchiopexy   _____

2. vasectomy   _____

3. TURP   _____

4. DRE   _____

5. semen analysis   _____

6. PSA test   _____

A. Measurement of the number, shape, and motility of sperm cells

B. Measures blood levels of prostate-specific antigen

C. Examination of the prostate gland with finger palpation through the rectum

D. Removal of portions of the prostate gland with an endoscope inserted into the urethra

E. Surgical fixation of an undescended testicle

F. Two tubes that carry sperm from the testicles are cut and tied off

Musculoskeletal System

ANATOMY

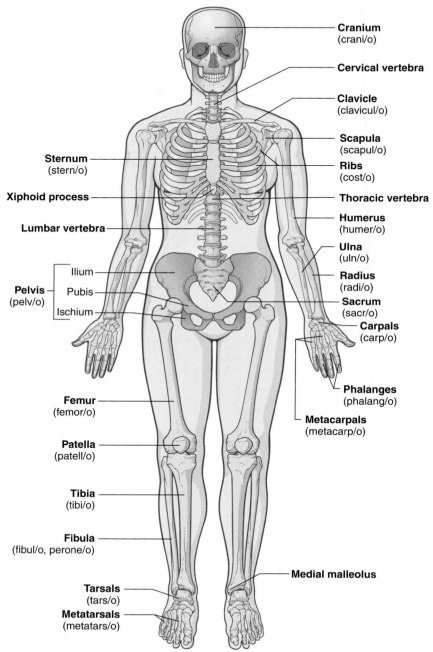

Cranium
(crani/o)

Cervical vertebra

Clavicle
(clavicul/o)

Scapula
(scapul/o)

Ribs
(cost/o)

Thoracic vertebra

Humerus
(humer/o)

Ulna
(uln/o)

Radius
(radi/o)

Sacrum
(sacr/o)

Carpals
(carp/o)

Phalanges
(phalang/o)

Metacarpals
(metacarp/o)

Sternum
(stern/o)

Xiphoid process

Lumbar vertebra

Ilium

Pelvis
(pelv/o)

Pubis

Ischium

Femur
(femor/o)

Patella
(patell/o)

Tibia
(tibi/o)

Fibula
(fibul/o, perone/o)

Medial malleolus

Tarsals
(tars/o)

Metatarsals
(metatars/o)

Bones are connected to muscles that contract to move the body. Joints are the spaces between bones. Near the joints are ligaments that connect bones to other bones and tendons that connect bones to muscles. *(Modified from Chabner D-E: The Language of Medicine, ed 9, Philadelphia, 2011, Saunders.)*

For your reference, included here are anterior and posterior views of superficial muscles in the body.

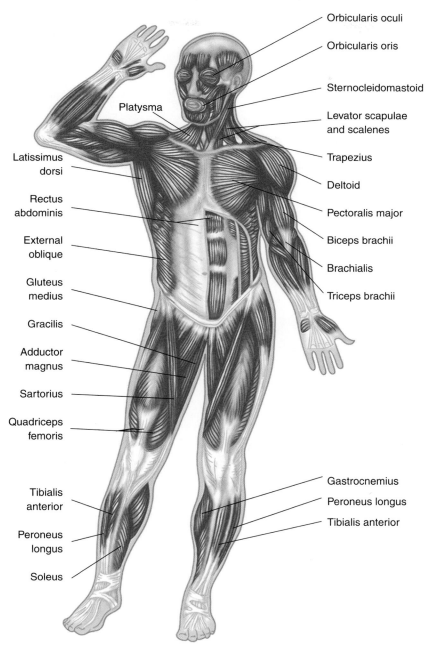

- Orbicularis oculi
- Orbicularis oris
- Sternocleidomastoid
- Levator scapulae and scalenes
- Trapezius
- Deltoid
- Pectoralis major
- Biceps brachii
- Brachialis
- Triceps brachii
- Platysma
- Latissimus dorsi
- Rectus abdominis
- External oblique
- Gluteus medius
- Gracilis
- Adductor magnus
- Sartorius
- Quadriceps femoris
- Tibialis anterior
- Peroneus longus
- Soleus
- Gastrocnemius
- Peroneus longus
- Tibialis anterior

The anterior superficial muscles. *(Modified from Miller-Keane:* Encyclopedia and Dictionary of Medicine, Nursing, and Allied Health, *ed 7, Philadelphia, 2003, Saunders.)*

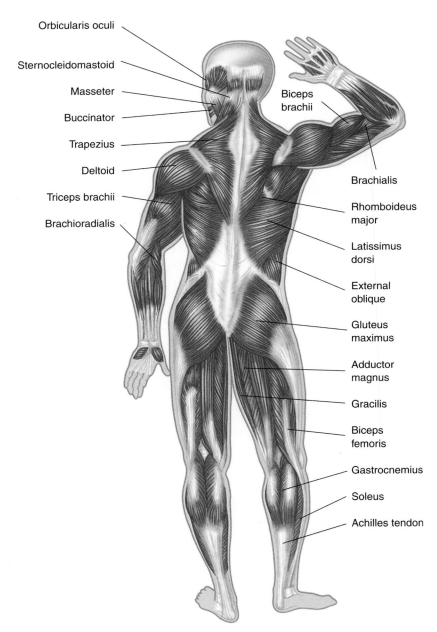

Orbicularis oculi
Sternocleidomastoid
Masseter
Buccinator
Trapezius
Deltoid
Triceps brachii
Brachioradialis

Biceps brachii
Brachialis
Rhomboideus major
Latissimus dorsi
External oblique
Gluteus maximus
Adductor magnus
Gracilis
Biceps femoris
Gastrocnemius
Soleus
Achilles tendon

The posterior superficial muscles. *(Modified from Miller-Keane:* Encyclopedia and Dictionary of Medicine, Nursing, and Allied Health, *ed 7, Philadelphia, 2003, Saunders.)*

TERMINOLOGY

Meanings for terminology are found in the *Mini-Dictionary: Glossary of Medical Terms.*

COMBINING FORM	MEANING	TERMINOLOGY	MEANING
arthr/o	joint	arthroscopy	
chondr/o	cartilage	chondroma	
cost/o	rib	costochondritis	
crani/o	skull	craniotomy	
ligament/o	ligament	ligamentous	
muscul/o	muscle	muscular	
my/o	muscle	myosarcoma	
myos/o	muscle	myositis	
myel/o	bone marrow	myelodysplasia	
oste/o	bone	osteomyelitis	
pelv/o	pelvis, hipbone	pelvic	
spondyl/o	vertebra	spondylosis	
vertebr/o	vertebra	intervertebral	
ten/o	tendon	tenorrhaphy	
tendin/o	tendon	tendinitis	

PATHOLOGY

Definitions for additional terms in **boldface** are found in the *Mini-Dictionary: Glossary of Medical Terms.*

Ankylosing spondylitis: Chronic, progressive **arthritis** with stiffening (**ankylosis**) of joints, primarily of the spine and hip.

Carpal tunnel syndrome: Compression of the median nerve as it passes between the ligament and the bones and tendons of the wrist.

Gouty arthritis: Inflammation of joints caused by excessive uric acid. Also called **gout.**

Muscular dystrophy: An inherited disorder characterized by progressive weakness and degeneration of muscle fibers.

Osteoporosis: Decrease in bone density with thinning and weakening of bone. -POROSIS means condition of containing passages or spaces.

Rheumatoid arthritis: Chronic inflammation of joints; pain, swelling, and stiffening, especially in the small joints of the hands and feet. RHEUMAT/O means flowing, descriptive of the swelling in joints.

LABORATORY TESTS AND DIAGNOSTIC PROCEDURES

Consult *Appendix 2* for pronunciation of terms and additional information.

Antinuclear antibody (ANA) test: Test in which a sample of plasma is tested for the presence of antibodies found in patients with systemic lupus erythematosus.

Arthrocentesis: Surgical puncture to remove fluid from a joint.

Arthrography: X-ray imaging of a joint.

Arthroscopy: Visual examination of a joint with an arthroscope.

Bone density test: Low-energy x-rays are used to image bones in the spinal column, pelvis, and wrist to detect areas of bone deficiency.

Bone scan: Procedure in which a radioactive substance is injected intravenously and its uptake in bones is measured with a special scanning device.

Calcium level: Measurement of the amount of calcium in a sample of blood (serum). This test is important in evaluating diseases of bone.

Electromyography (EMG): Recording of the strength of muscle contraction as a result of electrical stimulation.

Erythrocyte sedimentation rate (ESR): Measurement of the rate at which red blood cells fall to the bottom of a test tube. High sedimentation rates are associated with inflammatory diseases such as **rheumatoid arthritis.**

Muscle biopsy: The removal of muscle tissue for microscopic examination.

Uric acid test: Measurement of the amount of uric acid in a sample of blood. High uric acid levels are associated with gouty arthritis.

TREATMENT PROCEDURES

Arthroplasty: Surgical repair of a joint. Total hip arthroplasty is the replacement of the head of the femur (thigh bone) and acetabulum (cup-shaped portion of the hip socket) with artificial parts (**prostheses**) that are cemented into the bone.

Endoscopic diskectomy: Surgical removal of a herniated intervertebral disk with an endoscope.

Laminectomy: Surgical removal of a portion of a vertebra to allow visualization and removal of a portion of a protruding disk.

Microscopic diskectomy: Surgical removal of a herniated intervertebral disk with an incision that is 1 to 2 inches long and visualization of the surgical field with an operating microscope.

Vertebroplasty: Surgical repair of vertebrae. Special cement is injected into compressed backbones to strengthen them and to relieve pain.

USEFUL ABBREVIATIONS

ACL	Anterior cruciate ligament (of the knee)
ANA	Antinuclear antibody
C1-C7	Cervical vertebrae
Ca	Calcium
DOMS	Delayed-onset muscle soreness
EMG	Electromyography
ESR	Erythrocyte sedimentation rate
IM	Intramuscular
L1-L5	Lumbar vertebrae
NSAID	Nonsteroidal anti-inflammatory drug (prescribed to treat joint disorders)
Ortho	Orthopedics (*or* orthopaedics)
PT	Physical therapy
ROM	Range of motion
T1-T12	Thoracic vertebrae

MATCHING EXERCISES

The following exercises will help you review terminology related to the musculoskeletal system. Answers begin on page 288.

A Match the term in Column I with its description in Column II.

COLUMN I		COLUMN II
1. cranium	_____	A. Finger bones
2. clavicle	_____	B. Thigh bone
3. humerus	_____	C. Kneecap
4. radius	_____	D. Lower arm bone on the thumb side
5. ulna	_____	E. Collarbone
6. carpals	_____	F. Tailbone
7. metacarpals	_____	G. Breastbone
8. phalanges	_____	H. Skull
9. scapula	_____	I. Ankle bones
10. sternum	_____	J. Lower arm bone (little finger side)
11. tarsals	_____	K. Upper arm bone
12. metatarsals	_____	L. Smaller of the lower leg bones
13. fibula	_____	M. Hip bone
14. tibia	_____	N. Lower part of the backbone near the hip
15. patella	_____	O. Bones surrounding the chest cavity
16. sacrum	_____	P. Larger of the lower leg bones
17. coccyx	_____	Q. Hand bones
18. pelvis	_____	R. Wrist bones
19. femur	_____	S. Foot bones
20. ribs	_____	T. Shoulder bone

B Match the combining form in Column I with its meaning in Column II.

COLUMN I		COLUMN II
1. crani/o	_____	A. Backbone
2. arthr/o	_____	B. Cartilage
3. oste/o	_____	C. Joint
4. cost/o	_____	D. Skull
5. pelv/o	_____	E. Rib
6. my/o	_____	F. Muscle
7. ten/o	_____	G. Hip bone
8. chondr/o	_____	H. Bone
9. spondyl/o	_____	I. Connects muscles to bones
10. ligament/o	_____	J. Connects bones to other bones

C Match the medical term in Column I with its meaning in Column II.

COLUMN I		COLUMN II
1. myelodysplasia	_____	A. Incision of the skull
2. intervertebral	_____	B. Inflammation of cartilage attached to ribs
3. osteomyelitis	_____	C. Suture of a tendon
4. arthroscopy	_____	D. Inflammation of bone and bone marrow
5. costochondritis	_____	E. Pertaining to between the backbones
6. chondroma	_____	F. Benign tumor of cartilage tissue
7. tenorrhaphy	_____	G. Abnormal growth of bone marrow cells
8. myosarcoma	_____	H. Malignant tumor of muscle tissue
9. craniotomy	_____	I. Visual examination of a joint

(D) Match the pathologic condition in Column I with its meaning in Column II.

COLUMN I	COLUMN II
1. gouty arthritis _____	A. Chronic, progressive arthritis with stiffening of joints between the backbones
2. carpal tunnel syndrome _____	B. Compression of the median nerve in the wrist
3. rheumatoid arthritis _____	C. High levels of uric acid with inflammation of joints
4. osteoporosis _____	D. Weakness and degeneration of muscle fibers; congenital condition
5. ankylosing spondylitis _____	E. Chronic inflammation of joints, especially small bones in the hands and feet
6. muscular dystrophy _____	F. Decrease in bone density with thinning and weakening of bone

E Match the test or procedure in Column I with its description in Column II.

COLUMN I		COLUMN II

1. arthrocentesis   _____

2. serum calcium   _____

3. electromyography   _____

4. bone scan   _____

5. ESR   _____

6. ANA test   _____

7. muscle biopsy   _____

8. uric acid test   _____

9. arthroscopy   _____

10. arthrography   _____

A. Recording the strength of muscle contraction

B. Measures sedimentation rate of red blood cells; indicates inflammation

C. Plasma is tested for antibodies that are present in patients with systemic lupus erythematosus

D. Removal of muscle tissue for microscopic analysis

E. Surgical puncture to remove fluid from a joint

F. Radioactive substance is injected intravenously and uptake is measured in bone tissue

G. Measurement of an element in the blood that is necessary for normal bone formation

H. X-ray imaging of a joint

I. Measurement of the amount of a substance in blood that is associated with gouty arthritis

J. Visual examination of a joint using an endoscope

F Match the treatment procedure in Column I with its description in Column II.

COLUMN I		COLUMN II

1. laminectomy   _____

2. microscopic diskectomy   _____

3. arthroplasty   _____

4. vertebroplasty   _____

5. endoscopic diskectomy   _____

A. Surgical repair of a joint

B. Surgical repair of a backbone

C. Removal of a herniated disk using a tiny incision and an operating microscope

D. Surgical removal of a portion of a vertebra to allow visualization and removal of a portion of a disk

E. Surgical removal of a herniated disk with an endoscope

Nervous System

ANATOMY

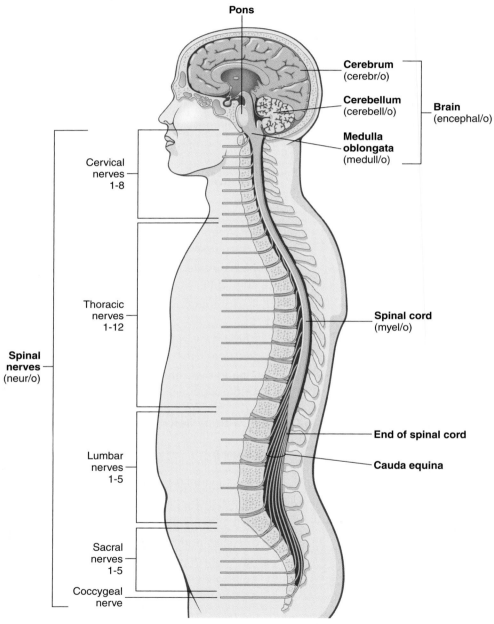

Pons

Cerebrum
(cerebr/o)

Cerebellum
(cerebell/o)

**Medulla
oblongata**
(medull/o)

Brain
(encephal/o)

Cervical
nerves
1-8

Thoracic
nerves
1-12

Spinal cord
(myel/o)

**Spinal
nerves**
(neur/o)

End of spinal cord

Cauda equina

Lumbar
nerves
1-5

Sacral
nerves
1-5

Coccygeal
nerve

The central nervous system consists of the brain and the spinal cord. The peripheral nervous system includes the nerves that carry messages to and from the brain and spinal cord. Spinal nerves carry messages to and from the spinal cord, and the cranial nerves *(not pictured)* carry messages to and from the brain.

TERMINOLOGY

Meanings for terminology are found in the ***Mini-Dictionary: Glossary of Medical Terms.***

COMBINING FORM	MEANING	TERMINOLOGY	MEANING
cerebell/o	cerebellum	cerebellar _____	
cerebr/o	cerebrum	cerebral _____	
encephal/o	brain	encephalitis _____	
medull/o	medulla oblongata	medullary _____	
myel/o	spinal cord	myelitis _____	
neur/o	nerve	neuropathy _____	

PATHOLOGY

Definitions for additional terms in **boldface** are found in the ***Mini-Dictionary: Glossary of Medical Terms.***

Alzheimer disease: Brain disorder marked by deterioration of mental capacity (**dementia**).

Cerebrovascular accident: Damage to the blood vessels of the cerebrum, leading to loss of blood supply to brain tissue; a **stroke.**

Concussion: Blunt injury to the brain severe enough to cause loss of consciousness.

Epilepsy: Chronic brain disorder characterized by recurrent **seizure** activity.

Glioblastoma: Malignant brain tumor arising from **glial cells.** BLAST means immature.

Hemiplegia: Paralysis (-PLEGIA) that affects the right or the left half of the body.

Meningitis: Inflammation of the **meninges** (membranes surrounding the brain and spinal cord).

Multiple sclerosis: Destruction of the **myelin sheath** on nerve cells in the central nervous system (brain and spinal cord), with replacement by plaques of sclerotic (hard) tissue.

Paraplegia: Paralysis that affects the lower portion of the body. From a Greek word meaning "to strike" (-PLEGIA) on one side (PARA-). This term was previously used to describe **hemiplegia.**

Syncope: Fainting; sudden and temporary loss of consciousness as a result of inadequate flow of blood to the brain.

LABORATORY TESTS AND DIAGNOSTIC PROCEDURES

Consult *Appendix 2* for pronunciation of terms and additional information.

Cerebral angiography: X-ray imaging of the blood vessels in the brain after the injection of contrast material into an artery.

Cerebrospinal fluid (CSF) analysis: Chemical tests (for sodium, chloride, protein, and glucose), cell counts, cultures, and bacterial smears on samples of CSF to detect diseases of the brain or meninges. A lumbar puncture is used to remove CSF for analysis.

Computed tomography (CT) scan: Cross-sectional x-ray images of the brain and spinal cord (with and without contrast).

Electroencephalography (EEG): Recording of the electrical activity within the brain.

Lumbar puncture (LP): Pressure of CSF is measured and contrast may be injected for imaging (**myelography**) after removal of CSF from a space between the lumbar vertebrae. An LP ("spinal tap") also provides a sample of CSF for analysis.

Magnetic resonance imaging (MRI): Magnetic waves and radiofrequency waves are used to create images of the brain and spinal cord.

Positron emission tomography (PET) scan: Uptake of radioactive material into the brain shows how the brain uses glucose and gives information about brain function.

TREATMENT PROCEDURES

Stereotactic radiosurgery: Placement in the skull of a stereotactic instrument that locates a target (such as a tumor) in the brain. Then a high-energy radiation beam (Gamma Knife) is delivered to that precise target to destroy the tissue.

Transcutaneous electrical nerve stimulation (TENS): A battery-powered device delivers stimulation to nerves to relieve acute and chronic pain.

USEFUL ABBREVIATIONS

AD	Alzheimer disease
CNS	Central nervous system
CSF	Cerebrospinal fluid
CVA	Cerebrovascular accident (stroke)
EEG	Electroencephalography
LP	Lumbar puncture
MS	Multiple sclerosis
TENS	Transcutaneous electrical nerve stimulation
TIA	Transient ischemic attack (temporary interference with blood supply to the brain)

MATCHING EXERCISES

The following exercises will help you review terminology related to the nervous system.
Answers begin on page 288.

(A) **Match the term in Column I with its description in Column II.**

COLUMN I		COLUMN II
1. cerebrum	_____	A. Lower part of the brain, nearest to the spinal cord; it controls breathing and heart beat
2. spinal cord	_____	
3. cerebellum	_____	B. Collection of nerves that are within the spinal cavity, surrounded by backbones
4. medulla oblongata	_____	
5. spinal nerves	_____	C. Largest part of the brain; controls body movements, thought, reasoning, vision, hearing, speech
		D. Nerves that transmit messages to and from the spinal cord
		E. Lower back part of the brain that controls muscular coordination and balance

(B) **Match the combining form in Column I with its meaning in Column II.**

COLUMN I		COLUMN II
1. cerebell/o	_____	A. Nerve
2. medull/o	_____	B. Cerebellum
3. myel/o	_____	C. Brain
4. cerebr/o	_____	D. Spinal cord
5. encephal/o	_____	E. Medulla oblongata
6. neur/o	_____	F. Cerebrum

C Match the medical term in Column I with its meaning in Column II.

COLUMN I		COLUMN II
1. myelitis	_____	A. Disease of nerves
2. cerebral	_____	B. Pertaining to the largest part of the brain
3. medullary	_____	C. Pertaining to the posterior portion of the brain that controls equilibrium
4. encephalitis	_____	D. Inflammation of the spinal cord
5. neuropathy	_____	E. Inflammation of the brain
6. cerebellar	_____	F. Pertaining to the lower part of the brain closest to the spinal cord

D Match the pathologic condition in Column I with its meaning in Column II.

COLUMN I		COLUMN II
1. cerebrovascular accident	_____	A. Inflammation of the membrane surrounding the brain and spinal cord
2. multiple sclerosis	_____	B. Brain disorder marked by deterioration in mental activity (dementia)
3. concussion	_____	C. Fainting
4. syncope	_____	D. Paralysis on one side of the body
5. epilepsy	_____	E. Damage to blood vessels in the brain; a stroke
6. meningitis	_____	F. Destruction of myelin sheath around nerve cells in the CNS
7. glioblastoma	_____	G. Blunt injury to the brain severe enough to cause loss of consciousness
8. paraplegia	_____	H. Paralysis of the lower portion of the body
9. hemiplegia	_____	I. Malignant tumor of the brain
10. Alzheimer disease	_____	J. Chronic brain disorder with seizure activity

E Match the test or procedure in Column I with its description in Column II.

COLUMN I		COLUMN II

1. lumbar puncture   _____

2. CSF analysis   _____

3. cerebral angiography   _____

4. electroencephalogram   _____

5. PET scan   _____

6. MRI   _____

7. stereotactic
   radiosurgery   _____

8. CT scan   _____

9. TENS   _____

A. Uptake of radioactive material in the brain shows how the brain uses glucose

B. Chemical tests, cell counts, cultures, and smears of fluid surrounding the brain and spinal cord

C. Record of the electrical activity in the brain

D. Procedure to remove cerebrospinal fluid; measurement of pressure and injection of contrast

E. X-ray image of blood vessels in the brain after injection of contrast

F. A battery-powered device delivers stimulation to nerves to relieve acute and chronic pain

G. Cross-sectional x-ray images of the brain and spinal cord

H. Magnetic and radiofrequency waves create images of the brain and spinal cord tissue

I. Gamma Knife is used to destroy brain tissue after a lesion is located with a special instrument

Respiratory System

ANATOMY

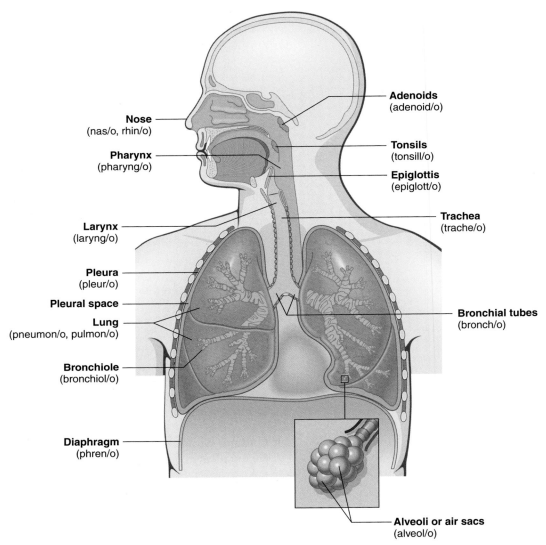

Adenoids
(adenoid/o)

Nose
(nas/o, rhin/o)

Tonsils
(tonsill/o)

Pharynx
(pharyng/o)

Epiglottis
(epiglott/o)

Larynx
(laryng/o)

Trachea
(trache/o)

Pleura
(pleur/o)

Pleural space

Bronchial tubes
(bronch/o)

Lung
(pneumon/o, pulmon/o)

Bronchiole
(bronchiol/o)

Diaphragm
(phren/o)

Alveoli or air sacs
(alveol/o)

Air enters the nose and travels to the pharynx (throat). From the pharynx, air passes through the epiglottis and larynx (voice box) into the trachea (windpipe). The trachea splits into two tubes, the bronchial tubes that carry air into the lungs. The bronchial tubes divide into smaller tubes, called bronchioles, that end in small alveoli, or air sacs. The thin walls of these sacs allow oxygen to pass through them into tiny capillaries containing red blood cells. Red blood cells transport the oxygen to all parts of the body. In a similar manner, gaseous waste (carbon dioxide) leaves the blood by entering the alveoli and traveling out of the body through bronchioles, bronchial tubes, trachea, larynx, pharynx, and the nose. *(Modified from Chabner D-E:* The Language of Medicine, *ed 9, Philadelphia, 2011, Saunders.)*

TERMINOLOGY

Meanings for terminology are found in the *Mini-Dictionary: Glossary of Medical Terms.*

COMBINING FORM	MEANING	TERMINOLOGY	MEANING
adenoid/o	adenoid	adenoidectomy _____	
alveol/o	alveoli (air sacs)	alveolar _____	
bronch/o	bronchial tube	bronchoscopy _____	
bronchiol/o	bronchiole	bronchiolitis _____	
cyan/o	blue	cyanosis _____	
epiglott/o	epiglottis	epiglottitis _____	
laryng/o	larynx	laryngeal _____	
nas/o	nose	nasal _____	
rhin/o	nose	rhinorrhea _____	
pharyng/o	pharynx	pharyngitis _____	
phren/o	diaphragm	phrenic _____	
pneumon/o	lung	pneumonectomy _____	
pulmon/o	lung	pulmonary _____	
tonsill/o	tonsils	tonsillitis _____	
trache/o	trachea	tracheostomy _____	

PATHOLOGY

Definitions for additional terms in **boldface** are found in the ***Mini-Dictionary: Glossary of Medical Terms.***

Asphyxia: Extreme decrease in the amount of **oxygen** in the body with increase of **carbon dioxide** leads to loss of consciousness or death.

Asthma: Spasm and narrowing of bronchi, leading to bronchial airway obstruction.

Atelectasis: Collapsed lung (ATEL/O means incomplete, and -ECTASIS indicates dilation or expansion).

Emphysema: Hyperinflation of air sacs with destruction of alveolar walls. Along with chronic **bronchitis** and **asthma,** emphysema is a type of **chronic obstructive pulmonary disease.**

Hemoptysis: Spitting up of blood.

Hemothorax: Blood in the pleural cavity (space between the **pleural membranes**).

Pneumoconiosis: Abnormal condition of dust (CONI/O) in the lungs.

Pneumonia: Inflammation and infection of alveoli, which fill with pus or products of the inflammatory reaction.

Tuberculosis: An infectious disease caused by bacteria (bacilli). The lungs and other organs are affected. Signs and symptoms are cough, weight loss, night sweats, **hemoptysis,** and pleuritic pain.

LABORATORY TESTS AND DIAGNOSTIC PROCEDURES

Consult ***Appendix II*** for pronunciation of terms and additional information.

Bronchoscopy: Visual examination of the bronchial tubes with an endoscope.

Chest x-ray film: X-ray image of the chest in an AP (anteroposterior), PA (posteroanterior), or lateral (side) view.

Computed tomography (CT) scan: Cross-sectional x-ray images of the chest.

Laryngoscopy: Visual examination of the larynx via the placement of a flexible tube (laryngoscope) through the nose or mouth and into the larynx.

Magnetic resonance imaging (MRI): Magnetic waves and radiofrequency waves create images of the chest in three planes of the body.

Pulmonary angiography: X-ray images are taken of the blood vessels in the lung after the injection of contrast material into a blood vessel. A blockage, such as a pulmonary embolism, can be located with this procedure.

Pulmonary function tests (PFTs): Measurement of the ventilation (breathing capability) of the lungs. A **spirometer** measures the air taken into and breathed out of the lungs.

Pulmonary ventilation-perfusion scans: Procedures that show air flow (ventilation) and blood supply (perfusion) to the lungs via the distribution of radioactive material in the lung tissue after the radioactive material is intravenously injected or is inhaled.

Sputum test: A patient expels sputum by coughing and the sputum is analyzed for bacterial content.

Tuberculin test: Agents are applied to the skin with punctures or injection and the reaction is noted. Redness and swelling result in people sensitive to the test substance and indicate previous or current infection with **tuberculosis.**

TREATMENT PROCEDURES

Endotracheal intubation: A tube is placed through the nose or mouth into the trachea to establish an airway during surgery and for placement on a respirator (a machine that moves air into and out of the lungs).

Thoracentesis: A needle is inserted through the skin between the ribs and into the pleural space to drain a **pleural effusion.**

Thoracotomy: Incision of the chest to remove a lung (**pneumonectomy**) or a portion of a lung (**lobectomy**).

Tracheostomy: Creation of an opening into the trachea through the neck and the insertion of a tube to create an airway.

USEFUL ABBREVIATIONS

ABG	Arterial blood gas
ARDS	Acute respiratory distress syndrome
CO$_2$	Carbon dioxide (gas expelled from the lungs)
COPD	Chronic obstructive pulmonary disease (chronic bronchitis and emphysema)
C-PAP	Continuous positive airway pressure
CPR	Cardiopulmonary resuscitation
CXR	Chest x-ray (film or image)
O$_2$	Oxygen (gas entering the bloodstream through the lungs)
MDI	Metered dose inhaler
PE	Pulmonary embolism (blockage of vessels in the lung by a blood clot)
PEEP	Positive end-expiratory pressure (method of mechanical ventilation)
PFTs	Pulmonary function tests
SOB	Shortness of breath
URI	Upper respiratory infection
VATS	Video-assisted thoracic surgery (using small incisions and an endoscope)
VQ	Ventilation-perfusion scan (also called VQ scans)

MATCHING EXERCISES

The following exercises will help you review terminology related to the respiratory system. Answers begin on page 288.

Ⓐ **Match the term in Column I with its description in Column II.**

COLUMN I	COLUMN II
1. nose _____	A. Throat
2. epiglottis _____	B. Windpipe
3. larynx _____	C. Muscle that separates the chest from the abdomen
4. pharynx _____	D. Flap of cartilage over the "mouth" of the trachea
5. lung _____	E. Small bronchial tube
6. diaphragm _____	F. Structure on the face that permits air to enter the body
7. trachea _____	G. Thin-walled sac through which gases can pass into and out of the bloodstream
8. bronchial tube _____	H. One of two tubes that carry air from the windpipe to the lungs
9. bronchiole _____	I. Voice box
10. air sac _____	J. One of two paired organs in the chest through which oxygen enters and carbon dioxide leaves the bloodstream

B Match the combining form in Column I with its meaning in Column II.

COLUMN I		COLUMN II
1. pharyng/o	_____	A. Diaphragm
2. bronch/o	_____	B. Air sac
3. bronchiol/o	_____	C. Windpipe
4. nas/o or rhin/o	_____	D. Nose
5. laryng/o	_____	E. Throat
6. phren/o	_____	F. Voice box
7. trache/o	_____	G. Tube that carries air from the windpipe to the lung
8. epiglott/o	_____	H. Lung
9. alveol/o	_____	I. Small bronchus
10. pneumon/o	_____	J. Epiglottis

C Match the medical term in Column I with its meaning in Column II.

COLUMN I		COLUMN II
1. pulmonary	_____	A. Discharge from the nose
2. rhinorrhea	_____	B. Pertaining to an air sac
3. pneumonectomy	_____	C. Inflammation of the throat
4. bronchoscopy	_____	D. Pertaining to a lung
5. laryngeal	_____	E. New opening of the windpipe to the outside of the body
6. pharyngitis	_____	F. Pertaining to the nose
7. phrenic	_____	G. Visual examination of the bronchus
8. tracheostomy	_____	H. Resection of a lung
9. alveolar	_____	I. Pertaining to the voice box
10. nasal	_____	J. Pertaining to the diaphragm

Ⓓ Match the pathologic condition in Column I with its meaning in Column II.

COLUMN I	COLUMN II
1. atelectasis _____	A. Collapsed lung
2. hemothorax _____	B. Condition of dust particles in the lung
3. asphyxia _____	C. Spitting up blood
4. emphysema _____	D. Infectious disease caused by bacilli; lungs and other organs are affected
5. asthma _____	E. Inflammation and infection of alveoli
6. hemoptysis _____	F. Blood in the pleural space
7. tuberculosis _____	G. Extreme decrease in oxygen and increase in carbon dioxide in the blood
8. pneumonia _____	H. Hyperinflation of air sacs and destruction of alveolar walls
9. pneumoconiosis _____	I. Spasm and narrowing of bronchial tubes leading to airway obstruction

E Match the test or procedure in Column I with its description in Column II.

COLUMN I		COLUMN II
1. pulmonary angiography	_____	A. Radiographic image in AP, PA, or lateral view
2. laryngoscopy	_____	B. Material expelled by coughing is analyzed
3. pulmonary ventilation-perfusion scans	_____	C. Visual examination of bronchial tubes
4. PFTs	_____	D. After administration of radioactive material (by injection or inhalation), images reveal distribution in lung tissue
5. chest x-ray	_____	E. Magnetic waves produce images of the chest in three planes
6. bronchoscopy	_____	F. Measurements of the ventilation capability of the lung using a spirometer
7. sputum test	_____	G. X-ray images of blood vessels in the lung
8. MRI	_____	H. Visual examination of the voice box
9. tuberculin test	_____	I. Cross-sectional x-ray images of the chest
10. chest CT scan	_____	J. Agents are applied to the skin with punctures, and reaction is noted

F Match the treatment procedure in Column I with its description in Column II.

COLUMN I		COLUMN II
1. tracheostomy	_____	A. A tube placed through the nose or mouth into the windpipe to establish an airway
2. thoracentesis	_____	B. Creation of an opening into the windpipe through the neck and insertion of a tube to create an airway
3. endotracheal intubation	_____	C. Incision of the chest to remove a lung or a portion of a lung
4. thoracotomy	_____	D. Insertion of a needle through the skin between the ribs and into the pleural space to drain a pleural effusion

Skin and Sense Organs

ANATOMY

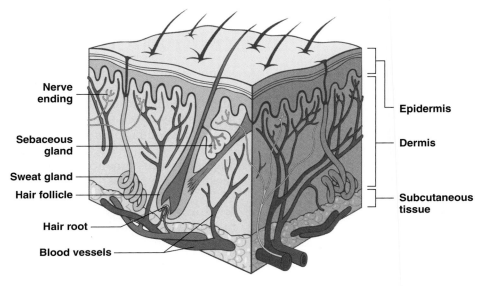

Nerve ending

Sebaceous gland

Sweat gland

Hair follicle

Hair root

Blood vessels

Epidermis

Dermis

Subcutaneous tissue

SKIN
(derm/o, dermat/o, cutane/o)

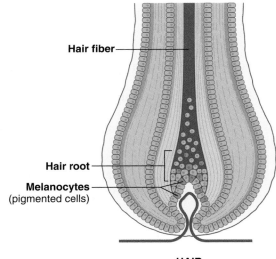

Hair fiber

Hair root

Melanocytes
(pigmented cells)

HAIR
(pil/o, trich/o)

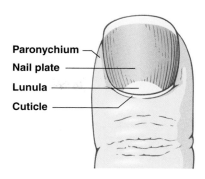

NAIL
(onych/o, ungu/o)

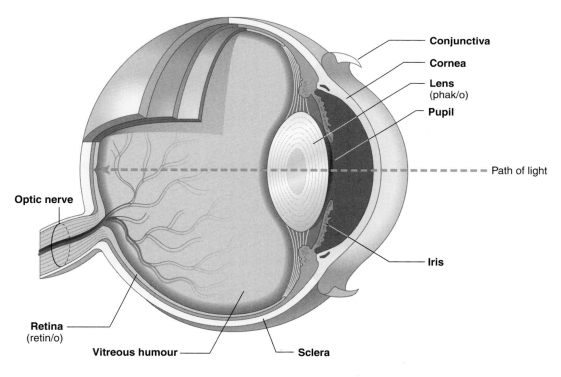

EYE
(ophthalm/o, ocul/o)

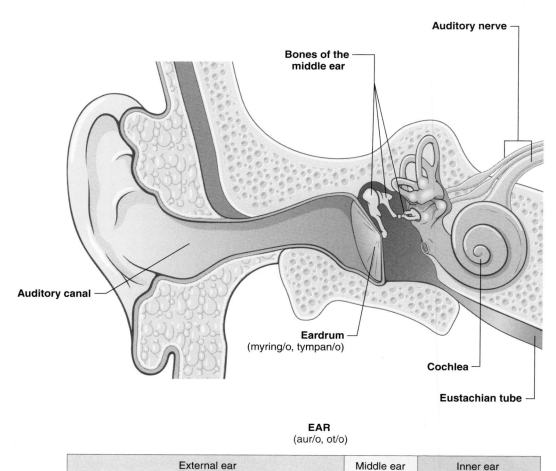

Auditory nerve

Bones of the middle ear

Auditory canal

Eardrum
(myring/o, tympan/o)

Cochlea

Eustachian tube

EAR
(aur/o, ot/o)

External ear	Middle ear	Inner ear

The skin and sense organs receive messages (touch sensations, light waves, sound waves) from the environment and send them to the brain via nerves. These messages are interpreted in the brain, making sight, hearing, and perception of the environment possible. *(Modified from Chabner D-E: The Language of Medicine, ed 9, Philadelphia, 2011, Saunders.)*

TERMINOLOGY

Meanings for terminology are found in the ***Mini-Dictionary: Glossary of Medical Terms.***

COMBINING FORM	MEANING	TERMINOLOGY	MEANING
aur/o	ear	aural discharge _____	
ot/o	ear	otitis _____	
cutane/o	skin	subcutaneous _____	
derm/o	skin	epidermis _____	
dermat/o	skin	dermatology _____	
myring/o	eardrum	myringotomy _____	
tympan/o	eardrum	tympanoplasty _____	
ocul/o	eye	ocular _____	
onych/o	nail	onycholysis _____	
ophthalm/o	eye	ophthalmoscope _____	
phak/o	lens of the eye	aphakia _____	
pil/o	hair	pilosebaceous _____	
retin/o	retina	retinopathy _____	
trich/o	hair	trichophagia _____	
ungu/o	nail	subungual _____	

PATHOLOGY

Definitions for additional terms in **boldface** are found in the ***Mini-Dictionary: Glossary of Medical Terms.***

Alopecia: Absence of hair from areas where it normally grows; baldness.
Cataract: Clouding (opacity) of the lens of the eye, causing impairment of vision or blindness.
Conjunctivitis: Inflammation of the **conjunctiva.**

Glaucoma: Increase in pressure (fluid accumulation) within the chamber at the front of the eye.

Melanoma: Malignant tumor of pigmented cells (MELAN/O means black) that arises from a **nevus** (mole) in the skin.

Nevus: Pigmented lesion in or on the skin; a mole.

Stye (sty): Pus-filled (purulent) infection of glands near the eyelid (most often caused by bacteria). Also called **hordeolum.**

Tinnitus: Abnormal noise (ringing, buzzing, roaring) sound in the ears.

LABORATORY TESTS AND DIAGNOSTIC PROCEDURES

Consult *Appendix 2* for pronunciation of terms and additional information.

Allergy test: Procedure in which allergy-causing substances are placed on the skin and a reaction is noted. In the patch test, a patch with a suspected allergen is placed on the skin. The scratch test involves making several scratches and inserting a small amount of allergen in the scratches.

Bacterial and fungal tests: Procedures in which samples from skin lesions are taken to determine the presence of bacterial infection or fungal growth.

Fluorescein angiography: Fluorescein (a contrast substance) is injected intravenously and the movement of blood is observed by ophthalmoscopy. It is used to detect diabetic or hypertensive retinopathy and also degeneration of the macular (central) area of the retina.

Ophthalmoscopy: Visual examination of the interior of the eye.

Otoscopy: Visual examination of the ear (to the eardrum).

Skin biopsy: Procedure in which samples of skin lesions are removed and sent to the pathology laboratory for microscopic examination.

Slit-lamp microscopy: Examination of the anterior eye structures (such as the cornea) using an instrument that projects intense light through a narrow opening for optimal visualization.

Tuning fork tests: Procedure in which a vibration source (tuning fork) is placed in front of the opening to the ear to test air conduction of sound waves. The tuning fork is also placed on the mastoid bone behind the ear to test bone conduction of sound waves.

USEFUL ABBREVIATIONS

AD	Right ear (Latin, *auris dexter*)
AS	Left ear (Latin, *auris sinister*)
ENT	Ears, nose, throat
HEENT	Head, eyes, ears, nose, throat
OD	Right eye (Latin, *oculus dexter*)
OS	Left eye (Latin, *oculus sinister*)
PERRLA	*P*upils *e*qual, *r*ound, *r*eactive to *l*ight and *a*ccommodation
VA	Visual acuity (clarity of vision)
VF	Visual field

MATCHING EXERCISES

The following exercises will help you review terminology related to the skin and sense organs. Answers begin on page 288.

A Match the term in Column I with its description in Column II.

COLUMN I		COLUMN II
1. epidermis	_____	A. Oil-producing gland in the skin
2. sebaceous gland	_____	B. Gland in the skin that produces a watery, salt-containing fluid
3. dermis	_____	C. Innermost layer of the skin, composed of fatty tissue
4. subcutaneous tissue	_____	D. Middle layer of the skin, containing hair follicles, connective tissue, blood vessels, and glands
5. sweat gland	_____	E. Outer layer of the skin

B Match the term in Column I with its description in Column II.

COLUMN I		COLUMN II
1. retina	_____	A. White, outer coat of the eyeball
2. conjunctiva	_____	B. Membrane that separates the outer and middle parts of the ear
3. pupil	_____	C. Transparent structure behind the pupil that bends light rays so that they focus on the back of the eye
4. lens	_____	D. Nerve that carries messages from the inner ear to the brain
5. cornea	_____	E. Transparent layer over the front of the eye that bends light so that it is focused on the back of the eye
6. sclera	_____	F. Black center of the eye through which light enters
7. iris	_____	G. Layer of sensitive cells (rods and cones) at the back of the eye
8. eardrum	_____	H. Nerve at the back of the eye that transmits light waves to the brain
9. auditory canal	_____	I. Colored, pigmented portion of the eye
10. auditory nerve	_____	J. Passageway leading into the ear from the outside of the body
11. optic nerve	_____	K. Thin, protective membrane over the front of the eye

C Match the combining form in Column I with its meaning in Column II.

COLUMN I		COLUMN II
1. derm/o	_____	A. Eye
2. phak/o	_____	B. Hair
3. retin/o	_____	C. Skin
4. myring/o	_____	D. Posterior, sensitive cell layer of the eye
5. aur/o	_____	E. Nail
6. ophthalm/o	_____	F. Eardrum
7. ungu/o	_____	G. Lens of the eye
8. pil/o	_____	H. Ear

D Match the medical term in Column I with its meaning in Column II.

COLUMN I		COLUMN II
1. ocular	_____	A. Disease of the rod and cone layer of eye (sensitive cells at the back of the eye)
2. otitis	_____	B. Pertaining to under the nail
3. subcutaneous	_____	C. Absence of the lens of the eye
4. myringotomy	_____	D. Inflammation of the ear
5. aphakia	_____	E. Pertaining to the eye
6. epidermis	_____	F. Pertaining to under the skin
7. retinopathy	_____	G. Incision of the eardrum
8. ophthalmoscope	_____	H. Outer layer of the skin
9. tympanoplasty	_____	I. Instrument to visually examine the eye
10. subungual	_____	J. Surgical repair of the eardrum

E Match the pathologic condition in Column I with its meaning in Column II.

COLUMN I	COLUMN II
1. melanoma _____	A. Clouding of the lens of the eye, causing impairment of vision
2. glaucoma _____	B. Absence of hair from areas where it normally grows
3. conjunctivitis _____	
4. tinnitus _____	C. Pigmented lesion on the skin; mole
5. cataract _____	D. Increase in pressure within the chamber at the front of the eye
6. nevus _____	E. Abnormal noise (ringing, buzzing) or sound in the ears
7. alopecia _____	F. Malignant tumor of pigmented cells in the skin
	G. Inflammation of the mucous membrane lining the inner surface of the eyelid

F Match the test or procedure in Column I with its description in Column II.

COLUMN I	COLUMN II
1. skin biopsy _____	A. Samples from skin lesions are examined to detect presence of microorganisms
2. slit-lamp microscopy _____	B. Visual examination of the interior of the eye
3. tuning fork tests _____	C. Patch test; scratch test
4. fluorescein angiography _____	D. Skin lesions are removed and sent to pathology laboratory for microscopic examination
5. otoscopy _____	E. A dye is injected intravenously, and movement of blood through blood vessels in the back of the eye is observed with an ophthalmoscope
6. allergy test _____	
7. bacterial and fungal tests _____	F. Visual examination of the ear to the eardrum
8. ophthalmoscopy _____	G. Microscopic examination of the anterior eye structures, such as the cornea, under intense light
	H. A vibration source is placed in front of the opening of the ear to test air conduction of sound waves

Urinary System

ANATOMY (FEMALE URINARY TRACT)

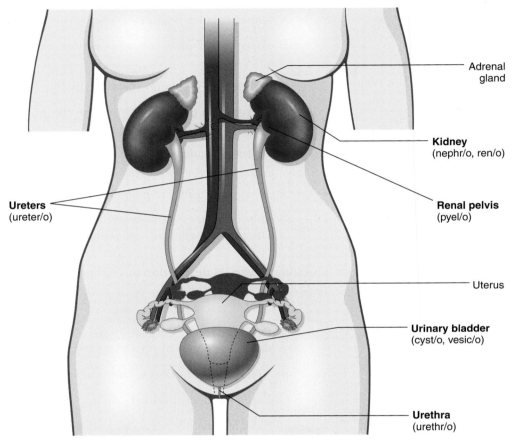

Adrenal
gland

Kidney
(nephr/o, ren/o)

Renal pelvis
(pyel/o)

Ureters
(ureter/o)

Uterus

Urinary bladder
(cyst/o, vesic/o)

Urethra
(urethr/o)

Urine is formed as waste materials, such as urea, are filtered from the blood into the tubules of the kidney. Urea is a nitrogenous waste product formed as proteins are used in cells. Urine passes from the kidney tubules into the central collecting section of the kidney, the renal pelvis. Each renal pelvis leads directly to a ureter, which takes the urine to the urinary bladder. The bladder releases urine to the urethra, and urine leaves the body. *(Modified from Chabner D-E: The Language of Medicine, ed 9, Philadelphia, 2011, Saunders.)*

TERMINOLOGY

Meanings for terminology are found in the **_Mini-Dictionary: Glossary of Medical Terms._**

COMBINING FORM	MEANING	TERMINOLOGY	MEANING
cyst/o	urinary bladder	cystoscopy	
vesic/o	urinary bladder	intravesical	
nephr/o	kidney	nephritis	
ren/o	kidney	renal	
pyel/o	renal pelvis	pyelogram	
ureter/o	ureter	ureterectomy	
urethr/o	urethra	urethritis	

PATHOLOGY

Definitions for additional terms in **boldface** are found in the **_Mini-Dictionary: Glossary of Medical Terms._**

Albuminuria: Abnormal condition of protein (albumin) in the urine.
Anuria: Abnormal condition of no urine production.
Dysuria: Painful urination.
Glycosuria: Abnormal condition of glucose in the urine.
Hematuria: Abnormal condition of blood in the urine.
Nephrolithiasis: Abnormal condition of stones in the kidney.
Renal failure: Condition in which the kidneys stop functioning and do not produce urine.
Uremia: Condition of high levels of **urea** (nitrogenous waste material) in the blood.

LABORATORY TESTS AND DIAGNOSTIC PROCEDURES

Consult **_Appendix 2_** for pronunciation of terms and additional information.

Blood urea nitrogen (BUN): Measures the amount of urea (nitrogenous waste) in the blood.
Cystoscopy: Visual examination of the urinary bladder with a cystoscope (endoscope).
Kidneys, ureters, bladder (KUB): X-ray images of the kidneys and urinary tract made without the use of contrast material.

Retrograde pyelogram (RP): Contrast material is injected through a catheter (a flexible, tubular instrument) into the urethra and bladder, and x-ray films are taken of the urethra, bladder, and ureters.

Voiding cystourethrogram (VCUG): X-ray films of the bladder and urethra taken after the bladder is filled with a contrast material and while the patient is expelling urine. Also called **cystogram.**

Urography: X-ray imaging of the urinary tract after injection of contrast material; pyelography.

TREATMENT PROCEDURES

Dialysis: Waste materials (**urea, creatinine,** and uric acid) are separated from the blood by a machine (**hemodialysis**). Alternatively, a peritoneal catheter (a flexible, tubular instrument) delivers a special fluid into the abdominal cavity, and then the fluid, which now contains waste materials that have seeped from the blood into it, is drained (**peritoneal dialysis**).

Lithotripsy: Shock waves are beamed into a patient to crush urinary tract stones. The stone fragments then pass out of the body with urine. Also called **extracorporeal shock wave lithotripsy (ESWL).**

Renal transplantation: A donor kidney is transferred to a recipient.

Urinary catheterization: A catheter (a flexible tubular instrument) is passed through the urethra and into the urinary bladder for short-term or long-term drainage of urine.

USEFUL ABBREVIATIONS

ARF	Acute renal failure
BUN	Blood urea nitrogen (measures kidney function)
CAPD	Continuous ambulatory peritoneal dialysis
CKD	Chronic kidney disease (rising BUN and serum creatinine levels affect many body systems)
CRF	Chronic renal failure (progressive loss of kidney function)
GFR	Glomerular filtration rate (measured to document stages of kidney disease)
HD	Hemodialysis
KUB	Kidneys, ureters, bladder (series of x-ray films made without contrast)
RP	Retrograde pyelogram
UA	Urinalysis
UTI	Urinary tract infection

MATCHING EXERCISES

The following exercises will help you review terminology related to the urinary system. Answers begin on page 288.

A Match the term in Column I with its description in Column II.

COLUMN I		COLUMN II
1. urinary bladder	_____	A. Tube that leads from the bladder to the outside of the body
2. kidney	_____	B. Central section of the kidney
3. renal pelvis	_____	C. Organ behind the abdomen that makes urine by filtering wastes from the blood
4. ureter	_____	D. One of two tubes that carry urine from the kidney to the urinary bladder
5. urethra	_____	E. Muscular sac that holds urine and releases it to leave the body through the urethra

B Match the combining form in Column I with its meaning in Column II.

COLUMN I		COLUMN II
1. ureter/o	_____	A. Urinary bladder
2. urethr/o	_____	B. Tube leading from the urinary bladder to the outside of the body
3. pyel/o	_____	C. Kidney
4. cyst/o, vesic/o	_____	D. Tube leading from the kidney to the urinary bladder
5. nephr/o, ren/o	_____	E. Renal pelvis (central collecting basin of the kidney)

C Match the medical term in Column I with its meaning in Column II.

COLUMN I		COLUMN II
1. pyelogram	_____	A. X-ray record of the renal pelvis
2. urethritis	_____	B. Visual examination of the urinary bladder
3. nephritis	_____	C. Resection of a ureter
4. intravesical	_____	D. Pertaining to within the urinary bladder
5. cystoscopy	_____	E. Inflammation of the kidney
6. ureterectomy	_____	F. Pertaining to the kidney
7. renal	_____	G. Inflammation of the urethra

D Match the pathologic condition in Column I with its meaning in Column II.

COLUMN I		COLUMN II
1. dysuria	_____	A. Kidneys stop functioning and fail to produce urine
2. hematuria	_____	B. Abnormal condition of protein in urine
3. uremia	_____	C. Blood in the urine
4. renal failure	_____	D. No urine production
5. nephrolithiasis	_____	E. High levels of urea in the bloodstream
6. albuminuria	_____	F. Sugar in the urine
7. glycosuria	_____	G. Painful urination
8. anuria	_____	H. Abnormal condition of kidney stones

E Match the test or procedure in Column I with its description in Column II.

COLUMN I		COLUMN II

1. KUB _____

2. dialysis _____

3. VCUG _____

4. lithotripsy _____

5. renal
   transplantation _____

6. cystoscopy _____

7. BUN _____

8. retrograde
   pyelogram _____

9. urinary
   catheterization _____

A. Measurement of amount of nitrogenous
   wastes in the blood

B. Visual examination of the urinary bladder

C. X-ray images of the kidneys and urinary
   tract without contrast

D. Tube is passed through the urethra into
   the urinary bladder for short- or long-
   term drainage of urine

E. Shock waves are beamed into the patient
   to crush stones in the kidney or ureter

F. Nitrogenous waste materials are
   separated from the blood by a machine

G. After the bladder is filled with contrast,
   x-ray images are taken of the bladder as
   the patient is expelling urine

H. Contrast material is injected via a
   catheter into the bladder, and x-ray
   images are taken of the ureters, bladder,
   and urethra

I. A kidney from a donor is surgically
   implanted in a patient whose kidneys
   have failed

ANSWERS TO MATCHING EXERCISES

Cardiovascular System

A
| 1. B | 3. F | 5. D | 7. J | 9. C |
| 2. I | 4. E | 6. A | 8. G | 10. H |

B
| 1. D | 2. E | 3. B | 4. F | 5. A | 6. C |

C
| 1. D | 3. G | 5. H | 7. A | 9. J |
| 2. F | 4. C | 6. E | 8. B | 10. I |

D
| 1. E | 3. D | 5. C | 7. F |
| 2. H | 4. G | 6. A | 8. B |

E
| 1. I | 3. C | 5. B | 7. D | 9. H |
| 2. J | 4. G | 6. E | 8. A | 10. F |

F
| 1. E | 2. B | 3. G | 4. F | 5. A | 6. C | 7. D |

Digestive System

A
| 1. G | 3. H | 5. F | 7. B |
| 2. C | 4. A | 6. D | 8. E |

B
| 1. C | 3. A | 5. D | 7. G |
| 2. H | 4. F | 6. B | 8. E |

C
| 1. D | 3. H | 5. J | 7. E | 9. C |
| 2. G | 4. I | 6. A | 8. F | 10. B |

D
| 1. C | 3. G | 5. D | 7. J | 9. A |
| 2. F | 4. H | 6. I | 8. E | 10. B |

E
| 1. D | 3. E | 5. A | 7. B | 9. J |
| 2. F | 4. G | 6. C | 8. I | 10. H |

F
| 1. G | 3. A | 5. C | 7. J | 9. E |
| 2. I | 4. D | 6. H | 8. F | 10. B |

Endocrine System

A
| 1. C | 3. A | 5. G | 7. F |
| 2. H | 4. E | 6. B | 8. D |

B
| 1. F | 3. E | 5. H | 7. B |
| 2. D | 4. G | 6. C | 8. A |

C
| 1. D | 3. F | 5. G | 7. A |
| 2. H | 4. B | 6. E | 8. C |

D
| 1. C | 2. D | 3. A | 4. B | 5. E |

E
| 1. B | 3. A | 5. F | 7. D |
| 2. E | 4. G | 6. C |

Female Reproductive System

A
| 1. C | 2. B | 3. D | 4. A | 5. F | 6. E |

B
| 1. D | 2. E | 3. B | 4. A | 5. C | 6. F |

C
| 1. D | 3. H | 5. G | 7. E |
| 2. F | 4. A | 6. B | 8. C |

D	1. C	3. D	5. A	7. B	
	2. E	4. G	6. F		

E	1. H	3. C	5. D	7. E	9. I
	2. F	4. A	6. G	8. B	

F	1. C	2. A	3. E	4. B	5. D

Lymphatic System

A	1. C	2. B	3. D	4. A	5. E

B	1. C	2. D	3. E	4. A	5. B

C	1. G	3. E	5. F	7. C	
	2. D	4. A	6. B		

D	1. D	2. C	3. E	4. B	5. A

Male Reproductive System

A	1. C	2. B	3. D	4. A	5. E	

B	1. B	2. E	3. D	4. F	5. C	6. A

C	1. D	3. F	5. A	7. B	
	2. E	4. C	6. G		

D	1. E	2. F	3. C	4. D	5. B	6. A

E	1. E	2. F	3. D	4. C	5. A	6. B

Musculoskeletal System

A	1. H	5. J	9. T	13. L	17. F
	2. E	6. R	10. G	14. P	18. M
	3. K	7. Q	11. I	15. C	19. B
	4. D	8. A	12. S	16. N	20. O

B	1. D	3. H	5. G	7. I	9. A
	2. C	4. E	6. F	8. B	10. J

C	1. G	3. D	5. B	7. C	9. A
	2. E	4. I	6. F	8. H	

D	1. C	2. B	3. E	4. F	5. A	6. D

E	1. E	3. A	5. B	7. D	9. J
	2. G	4. F	6. C	8. I	10. H

F	1. D	2. C	3. A	4. B	5. E

Nervous System

A	1. C	2. B	3. E	4. A	5. D	

B	1. B	2. E	3. D	4. F	5. C	6. A

C	1. D	2. B	3. F	4. E	5. A	6. C

D	1. E	3. G	5. J	7. I	9. D
	2. F	4. C	6. A	8. H	10. B

E	1. D	3. E	5. A	7. I	9. F
	2. B	4. C	6. H	8. G	

Respiratory System

A
| 1. F | 3. I | 5. J | 7. B | 9. E |
| 2. D | 4. A | 6. C | 8. H | 10. G |

B
| 1. E | 3. I | 5. F | 7. C | 9. B |
| 2. G | 4. D | 6. A | 8. J | 10. H |

C
| 1. D | 3. H | 5. I | 7. J | 9. B |
| 2. A | 4. G | 6. C | 8. E | 10. F |

D
| 1. A | 3. G | 5. I | 7. D | 9. B |
| 2. F | 4. H | 6. C | 8. E | |

E
| 1. G | 3. D | 5. A | 7. B | 9. J |
| 2. H | 4. F | 6. C | 8. E | 10. I |

F
| 1. B | 2. D | 3. A | 4. C |

Skin and Sense Organs

A
| 1. E | 2. A | 3. D | 4. C | 5. B |

B
| 1. G | 3. F | 5. E | 7. I | 9. J | 11. H |
| 2. K | 4. C | 6. A | 8. B | 10. D | |

C
| 1. C | 3. D | 5. H | 7. E |
| 2. G | 4. F | 6. A | 8. B |

D
| 1. E | 3. F | 5. C | 7. A | 9. J |
| 2. D | 4. G | 6. H | 8. I | 10. B |

E
| 1. F | 3. G | 5. A | 7. B |
| 2. D | 4. E | 6. C | |

F
| 1. D | 3. H | 5. F | 7. A |
| 2. G | 4. E | 6. C | 8. B |

Urinary System

A
| 1. E | 2. C | 3. B | 4. D | 5. A |

B
| 1. D | 2. B | 3. E | 4. A | 5. C |

C
| 1. A | 3. E | 5. B | 7. F |
| 2. G | 4. D | 6. C | |

D
| 1. G | 3. E | 5. H | 7. F |
| 2. C | 4. A | 6. B | 8. D |

E
| 1. C | 3. G | 5. I | 7. A | 9. D |
| 2. F | 4. E | 6. B | 8. H | |

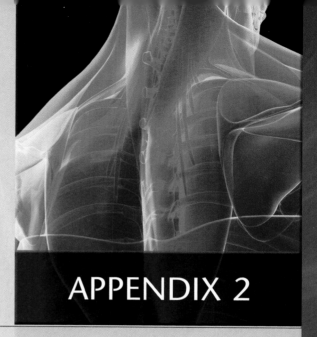

Diagnostic Tests and Procedures*

*Definitions of terms in this appendix are also included in the Student Evolve Resources.

Radiology, Ultrasound, and Imaging Procedures

In many of the following procedures, a *contrast* substance (sometimes referred to as a *dye*) is introduced into the bloodstream, the gastrointestinal tract, or spinal cord so that a body part can be viewed while x-ray pictures are taken. The contrast substance (often containing barium or iodine) appears dense on the x-ray image and outlines the body part that it fills.

The suffix -GRAPHY, meaning process of recording, is used in many terms describing imaging procedures. The suffix -GRAM, meaning record, also is used and describes the actual image that is produced by this procedure.

Pronunciation of each term is given with its meaning. The syllable that gets the accent is in CAPITAL LETTERS. *Italicized* terms indicate important additional terminology, and terms in SMALL CAPITAL LETTERS are defined elsewhere in this appendix.

Angiography (an-je-OG-rah-fe) or **angiogram** (AN-je-o-gram): X-ray imaging of blood vessels. A contrast substance is injected into a blood vessel (vein or artery), and x-ray images are taken of the vessel. In *cerebral angiography,* x-ray images show blood vessels in the brain. In *coronary angiography,* x-rays detect abnormalities in vessels that bring blood to the heart. Angiograms can detect blockage by clots, cholesterol plaques, or tumors or aneurysms (ballooning or dilating of the vessel wall). Angiography is performed most frequently to view arteries and is often used interchangeably with *arteriography.*

Arteriography (ar-teer-e-OG-rah-fe) or **arteriogram** (ar-TEER-e-oh-gram): X-ray recording of an artery and its branches after injection of a contrast substance into an artery. *Coronary arteriography* is the visualization of arteries that travel across the outer surface of the heart and bring blood to the heart muscle.

Arthrography (arth-ROG-rah-fe): X-ray examination of the inside of a joint with a contrast medium.

Barium enema: See LOWER GASTROINTESTINAL EXAMINATION and BARIUM TESTS.

Barium swallow: See ESOPHAGOGRAPHY, BARIUM TESTS, and UPPER GASTROINTESTINAL EXAMINATION.

Barium tests (BAH-re-um tests): X-ray examinations with a liquid barium mixture that is swallowed or given by enema to outline the surface of the gastrointestinal tract. It may locate disorders in the esophagus *(esophagogram),* duodenum, small intestine *(small bowel follow-through),* or colon *(barium enema).* Taken before or during the examination, barium causes the intestinal tract to stand out in silhouette when viewed through a *fluoroscope* (see FLUOROSCOPY) or seen on an x-ray film. The *barium swallow* is used to examine the upper gastrointestinal tract, and the *barium enema* is for examination of the lower gastrointestinal tract. These tests have largely been replaced by ENDOSCOPY (see page 299).

Bone density scan (bone DEN-sih-te scan): Low-energy x-rays are used for this study, which measures bone thickness and reveals areas of bone deficiency *(osteopenia)* and *osteoporosis* (bones become thinner, more fragile, and likely to break). This study is most often performed on the lower spine or hips. Also called *bone densitometry* or *DEXA* (dual-energy x-ray absorptiometry).

Cardiac catheterization (KAR-de-ak kath-eh-ter-ih-ZA-shun): Procedure in which a catheter (tube) is passed via vein or artery into the chambers of the heart to measure the blood flow out of the heart and the pressures and oxygen content in the heart chambers. Contrast material is also introduced into heart chambers, and x-ray pictures are taken to show heart and heart valve structure.

Cerebral angiography: See ANGIOGRAPHY.

Chest x-ray: An x-ray image of the chest wall, lungs, and heart. It may show infection (as in pneumonia or tuberculosis), emphysema, damage due to occupational exposure (asbestosis), lung tumors, fluid accumulation (PLEURAL EFFUSION), or heart enlargement. Also called *chest film* (or *chest x-ray film*) and *chest radiograph*.

Cholangiography (ko-lan-je-OG-rah-fe) or **cholangiogram** (ko-LAN-je-o-gram): X-ray recording or record of bile ducts. Contrast material is given by intravenous injection *(IV cholangiogram)* and collects in the gallbladder and bile ducts. Also, contrast can be introduced (through the skin) using a percutaneously placed needle inserted into an intrahepatic duct *(percutaneous transhepatic cholangiography)*. X-ray images of bile ducts are obtained to identify obstructions caused by tumors or stones. This procedure has largely been replaced by COMPUTED TOMOGRAPHY and MAGNETIC RESONANCE IMAGING, and by ULTRASONOGRAPHY for stones.

Computed tomography (kom-PU-ted to-MOG-rah-fe) or **CT** and **CT scan:** X-ray images that show the body in cross-section. Contrast material may be used (injected into the bloodstream) to highlight structures such as the liver, brain, or blood vessels, and barium can be swallowed to outline gastrointestinal organs. X-ray images, obtained as the x-ray tube rotates (helical CT) around the body, are processed by a computer to show "slices" of body tissues, most often within the head, chest, and abdomen.

Coronary arteriography: See ARTERIOGRAPHY.

Cystography (sis-TOG-rah-fe) or **cystogram** (SIS-to-gram): X-ray recording of the urinary bladder with a contrast medium so that the outline of the urinary bladder can be seen clearly. A contrast substance is injected via catheter into the urethra and urinary bladder, and x-ray images are made. A *voiding cystourethrogram* is an x-ray image of the urinary tract made while the patient is urinating.

Digital subtraction angiography (DIJ-ih-tal sub-TRAK-shun an-je-OG-rah-fe): A unique x-ray technique for viewing blood vessels by taking two images and subtracting one from the other. Images are first obtained without contrast material and then again after contrast is injected into blood vessels. The first image is then subtracted from the second so that the final image (sharp and precise) shows only contrast-filled blood vessels and not the surrounding tissue.

Doppler ultrasound (DOP-ler UL-trah-sownd): Technique that focuses sound waves on blood vessels and measures blood flow as echoes bounce off red blood cells. Arteries or veins in the arms, neck, legs, or abdomen are examined to detect vessels that are occluded (blocked) by clots or atherosclerosis.

Echocardiography (eh-ko-kar-de-OG-rah-fe) or **echocardiogram** (eh-ko-KAR-de-o-gram): Imaging of the heart by introducing high-frequency sound waves through the chest into the heart. The sound waves are reflected back from the heart, and echoes showing heart structure are displayed on a recording machine. It is a highly useful diagnostic tool in the evaluation of diseases of the valves that separate the heart chambers and diseases of the heart muscle.

Endoscopic retrograde cholangiopancreatography or **ERCP** (en-do-SKOP-ik REH-tro-grad kol-an-je-o-pan-kre-ah-TOG-rah-fe): X-ray recording of the bile ducts, pancreas, and pancreatic duct using radiopaque contrast injected through an endoscope, passed through the mouth, esophagus, and duodenum into the bile and pancreatic ducts, and x-ray images are then obtained.

Endoscopic ultrasonography or **E-US** (en-do-SKOP-ik ul-trah-so-NOG-rah-fe): Sound waves are generated from a tube inserted through the mouth and into the esophagus. The sound waves bounce off internal structures and are detected by surface coils. This study can detect enlarged cancerous lymph nodes and tumors in the chest and upper abdomen. This procedure is used for *staging* (evaluation of size and spread) of gastric and esophageal tumors.

Esophagography (eh-sof-ah-GOG-rah-fe) or **esophagogram** (eh-SOF-ah-go-gram): X-ray recording or record of the esophagus performed after barium sulfate is swallowed. This test is part of a BARIUM SWALLOW and UPPER GASTROINTESTINAL EXAMINATION.

Fluoroscopy (flur-OS-ko-pe): An x-ray examination that uses a fluorescent screen rather than a photographic plate to show images of the body in motion. X-rays that have passed through the body strike a screen covered with a fluorescent substance that emits yellow-green light. Internal organs are seen directly (still images are stored either on film or on a computer as digital images) and in motion. Fluoroscopy is used to guide the insertion of catheters and to direct organ biopsy and may be enhanced with barium ingestion. CT-guided biopsy is used most often now.

Gallbladder ultrasound (GAWL-blah-der UL-trah-sownd): Sound waves are used to visualize gallstones. This procedure has replaced the x-ray test known as cholecystography.

Hysterosalpingography (his-ter-o-sal-ping-OG-rah-fe) or **hysterosalpingogram** (his-ter-o-sal-PING-o-gram): X-ray recording or record of the uterus and fallopian tubes. Contrast material is inserted through the vagina into the uterus and fallopian tubes, and x-ray images are obtained to detect blockage or tumor.

Intravenous pyelography: See UROGRAPHY.

Kidneys, ureters, bladder (KID-nez, UR-eh-terz, BLA-der) or **KUB:** X-ray images of the kidney, ureters, and urinary bladder, made without contrast material.

Lower gastrointestinal examination (LO-wer gas-tro-in-TES-tin-al ek-zam-ih-NA-shun): X-ray pictures of the colon taken after a liquid contrast substance called barium sulfate is inserted through a plastic tube (enema) into the rectum and large intestine (colon). If tumor is present in the colon, it may appear as an obstruction or irregularity. Also known as a BARIUM ENEMA.

Magnetic resonance imaging or **MRI** (mag-NET-ik REZ-o-nans IM-ah-jing): A powerful magnetic field is created surrounding the whole patient, or only the head, and water molecules are aligned and then relaxed, generating electromagnetic currents that provide a detailed picture of organs and blood vessels. A computer produces images of body structures at successive depths (as with CT slices). This procedure is particularly useful for imaging tumors of the brain and spinal cord and abnormalities of the lungs and abdominal and pelvic organs. No x-rays are used, and the study may be performed with intravenous contrast material (gadolinium), depending on the purpose of the evaluation. In *magnetic resonance angiography (MRA* or *MR angiography)*, blood vessels are examined in key areas of the body such as the brain, kidneys, pelvis, legs, lungs, and heart.

Mammography (mah-MOG-rah-fe) or **mammogram** (MAM-o-gram): X-ray recording or record of the breast. X-rays of low voltage are beamed at the breast, and images are produced. Mammography detects abnormalities in breast tissue, such as breast cancer. In *stereotactic breast biopsy,* a hollow needle is passed through the skin into a suspicious lesion with the help of mammographic imaging. A specialized mammography machine uses intersecting coordinates to pinpoint an area of tissue (lesion) to be biopsied.

Myelography (mi-eh-LOG-rah-fe) or **myelogram** (MI-eh-lo-gram): X-ray recording of the spinal cord. This procedure has been largely replaced by MRI for detecting tumors or ruptured "slipped" disks between vertebrae (backbones).

Pulmonary angiography (PUL-mo-nair-e an-je-OG-rah-fe): X-ray images of blood vessels of the lung are obtained after injection of contrast. This procedure has been largely replaced by COMPUTED TOMOGRAPHY.

Pyelography or pyelogram: See UROGRAPHY.

Small bowel follow-through: See BARIUM TESTS and UPPER GASTROINTESTINAL EXAMINATION.

Sonography: See ULTRASONOGRAPHY.

Tomography (to-MOG-rah-fe) or **tomogram** (TO-mo-gram): X-ray recording or record that shows an organ in depth. Several pictures ("slices") are taken of an organ by moving the x-ray tube and film in sequence to blur out certain regions and bring others into sharper focus. Tomograms of the kidney and lung are examples.

Ultrasonography (ul-trah-so-NOG-rah-fe) or **ultrasound imaging** (UL-trah-sownd IM-a-jing): Images are produced by beaming high-frequency sound waves (not x-rays) into the body and capturing the echoes that bounce off organs. These echoes are then processed to produce an image showing the difference between fluid and solid masses and the general position of organs. Because ultrasound images are captured in real time, they can show structure and movement of internal organs, as well as blood flowing through blood vessels. Ultrasonography is particularly useful for detecting gallstones, fibroid tumors of the uterus and ovarian tumors and cysts *(pelvic ultrasonography),* enlargement of the heart or defects in heart valves *(echocardiography),* blood flow through major arteries and veins *(Doppler ultrasound),* and enlargement of lymph nodes in the abdomen and chest. Also called *sonography.*

Upper gastrointestinal examination (UP-er gas-tro-in-TES-tin-al ek-zam-ih-NA-shun): X-ray pictures are taken of the esophagus (BARIUM SWALLOW), duodenum, and small intestine after a liquid contrast substance (barium sulfate) is swallowed. In a *small bowel follow-through,* pictures are taken at increasing time intervals to follow the progress of barium through the small intestine. Identification of obstructions or ulcers is possible.

Urography (u-ROG-rah-fe) or **urogram** (U-ro-gram): X-ray recording of the kidney and urinary tract. If x-ray pictures are taken after contrast material is injected intravenously, the procedure is called *intravenous urography* (*descending* or *excretion urography*) or *intravenous pyelography (IVP)*. If x-ray pictures are taken after introduction of contrast directly into the bladder through the urethra, the study is called a *cystogram*. If contrast flows up the ureters into the kidneys, the procedure is called *retrograde urography* or *retrograde pyelography*. PYEL/O means renal pelvis (the collecting chamber of the kidney).

Nuclear Medicine: Radionuclide Scans

In the following diagnostic tests, radioactive material (*radionuclide* or *radioisotope*) is injected intravenously or inhaled and then detected with a scanning device in the organ in which it accumulates. X-rays, ultrasound waves, or magnetic waves are not used.

Bone scan: A radioactive substance (usually a TECHNETIUM isotope) is injected intravenously, and its uptake in bones is detected with a scanning device. Tumors in bone can be detected by increased uptake of the radioactive material in the areas of the lesions.

Brain scan: A radioactive substance is injected intravenously. It collects in any lesion that disturbs the natural barrier that exists between blood vessels and normal brain tissue (blood-brain barrier), allowing the radioactive substance to enter the brain tissue. A scanning device detects the presence of the radioactive substance and thus can identify an area of tumor, abscess, or hematoma. This procedure has largely been replaced by COMPUTED TOMOGRAPHY or MAGNETIC RESONANCE IMAGING.

Gallium scan (GAL-e-um scan): Radioactive gallium (gallium citrate) is injected into the bloodstream and is detected in the body with a scanning device that produces an image of the areas where gallium collects. The gallium collects in areas of certain tumors (Hodgkin disease) and in areas of infection.

MUGA scan (MUH-gah scan): Test that uses radioactive technetium to measure the rate of cardiac output of blood by a *multiple-gated acquisition* (MUGA) technique. Also called *technetium-99m ventriculography*.

Positron emission tomography or **PET scan** (POZ-ih-tron e-MISH-un to-MOG-rah-fe scan): A radioactive substance (usually an isotope incorporated into a sugar-like molecule) that releases radioactive particles called positrons is injected and travels to specialized areas of the body. Because of the way in which the positrons are released, cross-sectional color pictures can be made showing the location of the radioactive substance. The most common use for PET scans is to detect cancer and examine the effects of cancer therapy by showing biochemical changes in tumors.

Tumors pick up the radioactive substance (isotope) and appear as "hot spots" (areas of high glucose uptake) on the film. Also, PET scans can be performed on the heart to assess blood flow to heart muscle and to evaluate patients for coronary artery disease. PET scans of the brain are used to evaluate patients with memory disorders, seizure disorders, and brain tumors. *PET-CT* scans combine PET and CT imaging technology to aid localization of "hot" areas.

Pulmonary perfusion scan (PUL-mo-nair-e per-FU-shun scan): Radioactive particles are injected intravenously and travel rapidly to areas of the lung that are adequately filled with blood. Regions of obstructed blood flow caused by tumor, blood clot, swelling, and inflammation can be seen as nonradioactive areas on the scan.

Pulmonary ventilation scan (PUL-mo-nair-e ven-tih-LA-shun scan): Radioactive gas is inhaled, and a special camera detects its presence in the lungs. The scan is used to detect lung segments that fail to fill with the radioactive gas. Lack of filling is usually due to diseases that obstruct the bronchial tubes and air sacs. This scan is also used in the evaluation of lung function before surgery.

Technetium Tc-99m sestamibi scan (tek-NE-she-um Tc-99m ses-tah-MIH-be scan): The protein sestamibi, tagged with technetium-99, is injected, and the radioactivity is not taken up in areas of decreased blood flow (ischemia). This procedure can be used with an *exercise tolerance test (ETT-MIBI)* to help define areas of poor blood flow to heart muscle.

Thallium-201 scintigraphy (THAL-e-um-201 sin-TIH-grah-fe): Thallium-201 is injected into a vein, and images of blood flow through heart muscle are recorded. Cold spots correlate with areas of myocardial infarction. *Sestamibi scans* also are used to assess the status of blood flow through heart muscle during an *exercise tolerance test (ETT-MIBI)*. It also is useful in localizing disease of the parathyroid glands.

Thyroid scan and uptake (THI-royd scan and UP-take): In a thyroid scan, radioactive iodine (the radiotracer) is injected intravenously or swallowed and then collects in the thyroid gland. A scanning device (probe) detects the radiotracer in the gland tissue, producing an image that shows the size, shape, and position of the thyroid. The thyroid uptake test, or radioactive iodine uptake (RAIU) test, evaluates the function of the thyroid. Radioactive iodine is swallowed and a probe is placed over the thyroid gland to detect increased or decreased activity, as shown by the thyroid's ability to absorb the radiotracer. This test also can be used to detect areas of poor uptake (cold nodules), which may be cancerous.

Clinical Procedures

The following procedures are performed on patients to establish a correct diagnosis of an abnormal condition. In some instances, the procedure also may be used to treat the condition.

Abdominocentesis (ab-dom-in-o-sen-TE-sis): See PARACENTESIS.

Allergy test (AL-er-je test): A small quantity of suspected allergic substance is applied to the skin or injected under the skin, and any reaction is noted.

Amniocentesis (am-ne-o-sen-TE-sis): Surgical puncture to remove fluid from the sac (amnion) that surrounds the fetus in the uterus. The fluid contains cells from the fetus that can be examined with a microscope for chromosomal analysis. Levels of chemicals in amniotic fluid also can detect defects in the fetus.

Arthrocentesis (ar-thro-sen-TE-sis): Puncture to remove fluid from a joint. This usually is done through the skin with a *percutaneous* needle.

Aspiration (as-pih-RA-shun): Withdrawal of fluid by suction through a needle or tube. The term *aspiration pneumonia* refers to an infection caused by inhalation of food or an object into the lungs.

Audiometry (aw-de-OM-eh-tre): Test using sound waves of various frequencies (e.g., 500 Hz), up to 8000 Hz, to quantify the extent and type of hearing loss. An *audiogram* is the record produced by this test.

Auscultation (aw-skul-TA-shun): Process of listening for sounds produced within the body. This is most often performed with the aid of a stethoscope to determine the condition of the heart and lungs and blood vessels or to detect the fetal heartbeat.

Biopsy (BI-op-se): Removal of a piece of tissue from the body for subsequent examination under a microscope. The procedure is performed with a surgical knife or by needle aspiration, or *core biopsy*, or via an endoscopic approach (using a special forceps-like instrument inserted through a hollow flexible tube.) An *excisional biopsy* means that the entire tissue to be examined is removed. An *incisional biopsy* is the removal of only a small amount of tissue, and a *needle* or *core biopsy* indicates that tissue is pierced with a hollow needle and fluid and/or cells are withdrawn by aspiration for microscopic examination.

Bone marrow biopsy (bone MAH-ro BI-op-se): Removal of a small amount of bone marrow via a needle biopsy. The cells are then examined with a microscope. The liquid content of the marrow cavity is withdrawn by *aspiration* and examined separately from the rest of the biopsy sample. Often the hip bone (iliac crest) is used, and the biopsy is helpful in determining the number and type of blood cells in the bone marrow.

Bronchoscopy (brong-KOS-ko-pe): Visual examination of the bronchial passages through a flexible tube (endoscope) inserted into the airway. The lining of the bronchial tubes can be seen, and tissue may be removed for biopsy. The tube is usually inserted through the mouth but can also be directly inserted into the airway during mediastinoscopy. Sedation is required for this procedure.

Catheterization (kath-eh-ter-ih-ZA-shun): Introduction of a hollow, flexible tube into a vessel or cavity of the body to withdraw or instill fluids. Catheterization also is used to measure pressure in vessels and to inject contrast material for outlining vessels or heart chambers. Male and female *Foley catheters* are used for urinary catheterization. *Cardiac catheterization* involves insertion of a catheter into a large vein; from there, it is threaded through the circulation system to the heart. Contrast can be administered to visualize blood vessels for diagnosis and treatment procedures.

Chorionic villus sampling (kor-e-ON-ik VIL-us SAM-pling): Removal of a small piece of placental tissue for microscopic analysis to detect fetal abnormalities.

Colonoscopy (ko-lon-OS-ko-pe): Visual examination of the colon using a flexible tube (endoscope) inserted through the rectum and passed into the large bowel. Biopsy samples may be taken and benign growths, such as polyps, removed through the endoscope. The removal of a polyp is a *polypectomy* (pol-ih-PEK-to-me).

Colposcopy (kol-POS-ko-pe): Inspection of the vagina and cervix through a special microscope inserted into the vagina. The vaginal walls are held apart with a speculum so that all tissues can be viewed.

Conization (ko-nih-ZA-shun): Removal of a cone-shaped sample of uterine cervix tissue. This sample is then examined with a microscope for evidence of cancerous growth. The special shape of the tissue sample allows the pathologist to examine the transitional zone of the cervix, where cancers are most likely to develop.

Culdocentesis (kul-do-sen-TE-sis): Surgical puncture to remove fluid from the cul-de-sac (the space between the rectum and the uterus) through a thin, hollow needle inserted through the vagina into this space. The fluid is then analyzed for evidence of cancerous cells, infection, or blood cells.

Cystoscopy (sis-TOS-ko-pe): Visual examination of the urinary bladder through a thin tube or cystoscope (endoscope) inserted into the urethra and then passed into the bladder. This procedure is used to visualize inflammation and tumors of the bladder, to remove stones, and to perform a biopsy of suspicious areas.

Digital rectal examination or **DRE** (DIJ-ih-tal REK-tal eks-am-ih-NA-shun): The physician inserts a gloved finger into the patient's rectum to detect rectal cancer and as a primary method to detect prostate cancer.

Dilation and curettage or **D&C** (di-LA-shun and kur-eh-TAJ): A series of probes of increasing size are systematically inserted through the vagina into the opening of the cervix. The cervix is thus dilated (widened) so that a curette (spoon-shaped instrument) can be inserted to remove tissue from the lining of the uterus. The tissue is then examined with a microscope.

Electrocardiography or **ECG/EKG** (e-lek-tro-kar-de-OG-rah-fe): Connection of electrodes (wires or "leads") to the body to record electrical impulses from the heart. The *electrocardiogram* is the actual record produced. This test is useful in discovering abnormalities in heart rhythms and for diagnosing heart disorders.

Electroencephalography or **EEG** (e-lek-tro-en-sef-ah-LOG-rah-fe): Connection of electrodes (wires or "leads") to the scalp to record electricity coming from within the brain. The *electroencephalogram* is the actual record produced. This test is useful in the diagnosis and monitoring of epilepsy and in the investigation of neurologic disorders. It also is used to evaluate patients in coma (brain inactivity) and in the study of sleep disorders.

Electromyography or **EMG** (e-lek-tro-mi-OG-rah-fe): Insertion of needle electrodes into muscle to record electrical activity. This procedure detects injuries and diseases that affect muscles and nerves.

Endoscopy (en-DOS-ko-pe): Inspection of an organ or body cavity through a narrow, tube-like instrument (endoscope) inserted into the organ or cavity. The endoscope is placed through a natural opening (the mouth or anus) or into a surgical incision, such as through the abdominal wall. Endoscopes contain bundles of glass fibers that carry light (fiberoptic); some instruments are equipped with a small forceps-like device that withdraws a sample of tissue for microscopic study (biopsy). Examples of endoscopy are bronchoscopy, colonoscopy, esophagoscopy, gastroscopy, and laparoscopy.

Esophagogastroduodenoscopy or **EGD** (eh-SOF-ah-go-GAS-tro-du-o-den-NOS-ko-pe): Visual examination of the esophagus, stomach, and first part of the small intestine using an endoscope inserted through the mouth and down the throat.

Esophagoscopy (eh-sof-ah-GOS-ko-pe): Visual examination of the esophagus performed through an endoscope inserted into the mouth and down the throat. This procedure allows detection of ulcers, tumors, or other lesions.

Excisional biopsy (ek-SIH-zhin-al BI-op-se): See BIOPSY.

Exophthalmometry (eks-of-thal-MOM-eh-tre): Measurement of the extent of protrusion of the eyeball in *exophthalmos*. Exophthalmos may be caused by tumors behind the eye, or by an overactive thyroid gland.

Frozen section (fro-zen SEK-shun): Technique for (or method of) rapid preparation of a biopsy sample for examination during an actual surgical procedure. Tissue is taken from the operating room to the pathology laboratory and frozen. It is then thinly sliced, stained, and immediately examined with a microscope to determine whether the sample is benign or malignant and to determine the status of margins around a tumor.

Gastroscopy (gas-TROS-ko-pe): Visual examination of the stomach through an endoscope inserted down through the esophagus, for either diagnostic inspection or biopsy. When the upper portion of the small intestine is also visualized, the procedure is called *esophagogastroduodenoscopy (EGD)*.

Holter monitoring (HOL-ter MON-ih-ter-ing): Electrocardiographic recording of heart activity over an extended period of time. The Holter monitor device is worn by the patient as normal daily activities are performed. It detects heart rhythm abnormalities. Also called *ambulatory electrocardiography*.

Hysteroscopy (his-ter-OS-ko-pe): Visual examination of the uterus using an endoscope passed through the uterine neck or cervix into the uterus.

Incisional biopsy (in-SIZH-un-al BI-op-se): See BIOPSY.

Laparoscopy (lap-ah-ROS-ko-pe): Examination of the abdominal cavity through an endoscope inserted into the abdomen. After the patient receives a local anesthetic, a laparoscope is placed through an incision in the abdominal wall. This procedure gives the physician a view of the abdominal cavity, the surface of the liver and spleen, and the pelvic region. Laparoscopy can be used to remove some organs (such as the gallbladder, appendix, and ovary) and tumors and for fallopian tube ligation to prevent pregnancy.

Laryngoscopy (lah-rin-GOS-ko-pe): Visual examination of the voice box (larynx) through an endoscope inserted down the trachea (airway). The laryngoscope transmits a magnified image of the larynx through a system of lenses and mirrors. The procedure can reveal tumors and explain changes in the voice. Sputum samples and tissue biopsy specimens are obtained by using brushes or forceps attached to the laryngoscope.

Lumbar puncture or **LP** (LUM-bar PUNK-shur): Introduction of a hollow needle into a space surrounding the spinal cord to withdraw fluid for analysis. Later, contrast material may be injected for imaging.

Mediastinoscopy (me-de-ah-stih-NOS-ko-pe): Procedure for viewing structures in the mediastinum through an endoscope inserted into this space (in the chest between the lungs and in front of the heart). A *mediastinoscope* is introduced through a small incision in the neck while the patient is under anesthesia. This procedure is used to biopsy lymph nodes and and suspected tumors within the mediastinum.

Muscle biopsy (MUH-sl BI-op-se): A sample of muscle tissue is removed and analyzed microscopically.

Nasogastric intubation (na-zo-GAS-trik in-tu-BA-shun): Insertion of a tube through the nose into the stomach to withdraw fluid for analysis or to give nutrition directly into the stomach.

Needle biopsy (NE-dl BI-op-se): See BIOPSY.

Ophthalmoscopy (of-thal-MOS-ko-pe): A physician uses an *ophthalmoscope* to look directly into the eye, evaluating the optic nerve, retina, and blood vessels in the back of the eye and the lens in the front of the eye for cataracts. In *fluorescein angiography,* a contrast substance is injected intravenously, and movement of the dye through blood vessels in the back of the eye is observed with ophthalmoscopy.

Otoscopy (o-TOS-ko-pe): A physician uses an *otoscope* inserted into the ear canal to check for obstructions (e.g., wax), infection, fluid, and eardrum perforation or scarring.

Palpation (pal-PA-shun): Examination by touch. This is a technique of manual physical examination by which a doctor feels underlying tissues and organs through the skin.

Pap smear (pap smeer): Insertion of a cotton swab or wooden spatula into the vagina to obtain a sample of cells from the outer surface of the cervix (neck of the uterus). The cells are then smeared on a glass slide, preserved, and sent to the laboratory for microscopic examination. This test for cervical cancer was developed by and named after the late Dr. George Papanicolaou. Results are graded and reported as negative (no abnormalities) or ranging from mildly abnormal (presence of ASC or abnormal squamous cells) to high-grade squamous intraepithelial lesion (HSIL).

Paracentesis (pah-rah-sen-TE-sis): Surgical puncture of the membrane surrounding the abdomen (peritoneum) to remove fluid from the abdominal cavity. Fluid is drained for analysis and to prevent its accumulation in the abdomen. Also known as *abdominocentesis.*

Pelvic exam (PEL-vik ek-ZAM): Physician inserts fingers into the vagina while keeping the other hand over the abdomen to palpate the uterus and ovaries. This examination checks the uterus and ovaries for enlargement, cysts, tumors, or abnormal bleeding. It is also known as an "internal exam."

Percussion (per-KUSH-un): The technique of striking a part of the body with short, sharp taps of the fingers to determine the size, density, and position of the underlying parts by the sound obtained. Percussion is commonly used over the lungs to detect fluid, atelectasis, and infection, and on the abdomen to examine the liver.

Phlebotomy (fleh-BOT-o-me): Puncture of a vein to remove samples of blood for analysis. Also called *venipuncture.*

Proctosigmoidoscopy (prok-to-sig-moy-DOS-ko-pe): Examination of the first 10 to 12 inches of the rectum and colon using an endoscope inserted through the anus. When the sigmoid colon is visualized with a longer endoscope, the procedure is called *sigmoidoscopy.* The procedure detects polyps, malignant tumors, and sources of bleeding.

Pulmonary function test (PUL-mo-nair-e FUNG-shun test): Measurement of the air taken into and exhaled from the lungs by means of an instrument called a *spirometer.* The test results may be abnormal in patients with asthma, chronic bronchitis, emphysema, or occupational exposures to asbestos, chemicals, and dusts.

Sigmoidoscopy (sig-moy-DOS-ko-pe): See PROCTOSIGMOIDOSCOPY.

Skin tests: Tests in which substances are applied to the skin or injected under the skin and the reaction of immune cells in the skin is observed. These tests detect the patient's sensitivity to substances such as dust or pollen. They also can indicate whether the person has been exposed to the bacteria that cause tuberculosis or diphtheria.

Slit-lamp microscopy (slit-lamp mi-KROS-ko-pe): Examination of the anterior eye structures (such as the cornea) using an instrument that projects intense light through a narrow opening for optimal visualization.

Stool culture (stool KUL-chur): Feces (stools) placed in a growth medium (culture) are analyzed microscopically for evidence of microorganisms (bacteria).

Stress test: Electrocardiography performed during exercise. With intense exercise, the ECG may become abnormal as a result of poor blood flow through blocked arteries. This study may reveal hidden heart disease or confirm the cause of cardiac signs and symptoms.

Thoracentesis (thor-ah-sen-TE-sis): Insertion of a needle into the chest to remove fluid from the space surrounding the lungs (pleural cavity). After injection of a local anesthetic, a hollow needle is placed through the skin and muscles of the back and into the space between the lungs and chest wall. Fluid is then withdrawn by applying suction. Excess fluid *(pleural effusion)* may be a sign of infection, heart failure, or malignant disease. This procedure is used to diagnose conditions, to drain a pleural effusion, or to reexpand a collapsed lung *(atelectasis).*

Thoracoscopy (thor-ah-KOS-ko-pe): Visual examination of the surface of the lungs using an endoscope inserted through an incision in the chest. *VATS* is *video-assisted thoracoscopy* (or *thorascopy*).

Tuning fork tests (TOO-ning fork tests): Tests of hearing using a vibrating tuning fork of known frequency as a source of sound.

Venography (ve-NOG-rah-fe): X-ray examination of veins performed after contrast material is injected into veins. It is used to detect *deep vein thrombosis* or *venous insufficiency.*

Laboratory Tests

The following laboratory tests are performed on samples of a patient's blood, *plasma* (fluid portion of the blood), *serum* (plasma minus clotting proteins and produced after blood has clotted), urine, feces, *sputum* (mucus coughed up from the lungs), *cerebrospinal fluid* (fluid within the spaces around the spinal cord and brain), and skin.

Acid phosphatase (AH-sid FOS-fah-tas): Measurement of the amount of an enzyme called *acid phosphatase* in serum. Enzyme levels are elevated in metastatic prostate cancer. Moderate elevations occur in bone disease and metastatic breast cancer.

Albumin (al-BU-min): Measurement of the amount of albumin (a large protein found in blood and tissues) in both serum and urine. A decreased albumin level in serum indicates malnutrition or liver disease or may occur with extensive loss of protein in the urine or intestines, or from the skin, as in a burn. The presence of albumin in the urine *(albuminuria)* indicates malfunction of the kidney.

Alkaline phosphatase (AL-kah-lin FOS-fah-tase): Measurement of the amount of *alkaline phosphatase* (an enzyme found in cells) in serum. Levels are elevated in liver diseases (such as hepatitis and hepatoma) and in bone disease and cancer metastatic to bone or liver. On laboratory reports, usually abbreviated *alk phos* or *ALK PHOS*.

Alpha-fetoprotein (al-fah-fe-to-PRO-teen): Determination of the presence of a protein called alpha-globulin in serum. The protein normally is present in the serum of the fetus, infant, and pregnant woman. In fetuses with abnormalities of the brain and spinal cord, the protein leaks into the amniotic fluid surrounding the fetus, so it is an indicator of a spinal tube defect (spina bifida) or anencephaly (lack of brain development). High levels are found in patients with cancer of the liver and other malignant diseases (testicular and ovarian cancers). Serum levels monitor the effectiveness of cancer treatment. Elevated levels are also seen in benign liver disease such as cirrhosis and viral hepatitis. On laboratory reports, usually abbreviated *AFP*.

ALT: Measurement of the amount of the enzyme called *alanine transaminase* in serum. The enzyme is normally present in blood but accumulates in blood with damage to liver cells. Formerly called *SGPT*.

ANA: See ANTINUCLEAR ANTIBODY TEST.

Antinuclear antibody test (an-tih-NU-kle-ar AN-tih-bod-e test): A sample of plasma is tested for the presence of antibodies that are found in patients with systemic lupus erythematosus. On laboratory reports, usually abbreviated *ANA*.

AST: Measurement of the enzyme *aspartate transaminase* in serum. The enzyme normally is present in blood but accumulates when there is damage to the heart or to liver cells. Formerly called *SGOT*.

Bacterial and fungal tests (bak-TER-e-al and FUNG-al tests): Samples from skin lesions are cultured in a laboratory or analyzed microscopically to diagnose bacterial or fungal conditions.

Bence Jones protein (bens jonz PRO-teen): Measurement of the Bence Jones protein in serum or urine. Bence Jones protein is a fragment of a normal serum protein, an immunoglobulin, produced in greatly excessive amounts by cancerous bone marrow cells (myeloma cells). Normally it is not found in either blood or urine, but in *multiple myeloma* (a malignant condition of bone marrow), high levels of Bence Jones protein may be detected in urine.

Bilirubin (bil-ih-RU-bin): Measurement of the amount of bilirubin, an orange-brown pigment, in serum and urine. Bilirubin is derived from hemoglobin, the oxygen-carrying protein in red blood cells. Its presence in high concentration in serum and urine causes *jaundice* (yellow coloration of the skin) and may indicate disease of the liver, obstruction of bile ducts, or a type of anemia due to excessive destruction of red blood cells.

Blood chemistry profile: A comprehensive blood test that is a biochemical examination of various substances in the blood using a computerized laboratory analyzer. Tests include measurements of calcium (bones), phosphorus (bones), urea (kidney), creatinine (kidney), bilirubin (liver), AST (liver and heart muscle) and ALT (liver), alkaline phosphatase (liver and bone), globulin (liver and immune disorders), and albumin (liver and kidney). Also called *sequential multiple analysis* (SMA). SMA-6, SMA-12, and SMA-18 indicate the number of blood tests performed.

Blood culture (blud KUL-chur): Test to determine whether infection is present in the bloodstream. A sample of blood is added to a special medium (food) that promotes the growth of microorganisms. The medium is then examined by a medical technologist for evidence of bacteria or other microbes.

Blood urea nitrogen (blud u-RE-ah NI-tro-jen): Measurement of the amount of urea (nitrogen-containing waste material) in serum. A high level of serum urea indicates poor kidney function because it is the kidney's job to remove urea from the bloodstream and filter it into urine. On laboratory reports, usually abbreviated *BUN*.

CA-125: Protein released into the bloodstream by ovarian cancer cells. Measurement of CA-125 determines response to treatment.

Calcium (KAL-se-um): Measurement of the amount of calcium in serum, plasma, or whole blood. Low blood levels cause abnormal functioning of nerves and muscles, and high blood levels may be due to loss of calcium from bones, excessive intake of calcium, disease of the parathyroid glands, or cancer. On laboratory reports, usually given as the symbol *Ca*.

Carbon dioxide (KAR-bon di-OK-side): Blood test that measures all forms of carbon dioxide (gas produced by cells and eliminated by the lungs) in blood. On laboratory reports, abbreviated CO_2.

Carcinoembryonic antigen (kar-sih-no-em-bree-ON-ik AN-ti-jen): A plasma test for a protein normally found in the blood of human fetuses and produced in healthy adults in only a very small amount. High levels of this antigen may be a sign of one of a variety of cancers, especially colon or pancreatic cancer. This test monitors the response of patients to cancer treatment. On laboratory reports, usually abbreviated *CEA*.

Cardiac enzyme tests (CAR-dee-ak EN-zim tests): Measurements of enzymes released into the bloodstream after a heart attack. Examples are creatine kinase (CK) and troponin I and troponin T.

Cerebrospinal fluid (seh-re-bro-SPI-nal FLU-id): Measurement of cerebrospinal fluid for pressure, protein and sugar content, blood cells, and malignant cells. The fluid also is cultured to detect microorganisms. Chemical tests are performed on specimens of the fluid removed by *lumbar puncture*. Abnormal conditions such as meningitis, tumor involving the spinal canal, and encephalitis are detected by analysis of the spinal fluid. On laboratory reports, usually abbreviated *CSF*.

Cholesterol (ko-LES-ter-ol): Measurement of the amount of cholesterol (substance found in animal fats and oils, egg yolks, and milk and produced by the liver) in serum. Normal values for adults are 120 to 200 mg/dL. Levels above 200 mg/dL indicate a need for further testing and efforts to reduce cholesterol level, because high levels are associated with blockage of arteries and heart disease. Blood also is tested for the presence of a lipoprotein substance that is a combination of cholesterol and protein. High levels (optimal level is 60 to 100 mg/dL) of high-density lipoprotein (*HDL*) cholesterol in the blood are beneficial because HDL cholesterol promotes the removal and excretion of excess cholesterol from the blood serum, whereas high levels of low-density lipoprotein (*LDL*) are associated with the development of atherosclerosis (optimal level is 100 mg/dL or less). The ratio of HDL to LDL is most important.

Complete blood count (CBC): Determination of the numbers of leukocytes (white blood cells), erythrocytes (red blood cells), and platelets (clotting cells). The CBC is useful in diagnosis of anemia, infection, and blood cell disorders, such as leukemia.

Creatine kinase (KRE-ah-tin KI-nas): Measurement of levels of creatine kinase, a blood enzyme. Creatine kinase is normally found in heart muscle, brain tissue, and skeletal muscle. The presence of one form *(isoenzyme)* of creatine kinase (either CK-MB or CK2) in the blood is strongly indicative of recent myocardial infarction (heart attack) because the enzyme is released from heart muscle when the muscle is damaged or dying.

Creatinine (kre-AT-tih-nin): Measurement of the amount of creatinine, a nitrogen-containing waste material, in serum or plasma. It is the most commonly used test for kidney function. Because creatinine normally is produced as a protein breakdown product in muscle and is excreted by the kidney in urine, an elevation in the creatinine level in the blood indicates an abnormality of kidney function. Elevations also are seen in patients on high-protein diets and with dehydration.

Creatinine clearance (kre-AT-tih-nin KLEER-ans): Measurement of the rate at which creatinine is cleared (filtered) by the kidneys from the blood. A low creatinine clearance indicates that the kidneys are not functioning effectively to clear creatinine from the bloodstream and filter it into urine.

Culture (KUL-chur): Test in which a sample of body fluids (such as urine, blood, sputum) is mixed with or applied to a sterile growth medium, and if present, bacteria, fungi, or viruses are allowed to grow for several days. Microorganisms that grow out are then identified. In *sensitivity* testing, culture plates containing a specific microorganism are prepared and antibiotic-containing disks are applied to the culture surface. After overnight incubation, the area surrounding the disk (where growth was inhibited) is measured to determine whether the antibiotic is effective against the specific organism. Stool samples may also be cultured.

Differential (dih-fer-EN-shul): See WHITE BLOOD CELL (WBC) COUNT.

Electrolytes (e-LEK-tro-litz): Determination of the concentrations of *electrolytes* (chemical substances capable of conducting an electric current) in serum or whole blood. When dissolved in water, salts, such as sodium chloride, break apart into charged particles *(ions)*. The common positively charged electrolytes are *sodium* (Na^+), *potassium* (K^+), *calcium* (Ca^{2+}), and *magnesium* (Mg^{2+}). The common negatively charged electrolytes are *chloride* (Cl^-) and *bicarbonate* (HCO_3^-). These charged particles should be present at all times for proper functioning of cells. An electrolyte imbalance occurs when serum concentration is either too high or too low. Calcium imbalance can affect the bones, kidneys, gastrointestinal tract, and neuromuscular activity, and sodium imbalance will affect blood pressure, nerve functioning, and fluid levels surrounding cells. Potassium ion imbalance impairs heart and muscular activity.

Electrophoresis: See SERUM PROTEIN ELECTROPHORESIS.

ELISA (eh-LI-zah): A laboratory assay (test) for the presence of antibodies to abnormal proteins such as tumor antigens or viruses, such as HIV. ELISA is an acronym for *enzyme-linked immunosorbent assay*. It also is known as *EIA* or *enzyme immunoassay*.

Erythrocyte sedimentation rate (eh-RITH-ro-sit sed-ih-men-TA-shun rate): Measurement of the rate at which red blood cells (erythrocytes) in well-mixed venous blood settle to the bottom (sediment) of a test tube. If the rate of sedimentation is markedly rapid (elevated rate), it may indicate inflammatory conditions, such as rheumatoid arthritis, or conditions that produce excessive proteins in the blood. On laboratory reports, usually abbreviated *ESR* or *sed rate*.

Estradiol assay (es-trah-DI-ol AS-a): Test for the concentration of estradiol, which is the predominant form of estrogen (female hormone) in serum, plasma, or urine.

Estrogen receptor assay (ES-tro-jen re-SEP-tor AS-a): Test performed on a breast biopsy specimen to determine whether a sample of tumor contains an estrogen receptor protein. If the protein is present (positive result) on breast cancer cells, this indicates that estrogens in the tumor tissue can stimulate growth of the tumor. Then treatment with an antiestrogen drug would retard tumor growth. If the assay result is negative (the protein is not present), then the tumor cells would not be killed by antiestrogen drug treatment.

Glucose (GLU-kos): Measurement of the amount of glucose (sugar) in serum and plasma. High levels of glucose *(hyperglycemia)* indicate the presence of diabetes mellitus. Glucose also is measured in urine, where its presence also usually indicates diabetes mellitus. The *fasting blood sugar test* is measurement of blood sugar after a patient has fasted.

Glucose tolerance test (GLU-kos TOL-er-ans test): Test to determine how the body responds to glucose. In the first part of this test, blood and urine samples are taken after the patient has fasted. Then a solution of glucose is given by mouth. Additional blood and urine samples are obtained a half hour after the glucose is taken and again at intervals of 4 to 5 hours to determine the rate of rise in and then the fall of glucose in the blood. This test will diagnose diabetes mellitus.

Hematocrit (he-MAT-o-krit): Measurement of the percentage blood volume occupied by red blood cells. The normal range is 40% to 50% in males and 37% to 47% in females. A low hematocrit indicates anemia. On laboratory reports, usually abbreviated *Hct* or *HCT*.

Hemoccult test (he-mo-KULT test): Examination of small sample of stool for otherwise inapparent occult (hidden) traces of blood. The sample is placed on the surface of a collection kit and reacts with a chemical (e.g., guaiac). A positive result may indicate bleeding from polyps, ulcers, or malignant tumors. This is an important screening test for colon cancer. Also called a STOOL GUAIAC TEST.

Hemoglobin assay (HE-mo-glo-bin AS-a): Measurement of the concentration of hemoglobin (protein that carries oxygen in red blood cells) in blood. The normal blood hemoglobin ranges are 13.0 to 17.0 g/dL in adult males and 12.0 to 15.0 g/dL in adult females. On laboratory reports, usually abbreviated *Hb* (or *hgb* or *Hgb).*

Human chorionic gonadotropin assay (HU-man kor-e-ON-ik go-nad-o-TRO-pin AS-a): Measurement of the concentration of human chorionic gonadotropin (a hormone secreted by cells of the fetal placenta) in urine. It is detected in urine within days after fertilization of egg and sperm cells and provides the basis of the most commonly used pregnancy test. It also is elevated in patients with certain tumors. On laboratory reports, usually abbreviated *HCG* or *hCG.*

Immunoassay (im-u-no-AS-a): A method of testing blood and urine for the concentration of various chemicals, such as hormones, drugs, or proteins. The technique makes use of the immunological reaction between antigens and antibodies. An *assay* is a determination of the amount of any particular substance in fluid or tissue.

Immunoglobulin (im-u-no-GLOB-u-lin): Measurement (in serum) of proteins (antibodies) that bind to and destroy foreign substances (antigens). Immunoglobulins are made by cells of the immune system.

Immunohistochemistry (im-u-no-his-to-KEM-is-tre): An antibody tagged with a fluorescent label or dye is spread over a tissue biopsy specimen and used to detect the presence of a particular antigen (protein) produced by the tissue or a tumor or infection.

Lipid tests (LIP-id tests): Lipids are fatty substances such as cholesterol and triglycerides. See CHOLESTEROL and TRIGLYCERIDE.

Lipoprotein tests (li-po-PRO-teen tests): See CHOLESTEROL.

Liver function tests (LIV-er FUNG-shun tests): See ALKALINE PHOSPHATASE, BILIRUBIN, ALT, and AST.

Occult blood test: See HEMOCCULT TEST.

PCR test: Blood test to find and analyze DNA and RNA in viruses, diagnose genetic diseases, and do DNA fingerprinting. Multiple copies of DNA or RNA are made. PCR stands for *p*olymerase *c*hain *r*eaction.

PKU test: Test that determines whether the urine of a newborn baby contains substances called *phenylketones*. If these ketones are present, the baby is diagnosed with a condition called *phenylketonuria (PKU)*. PKU affects infants who lack a specific enzyme. When the enzyme is missing, high levels of *phenylalanine* (an amino acid) accumulate in the blood, affecting the infant's brain and causing mental retardation. This situation is prevented by placing the infant on a special diet that prevents accumulation of phenylalanine in the bloodstream.

Platelet count (PLAYT-let kownt): Determination of the number of clotting cells (platelets) in a sample of blood.

Potassium (po-TAS-e-um): Measurement of the concentration of potassium in serum. Potassium is an important chemical for regulating electrical currents and maintaining the cell membrane charge. Muscle and nerve function depends on movement of potassium and other electrolytes across the cell membrane. On laboratory reports, usually given as the symbol $K+$. See also ELECTROLYTES.

Pregnancy test (PREG-nan-se test): Measurement in blood or urine of *human chorionic gonadotropin,* or hCG, a hormone secreted by the placenta early in pregnancy.

Progesterone receptor assay (pro-JES-teh-rone re-SEP-tor AS-a): Test to determine whether a sample of tumor contains a progesterone receptor protein. A positive test result identifies that a breast cancer tumor would be responsive to antihormone therapy.

Prostate-specific antigen (PROS-tat speh-SIH-fic AN-tih-jen): Blood test that measures the amount of an antigen elevated in all patients with prostatic cancer and in some with an inflamed prostate gland. On laboratory reports, usually abbreviated *PSA.*

Protein electrophoresis: See SERUM PROTEIN ELECTROPHORESIS.

Prothrombin time (pro-THROM-bin time): Measurement of the activity of factors in the blood that participate in clotting. Deficiency of any of these factors can lead to a prolonged prothrombin time and difficulty in blood clotting. The test is important as a monitor for patients taking anticoagulants, substances that block the activity of blood clotting factors but increase the risk of bleeding.

PSA: See PROSTATE-SPECIFIC ANTIGEN.

Red blood cell (RBC) count: Test in which the number of erythrocytes in a sample of blood is counted. A low RBC count may indicate anemia. A high count can indicate *polycythemia vera.*

Rheumatoid factor assay (ROO-mah-toyd FAK-tor AS-a): Detection of the abnormal protein *rheumatoid factor* in the serum. This factor is found in patients with rheumatoid arthritis.

Semen analysis (SE-men ah-NAL-ih-sis): Microscopic examination of sperm cells to detect viability and motility of sperm cells.

Serum enzyme tests (SE-rum EN-zim tests): see CARDIAC ENZYME TESTS.

Serum protein electrophoresis (SE-rum PRO-teen e-lek-tro-for-E-sis): A procedure that separates proteins through their migration in an electric current. The material tested, such as serum, containing various proteins, is placed on gel or in liquid, and under the influence of an electric current, the proteins separate (-PHORESIS means separation) so that they can be identified and measured. The procedure is also known as *protein electrophoresis.*

SGOT: See AST.

SGPT: See ALT.

SMA: See BLOOD CHEMISTRY PROFILE.

Sodium level: Measurement of the concentration of sodium (Na^+) in serum. Sodium is one of the most important elements in the body. It is the chief *electrolyte* in fluid outside cells, and it exchanges with potassium within cells during muscle contraction or nerve conduction. Excess sodium is excreted by the kidneys, and sodium is thus involved in water (fluid) balance and acid-base chemical balance during muscle contraction or nerve conduction.

Sputum test (SPU-tum test): Examination of mucus coughed up from the patient's lungs to detect tumor or infection. The sputum is examined microscopically, analyzed chemically, and cultured for the presence of microorganisms.

Stool guaiac test (stool GWI-ak test): See HEMOCCULT TEST.

Thyroid function tests (THI-royd FUNG-shun tests): Tests that measure the levels of thyroid hormones, such as *thyroxine* (T_4) and *triiodothyronine* (T_3), in serum. *Thyroid-stimulating hormone* (TSH), which is produced by the pituitary gland and stimulates the release of T_4 and T_3 from the thyroid gland, is also measured in serum. These tests diagnose hypothyroidism and hyperthyroidism and are helpful in monitoring response to thyroid treatment.

Triglycerides (tri-GLIS-er-ides): Determination of the amount of triglycerides (fatty substances) in the serum. Elevated triglyceride levels (normal is 150 to 200 mg/dL) are considered to be an important risk factor for the development of heart disease.

Troponin (tro-PO-nin): Measurement of levels of proteins troponin I and troponin T in blood is used to indicate the presence and degree of myocardial injury, as from a heart attack.

Uric acid (UR-ik AS-id): Measurement of the amount of uric acid (a nitrogen-containing waste material) in the serum. High serum levels are associated with a type of arthritis called *gout*. In gout, uric acid accumulates as crystals in joints and in tissues. High levels of uric acid may also cause kidney stones.

Urinalysis (u-rih-NAL-ih-sis): Examination of urine as an aid in the diagnosis of disease. Routine urinalysis involves the observation of unusual color or odor; determination of specific gravity (amount of materials dissolved in urine); chemical tests (for protein, sugar, acetone); and microscopic examination for bacteria, blood cells, and sediment. Urinalysis is used to detect abnormal functioning of the kidneys and bladder, infections, and diabetes mellitus. On laboratory reports, usually abbreviated *UA*.

Western blot (WES-tern blot): Test used to detect infection by *HIV* (the AIDS virus). It is more specific than the ELISA. A patient's serum is mixed with purified proteins from HIV, and the reaction is examined. If the patient has made antibodies to HIV, those antibodies react with the purified HIV proteins, and the test result is positive.

White blood cell (WBC) count: Determination of the number of leukocytes in the blood. Higher-than-normal counts can indicate the presence of infection or leukemia. A *differential* (differential count) is the percentages of different types of white blood cells (neutrophils, eosinophils, basophils, lymphocytes, and monocytes) in a sample of blood. It gives more specific information about leukocytes and aids in the diagnosis of infection, allergic diseases, disorders of the immune system, and various forms of leukemia.

Viral load test for HIV: Measures the number of viral particles in the blood. It is used to determine the effectiveness of antiviral treatment.

Abbreviations, Acronyms, Symbols, and Eponyms

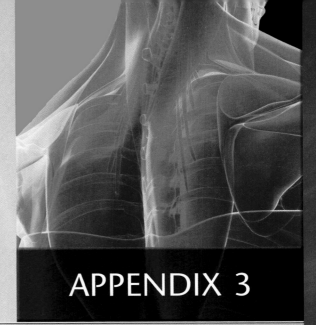

APPENDIX 3

Abbreviations

Ⓐ

AB	abortion
Ab	antibody
ABC	aspiration, biopsy, cytology
abd	abdomen
a.c., ac	before meals *(ante cibum)*
ACE	angiotensin-converting enzyme (ACE inhibitors treat hypertension)
ACL	anterior cruciate ligament (of knee)
ACS	acute coronary syndrome (myocardial infarction, unstable angina)
ACTH	adrenocorticotropic hormone (secreted by the pituitary gland)
a.d.	right ear *(auris dexter)*; because "a" can be misread as "o,", better to write out "right ear" instead of abbreviating
AD	Alzheimer disease
ADD	attention deficit disorder
ADH	antidiuretic hormone (secreted by the pituitary gland)
ADHD	attention deficit/hyperactivity disorder
ad lib	freely as desired *(ad libitum)*
AED	automated external defibrillator
AICD	automatic implantable cardioverter-defibrillator
AIDS	acquired immunodeficiency syndrome
alb	albumin (protein)
ALL	acute lymphocytic leukemia
alk phos	alkaline phosphatase (enzyme elevated in liver disease)
ALS	amyotrophic lateral sclerosis (Lou Gehrig disease)
ALT	alanine transaminase (enzyme elevated in liver disease); formerly called SGPT
AMI	acute myocardial infarction
AML	acute myelocytic (myelogenous) leukemia
AP *or* A/P	anteroposterior (front to back)
A&P	auscultation and percussion
aq	water *(aqua)*
a.s.	left ear *(auris sinister)*; better to write out "left ear" instead of abbreviating
AS	aortic stenosis
ASD	atrial septal defect
ASHD	arteriosclerotic heart disease
AST	aspartate transaminase (elevated in liver and heart disease); formerly called SGOT
a.u.	each ear *(auris uterque)*; better to write out "in each ear/for both ears," rather than abbreviating
AV	arteriovenous; atrioventricular
A&W	alive and well

B

BE	barium enema
B cells	white blood cells (lymphocytes) produced in bone marrow
b.i.d., bid	twice a day *(bis in die)*
BM	bowel movement; bone marrow
BMT	bone marrow transplant
BP, B/P	blood pressure
BPH	benign prostatic hypertrophy (hyperplasia)
Bronch	bronchoscopy
bs	blood sugar; bowel sounds; breath sounds
BSE	breast self-examination
BSO	bilateral salpingo-oophorectomy
BUN	blood urea nitrogen (test of kidney function)
BW	birth weight
Bx, bx	biopsy

C

c̄	with *(cum)*
C1, C2	first cervical vertebra, second cervical vertebra
CA	cancer; carcinoma; cardiac arrest; chronologic age
Ca	calcium
CABG	coronary artery bypass graft
CAD	coronary artery disease
CAPD	continuous ambulatory peritoneal dialysis
cap	capsule
cath	catheter; catheterization
CBC	complete blood count
cc	cubic centimeter (1 cc equals 1/1000 liter, or 1 mL)
CC	chief complaint
CCU	coronary care unit; critical care unit
CF	cystic fibrosis
Chemo	chemotherapy
CHF	congestive heart failure
Chol	cholesterol
CIN	cervical intraepithelial neoplasia
CIS	carcinoma in situ
CKD	chronic kidney disease
cm	centimeter (1 cm is 1/100 meter)
CLL	chronic lymphocytic leukemia
CML	chronic myelocytic (myelogenous) leukemia
CNS	central nervous system
c/o	complains of
CO$_2$	carbon dioxide
COPD	chronic obstructive pulmonary disease
CP	cerebral palsy; chest pain

CPAP	continuous positive airway pressure (provided by machine to aid breathing in patients with sleep apnea)
CPD	cephalopelvic disproportion
CPR	cardiopulmonary resuscitation
C&S, C+S	culture and sensitivity (testing)
C-section, CS	cesarean section
CSF	cerebrospinal fluid
CT scan	computed tomography scan (x-ray images in cross-sectional view)
CVA	cerebrovascular accident (stroke)
c/w	compare with; consistent with
CX, CXR	chest x-ray (image)
Cx	cervix
cysto	cystoscopy

Ⓓ

D&C	dilation (dilatation) and curettage (of the uterine lining)
DES	diethylstilbestrol (estrogen causing defects in children whose mothers took the drug during pregnancy)
DEXA (DXA)	dual-energy x-ray absorptiometry
DIC	disseminated intravascular coagulation
diff.	differential (percentages of types of white blood cells)
DKA	diabetic ketoacidosis
DM	diabetes mellitus
DNA	deoxyribonucleic acid
DNR	do not resuscitate
DOB	date of birth
DOE	dyspnea on exertion
DRE	digital rectal examination
DT	delirium tremens (caused by alcohol withdrawal)
DTR	deep tendon reflex
DVT	deep vein thrombosis
Dx	diagnosis

Ⓔ

EBV	Epstein-Barr virus (cause of mononucleosis)
ECC	emergency cardiac care
ECG	electrocardiography
ECHO	echocardiography
ECMO	extracorporeal membrane oxygenator
ECT	electroconvulsive therapy
ED	emergency department
EDD	expected date of delivery
EEG	electroencephalography
EENT	eyes, ears, nose, throat
EGD	esophagogastroduodenoscopy

EKG	electrocardiography (*ECG* is preferred)
ELISA	enzyme-linked immunosorbent assay (an AIDS test)
EMG	electromyography
ENT	ears, nose, throat
eos.	eosinophils (type of white blood cell)
ER	emergency room; estrogen receptor
ERCP	endoscopic retrograde cholangiopancreatography
ESR	erythrocyte sedimentation rate; see *sed rate*
ESRD	end-stage renal disease
ESWL	extracorporeal shock wave lithotripsy
ETOH	ethyl alcohol (ethanol)
ETT	exercise tolerance test; endotracheal tube

F

FBS	fasting blood sugar
FDA	U.S. Food and Drug Administration
FDG-PET	fluorodeoxyglucose positron emission tomography (nuclear medicine test)
Fe	iron
FEV	forced expiratory volume
FH	family history
FHR	fetal heart rate
FSH	follicle-stimulating hormone (secreted by the pituitary gland)
F/U, f/u	follow-up
FUO	fever of unknown (undetermined) origin
Fx	fracture

G

G	gravida (a pregnant woman)
g, gm	gram
Ga	gallium (element used in nuclear medicine diagnostic tests)
GB	gallbladder
GC	gonococcus (bacterial cause of gonorrhea; another name for *Neisseria gonorrhoeae*)
Gd	gadolinium (widely used MRI contrast agent)
GERD	gastroesophageal reflux disease
GH	growth hormone (secreted by the pituitary gland)
GI	gastrointestinal
Grav. 1, 2, 3	gravida—a woman who has had a first, second, or third pregnancy of any duration
GFR	glomerular filtration rate
gt, gtt	drop, drops
GTT	glucose tolerance test
GU	genitourinary
GVHD	graft-versus-host disease

Gy	gray (unit of irradiation)
GYN, gyn	gynecology

H

H	hydrogen
h, hr	hour
HAART	highly active antiretroviral therapy (for AIDS)
Hb, hgb, Hgb	hemoglobin
HbA1$_c$	glycosylated hemoglobin (measured to test for diabetes)
HBV	hepatitis B virus
HCG, hCG	human chorionic gonadotropin (secreted during pregnancy)
Hct, HCT	hematocrit
HCV	hepatitis C virus
HD	hemodialysis (performed by artificial kidney machine)
HDL	high-density lipoprotein (associated with decreased incidence of coronary artery disease)
HEENT	head, ears, eyes, nose, throat
Hg	mercury
Hgb, hgb, Hb	hemoglobin
HIPAA	Health Insurance Portability and Accountability Act (of 1996)
HIV	human immunodeficiency virus
h/o	history of
H$_2$O	water
H&P	history and physical (examination)
HPV	human papillomavirus
HRT	hormone replacement therapy
h.s.	at bedtime *(hora somni);* write out so as not to confuse with hs (half strength)
HSG	hysterosalpingography
HSV-1, HSV-2	herpes simplex virus type 1, type 2
HTN	hypertension (high blood pressure)
Hx	history

I

I	iodine
^{131}I	radioactive isotope of iodine
I&D	incision and drainage
IBD	inflammatory bowel disease (ulcerative colitis and Crohn disease)
IBS	irritable bowel syndrome (of unknown etiology)
ICD	implantable cardioverter-defibrillator
ICU	intensive care unit
ID	infectious disease
IgA, IgD, IgE, IgG, IgM	immunoglobulins (antibodies)
IM	intramuscular; infectious mononucleosis

INH	isoniazid (drug to treat tuberculosis)
INR	international normalized ratio (system for reporting results of blood coagulation tests)
I&O	intake and output (measurement of patient's fluids)
IOL	intraocular lens (implant)
IUD	intrauterine device (contraceptive)
IV	intravenous
IVP	intravenous pyelography

K

K	potassium
kg	kilogram (1 kg is 1000 grams)
KS	Kaposi sarcoma (malignant lesion associated with AIDS)
KUB	kidneys, ureters, bladder (x-ray study without contrast)

L

L, l	left; liter; lower
L1, L2	first lumbar vertebra, second lumbar vertebra
LA	left atrium
LAD	left anterior descending artery (of the heart); lymphadenopathy
lat	lateral
LBP	low back pain; low blood pressure
LDH	lactate dehydrogenase (elevations associated with heart attacks)
LDL	low-density lipoprotein (high levels associated with heart disease)
LE	lupus erythematosus
LEEP	loop electrocautery excision procedure
LES	lower esophageal sphincter
LFTs	liver function tests
LLQ	left lower quadrant (of the abdomen)
LMP	last menstrual period
LP	lumbar puncture
LPN	licensed practical nurse
LTB	laryngotracheal bronchitis (croup)
LUQ	left upper quadrant (of the abdomen)
LV	left ventricle
LVAD	left ventricular assist device (bridge to cardiac transplantation)
L&W	living and well
lymphs	lymphocytes
lytes	electrolytes

M

m	meter; milli (one thousandth)
MAC	monitored anesthesia care
MCH	mean corpuscular hemoglobin (amount in each red blood cell)

MCHC	mean corpuscular hemoglobin concentration (amount per unit of blood)
MCV	mean corpuscular volume (size of individual red blood cell)
MD, M.D.	doctor of medicine; muscular dystrophy
MDS	myelodysplastic syndrome (a bone marrow disorder)
mets	metastases
mg	milligram (1 mg is 1/1000 gram)
Mg	magnesium
MH	marital history; mental health
MI	myocardial infarction (heart attack)
mL	milliliter (1 mL is 1/1000 liter)
mm	millimeter (1 mm is 1/1000 meter)
mm Hg	millimeters of mercury (units for measurement of blood pressure)
mono	monocytes (type of white blood cell)
MRA	magnetic resonance angiography
MRI	magnetic resonance imaging
MRSA	methicillin-resistant *Staphylococcus aureus*
MS	mental status; mitral stenosis; multiple sclerosis
MSW	medical social worker
MTD	maximum tolerated dose
MVP	mitral valve prolapse
myop	myopia (nearsightedness)

Ⓝ

N	nitrogen
Na	sodium
NB	newborn
NED	no evidence of disease
NG tube	nasogastric tube
NICU	neonatal intensive care unit
NKA	no known allergies
NPO	nothing by mouth *(nil per os)*
NSAID	nonsteroidal anti-inflammatory drug
NSR	normal sinus rhythm (of the heart)
NT	not tender (to touch)
NTP	normal temperature and pressure
N+V	nausea and vomiting

Ⓞ

O_2	oxygen
OA	osteoarthritis
OB	obstetrics
OD	doctor of optometry
o.d.	right eye *(oculus dexter)*; better to write out "right eye" so as not to confuse "o" with "a" (for ear)

OR	operating room
ORIF	open reduction plus internal fixation (to set a broken bone)
ORTH, ortho.	orthopedics *or* orthopaedics
os	mouth
o.s.	left eye *(oculus sinister)*; better to write out "left eye"
OSA	obstructive sleep apnea
OT	occupational therapy
o.u.	each eye *(oculus uterque);* better to write out "each eye"
OV	office visit

℗

p̄	after; following
P	phosphorus; plan; posterior; pressure; pulse; pupil
PA	posteroanterior (back to front); pulmonary artery
PAC	premature atrial contraction
PaCO₂, Paco₂	arterial pressure of carbon dioxide in the blood; may also be written "arterial PCO_2"
PACS	picture archival communications system
palp	palpable; palpation (examine by touch)
PaO₂, Pao₂	arterial pressure of oxygen in the blood; may also be written "arterial PO_2"
Pap smear	Papanicolaou smear (preparation of cells from the cervix and vagina for microscopic examination)
para	paracentesis (abdominocentesis)
Para 1, 2, 3	A woman who has produced one, two, or three viable offspring; unipara, bipara, tripara
p.c., pc	after meals *(post cibum)*
PCI	percutaneous coronary intervention
PE	physical examination; pulmonary embolus
PEEP	positive end-expiratory pressure
per	by
PERRLA	pupils equal, round, reactive to light and accommodation
PET	positron emission tomography
PE tube	pressure-equalizing tube (ventilating tube for the eardrum)
PFT	pulmonary function test
pH	hydrogen ion concentration (measurement of acidity or alkalinity of a solution)
PH	past history
PI	present illness
PID	pelvic inflammatory disease
PKU	phenylketonuria (disease due to lack of an enzyme in infants)
PM	afternoon *(post meridiem)*; postmortem
PMH	past medical history
PMS	premenstrual syndrome
PND	paroxysmal nocturnal dyspnea; postnasal drip
p/o	postoperative

p.o., po	by mouth *(per os)*
polys	polymorphonuclear leukocytes (neutrophils)
poplit	popliteal (behind the knee)
post-op	after operation
PP	after meals *(postprandial)*; after birth *(postpartum)*
PPD	purified protein derivative (skin test for tuberculosis)
pre-op	before operation (preoperative)
prep	prepare for
p.r.n., prn	as needed *(pro re nata)*
procto	proctoscopy (visual examination of the anus and rectum)
pro time	prothrombin time (test of blood clotting)
PSA	prostate-specific antigen (screening test for prostate cancer)
pt	patient
PT	physical therapy; prothrombin time
PTA	prior to admission (to hospital)
PTCA	percutaneous transluminal coronary angioplasty (balloon angioplasty)
PTH	parathyroid hormone
PTR	patient to return
PTSD	post-traumatic stress disorder
PTT	partial thromboplastin time (test of blood clotting)
PVC	premature ventricular contraction (abnormal heart rhythm)
PVD	peripheral vascular disease
PVT	paroxysmal ventricular tachycardia
PWB	partial weight bearing
Px	prognosis

Q

q	every *(quaque)*
q.d.	each (every) day *(quaque die)*; better to write out "each day," because can be misread as q.i.d.
q.h.	each (every) hour *(quaque hora)*
q2h	each (every) two hours *(quaque secunda hora)*
q.i.d.	four times a day *(quater in die)*
q.n.	each (every) night *(quaque nox)*
q.n.s.	quantity not sufficient *(quantum non sufficit)*
q.s.	quantity sufficient *(quantum sufficit)*
qt	quart

R

R, r	respiration; right
RA	rheumatoid arthritis; right atrium
rad	radiation absorbed dose
RBC, rbc	red blood cell (count)
REM	rapid eye movement
RIA	radioimmunoassay (minute quantities are measured)

RLQ	right lower quadrant (of the abdomen)
R/O, r/o	rule out
ROM	range of motion
ROS	review of systems
RP	retrograde pyelography (urography)
RR	recovery room; respiration rate
RRR	regular rate and rhythm (of the heart)
RT	radiation therapy; recreational therapy; radiologic technologist
RUQ	right upper quadrant (of the abdomen)
RV	right ventricle (of the heart)
Rx	treatment; therapy; prescription (*recipe*, "take"; therapy; treatment)

S

s̄	without *(sine)*
S1, S2	first sacral vertebra, second sacral vertebra
S-A node	sinoatrial node (pacemaker of the heart)
SAD	seasonal affective disorder
SARS	severe acute respiratory syndrome
SBFT	small bowel follow-through (x-ray study of the small intestine with contrast)
sed rate	erythrocyte sedimentation rate (time it takes red blood cells to settle out of blood)
segs	segmented white blood cells (granulocytes)
SERM	selective estrogen receptor modulator (tamoxifen is an example)
s.gl.	without glasses
SGOT	see *AST*
SGPT	see *ALT*
SH	serum hepatitis; social history
sig.	"let it be labeled" (directions or medical instructions)
SIDS	sudden infant death syndrome
SIRS	systemic inflammatory response syndrome (severe bacteremia)
SLE	systemic lupus erythematosus
SMA-12	blood chemistry profile including 12 different studies or assays (*sequential multiple analysis*)
SOAP	subjective (symptoms perceived by the patient) data, objective (exam findings) data, assessment (evaluation of condition), plan (goals for treatment)
SOB	shortness of breath
S/P, s/p	status post (previous disease condition)
SPECT	single-photon emission computed tomography
sp. gr.	specific gravity
SSRI	selective serotonin reuptake inhibitor (antidepressant drug)
staph	staphylococci (bacteria)
STAT, stat	immediately *(statim)*
STD	sexually transmitted disease (older name for STI)
STI	sexually transmitted infection

strep	streptococci (bacteria)
sub-Q	subcutaneous (under the skin)
Sx	signs and symptoms
Sz	seizure

T

T	temperature; time
T1, T2	first thoracic vertebra, second thoracic vertebra
T$_3$	triiodothyronine (thyroid gland hormone)
T$_4$	thyroxine (thyroid gland hormone)
T&A	tonsillectomy and adenoidectomy
tab	tablet
TAB	therapeutic abortion
TAH-BSO	total abdominal hysterectomy–bilateral salpingo-oophorectomy
TB	tuberculosis
T cells	lymphocytes originating in the thymus gland
TEE	transesophageal echocardiography
TENS	transcutaneous electrical nerve stimulator
TFT	thyroid function test
THR	total hip replacement
TIA	transient ischemic attack
t.i.d., tid	three times a day *(tris in die)*
TLC	total lung capacity
TM	tympanic membrane
TMJ	temporomandibular joint
TNM	tumor-node-metastasis (staging system for cancer)
TPN	total parenteral nutrition (administration of IV solution to maintain nutrition)
TPR	temperature, pulse, respiration
TSH	thyroid-stimulating hormone (secreted by the pituitary gland)
TUR, TURP	transurethral resection of the prostate gland
TVH	total vaginal hysterectomy
Tx	treatment

U

UA, U/A	urinalysis
UE	upper extremity
UGI	upper gastrointestinal
umb	navel (umbilical cord region)
ung	ointment
U/O	urine output
URI	upper respiratory infection
U/S, u/s	ultrasound (imaging examination)
UTI	urinary tract infection
UV	ultraviolet

V

VA	visual acuity
VATS	video-assisted thoracoscopy
VC	vital capacity (of lungs)
VCUG	voiding cystourethrogram
VEGF	vascular endothelial growth factor
VF	visual field; ventricular fibrillation
VS, V/S	vital signs; versus
VSD	ventricular septal defect
VSS	vital signs stable
V tach, VT	ventricular tachycardia (abnormal heart rhythm)

W

WBC, wbc	white blood cell (count)
W/C	wheelchair
wd	wound
WDWN	well-developed and well-nourished
WNL	within normal limits
WT, wt	weight
w/u	workup

X

XRT	radiation therapy

Y

y, yr	year(s)
y/o	year(s) old

Acronyms*

An *acronym* is the name for an abbreviation that forms a pronounceable "word."

ACE (ace)	**a**ngiotensin-**c**onverting **e**nzyme
AIDS (aydz)	**a**cquired **i**mmune **d**eficiency **s**yndrome
Apgar (apgahr)	**a**ppearance, **p**ulse, **g**rimace, **a**ctivity, **r**espiration (letters spell out name of originator of scoring system, Virginia Apgar)
BUN (bun)	**b**lood **u**rea **n**itrogen
CABG (cabbage)	**c**oronary **a**rtery **b**ypass **g**raft (grafting)
CAT (cat)	**c**omputerized **a**xial **t**omography (older name for CT)
CPAP (seepap)	**c**ontinuous **p**ositive **a**irway **p**ressure
ELISA (eliza)	**e**nzyme-**l**inked **i**mmuno**s**orbent **a**ssay

---

*Modified from Chabner D-E: *The Language of Medicine,* ed 9, Philadelphia, 2011, Elsevier.

GERD (gird)	gastroesophageal reflux disease
HAART (heart)	highly active antiretroviral therapy
HIPAA (hippah)	Health Insurance Portability and Accountability Act of 1996
LASER (layzer)	light amplification by stimulated emission of radiation
LASIK (laysick)	laser in situ keratomileusis
LEEP (leap)	loop electrocautery excision procedure
MAC (mack)	monitored anesthesia care
MICU (mickyou)	medical intensive care unit
MIS (miss)	minimally invasive surgery
MODS (modz)	multiorgan dysfunction syndrome
MUGA (myougah)	multiple-gated acquisition (scan)
NICU (nickyou)	neonatal intensive care unit
NSAID (ensayd)	nonsteroidal anti-inflammatory drug
PACS (packs)	picture archival communications system
PALS (pals)	pediatric advanced life support
PEEP (peep)	positive end-expiratory pressure
PEG (peg)	percutaneous endoscopic gastrostomy
PERRLA (perlah)	pupils equal, round, reactive to light and accommodation
PET (pet)	positron emission tomography
PICU (pickyou)	pediatric intensive care unit
PIP (pip)	proximal interphalangeal (joint)
pixel (picksul)	picture element
PUVA (poovah)	psoralen ultraviolet A
REM (rem)	rapid eye movement
SAD (sad)	seasonal affective disorder
SARS (sarz)	severe acute respiratory syndrome
SERM (serm)	selective estrogen receptor modulator
SICU (sickyou)	surgical intensive care unit
SIDS (sidz)	sudden infant death syndrome
SIRS (sirz)	systemic inflammatory response syndrome
SMAC (smack)	sequential multiple analyzer computer (for blood testing)
SOAP (soap)	subjective, objective, assessment, plan (formatted approach to nursing care)
SPECT (spekt)	single-photon emission computed tomography
SPORE (spore)	specialized program of research excellence
TENS (tenz)	transcutaneous electrical nerve stimulation
TRUS (truss)	transrectal ultrasound
TURP (turp)	transurethral resection of the prostate
VATS (vatz)	video-assisted thoracoscopy
voxel (vocksul)	volume element (of CT scan)

Symbols*

Symbol	Meaning
=	equals
≠	does not equal
+	positive
−	negative
↑	above, increase
↓	below, decrease
♀	female
♂	male
→	to (in the direction of)
>	is greater than
<	is less than
1°	first-degree (burn, heart block); primary
2°	second-degree (burn, heart block); secondary
℥	dram
℥	ounce
%	percent
°	degree; hour
:	ratio ("is to")
±	plus or minus (either positive or negative)
′	foot
″	inch
∴	therefore
@	at, each
c̄	with (cum)
s̄	without (sine)
#	pound; number
≈	approximately, about
Δ	change, change in
p	short arm of a chromosome
q	long arm of a chromosome

*Modified from Chabner D-E: *The Language of Medicine,* ed 9, Philadelphia, 2011, Elsevier.

Eponyms

Achilles tendon
(Achilles, Greek mythologic hero)

This tendon connects the calf muscles to the heel. It lies at the only part of Achilles' body that was still vulnerable after his mother dipped him as an infant into the river Styx, when she held him by the heel.

Alzheimer disease
(Alois Alzheimer, German neurologist, 1864-1915)

Progressive mental deterioration marked by confusion, memory failure, and disorientation.

Apgar score
(Virginia Apgar, American anesthesiologist, 1909-1974)

Evaluation of an infant's physical condition, usually performed 1 minute and then 5 minutes after birth. Highest score is 10. An Apgar rating of 9/10 is a score of 9 at 1 minute and 10 at 5 minutes.

Asperger syndrome
(Hans Asperger, Austrian psychiatrist, 1906-1980)

A developmental disorder characterized by impairment of social interactions (resembling autism) but lacking in delays in language development and mental functioning.

Bell palsy
(Charles Bell, Scottish surgeon, 1774-1842)

Unilateral (one-sided) paralysis of the facial nerve.

Barlow syndrome
(John Barlow, South African cardiologist, born 1924)

Mitral valve prolapse.

Barrett esophagus
(Norman Barrett, Australian thoracic surgeon, 1903-1979)

Abnormal changes in the lining of the esophagus, resulting from acid reflux from the stomach.

Burkitt lymphoma
(Denis Burkitt, English surgeon in Africa, 1911-1993)

Malignant tumor of lymph nodes; chiefly seen in central Africa. The Epstein-Barr virus is associated with this lymphoma.

Cheyne-Stokes respiration
(John Cheyne, Scottish physician, 1777-1836; William Stokes, Irish physician, 1804-1878)

Abnormal pattern of breathing with alternating periods of stoppage of breathing and deep, rapid breathing.

Colles fracture
(Abraham Colles, Irish surgeon, 1773-1843)

A break (fracture) of the radius (bone near the wrist).

Crohn disease
(Burrill B. Crohn, American physician, 1884-1983)

Chronic inflammatory bowel disease of unknown origin; usually affecting the ileum (last part of the small intestine), colon, or any part of the gastrointestinal tract.

Cushing syndrome
(Harvey W. Cushing, American surgeon, 1869-1939)

A disorder resulting from chronic, excessive production of cortisol from the adrenal cortex. It can also result from administration of glucocorticoids (cortisone) in large doses for long periods of time.

Duchenne muscular dystrophy
(Guillaume Benjamin Amand Duchenne, French neurologist, 1806-1875)

Abnormal, inherited condition that infants are born with; marked by progressive hardening of muscles in the leg and hips (pelvis).

Epstein-Barr virus
(Michael A. Epstein, English pathologist, born 1921; Yvonne M. Barr, English virologist, born 1932)

The herpesvirus that causes infectious mononucleosis and is associated with malignant conditions such as nose and throat cancer, Burkitt lymphoma, and Hodgkin disease.

eustachian tube
(Bartolomeo Eustachio, Italian anatomist, 1524-1574)

A tube that joins the throat and the middle ear cavity.

Ewing sarcoma
(James Ewing, American pathologist, 1866-1943)

Malignant tumor that develops from bone marrow, usually in long bones or the hip (pelvis).

fallopian tube
(Gabriele Falloppio, Italian anatomist, 1523-1562)

One of a pair of tubes or ducts leading from the ovary to the upper portion of the uterus.

Foley catheter
(Frederic Foley, American physician, 1891-1966)

Rubber tube that is placed in the urethra to provide drainage of urine.

Giardia
(Alfred Giardia, French biologist, 1846-1908)

One-celled organism (protozoan) that causes gastrointestinal infection with diarrhea, abdominal cramps, and weight loss. Cause of infection usually is fecally contaminated water.

Hodgkin disease
(Thomas Hodgkin, English physician, 1798-1866)

Malignant tumor of the lymph nodes.

Horner syndrome
(Johann Friedrich Horner, Swiss ophthalmologist, 1831-1886)

Partial ptosis (prolapse or drooping) of the upper eyelid, along with other signs of damage to nerves controlling the eye muscles and face.

Huntington disease
(George S. Huntington, American physician, 1851-1916)

Rare, hereditary condition marked by chronic, progressively worsening dance-like movements (chorea) and mental deterioration, resulting in dementia.

Kaposi sarcoma
(Moricz Kaposi, Austrian dermatologist, 1837-1902)

Malignant neoplasm of cells that line blood and lymph vessels. Soft brownish or purple papules appear on the skin. The tumor can metastasize to lymph nodes and internal organs. It often is associated with AIDS.

Marfan syndrome
(Bernard-Jean A. Marfan, French pediatrician, 1858-1942)

Hereditary condition that affects bones, muscles, the cardiovascular system (leading to aneurysms) and eyes (lens dislocation). Affected people have long, "spidery" extremities, underdeveloped muscles, and easily movable joints.

Meniere disease
(Prosper Meniere, French physician, 1799-1862)

Chronic disease of the inner ear with recurrent episodes of dizziness (vertigo), hearing loss, and ringing in the ears (tinnitus).

Neisseria gonorrhoeae
(Albert L. S. Neisser, Polish dermatologist, 1855-1916)

A type of bacterium that causes gonorrhea (sexually transmitted infection).

Paget disease
(James Paget, English surgeon, 1814-1899)

Disease of bone, often affecting middle-aged or elderly people; marked by bone destruction and poor bone repair.

Pap test
(George Papanicolaou, Greek physician in the United States, 1883-1962)

Method of examining stained cells obtained from the cervix and vagina. It is a common way to detect cervical cancer.

Parkinson disease
(James Parkinson, English physician, 1755-1824)

Slowly progressive degenerative neurological disorder marked by tremors, mask-like facial appearance, shuffling gait (manner of walking), and muscle rigidity and weakness.

Raynaud phenomenon
(Maurice Raynaud, French physician, 1834-1881)

Intermittent attacks of loss of blood flow (ischemia) in the extremities of the body (fingers, toes, ears, and nose). Episodes most often are caused by exposure to cold.

Reye syndrome
(R. Douglas Reye, Austrian pathologist, 1912-1978)

Acute brain disease (encephalopathy) and disease of internal organs following an acute viral infection.

Rinne test
(Heinrich A. Rinne, German otologist, 1819-1868)

Hearing test using a vibrating tuning fork placed against a bone behind the patient's ear (mastoid bone).

Rorschach test
(Herman Rorschach, Swiss psychiatrist, 1884-1922)

Personality test based on a patient's interpretation of 10 inkblots.

Salmonella
(Daniel E. Salmon, American pathologist, 1850-1914)

A type of bacterium (rod-shaped) that causes typhoid fever and types of gastroenteritis (inflammation of the stomach and intestines).

Shigella
(Kiyoshi Shiga, Japanese bacteriologist, 1870-1957)

A type of bacterium that causes severe infectious gastroenteritis (inflammation of stomach and intestines) and dysentery (diarrhea, abdominal pain, and fever).

Sjögren syndrome
(Heinrik S.C. Sjögren, Swedish ophthalmologist, 1899-1986)

Abnormal dryness of the mouth, eyes, and mucous membranes, caused by deficient fluid production. It is a disorder of the immune system.

Snellen test
(Herman Snellen, Dutch ophthalmologist, 1834-1908)

Test of visual clarity (acuity) using a special chart. Letters, numbers, or symbols are arranged on the chart in decreasing size from top to bottom.

Tay-Sachs disease
(Warren Tay, English ophthalmologist, 1843-1927; Bernard Sachs, American neurologist, 1858-1944)

Inherited disorder of nerve degeneration caused by deficiency of an enzyme. Most affected children die between the ages of 2 and 4 years.

Tourette syndrome
(George Gilles de la Tourette, French neurologist, 1857-1927)

Condition marked by abnormal facial grimaces, inappropriate speech, involuntary movements (tics) of eyes, arms, and shoulders.

von Willebrand disease
(Erick A. von Willebrand, Finnish physician, 1870-1949)

Inherited blood disorder marked by abnormally slow blood clotting; caused by deficiency in a blood clotting factor (factor VIII).

Weber tuning fork test
(Hermann D. Weber, English physician, 1823-1918)

Test of hearing by placing the stem of vibrating tuning fork in the center of the person's forehead.

Whipple procedure
(Allen O. Whipple, American surgeon, 1881-1963)

A surgical procedure to remove a portion of the pancreas and the stomach and the entire first part of the small intestine (duodenum). Used in the treatment of pancreatic cancer and other conditions.

Wilms tumor
(Max Wilms, German surgeon, 1867-1918)

Malignant tumor of the kidney occurring in young children.

Allied Health Careers

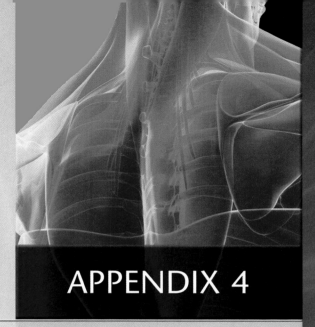

Title/Description	Education Requirements	Certification or Licensure Requirements	National Association or Additional Information
Audiologist Works with people who have hearing problems by using testing devices to measure hearing loss.	Clinical doctoral degree—Doctor of Audiology (AuD) graduate degree including 9 to 12 months of clinical experience.	In addition to complying with state license requirements (which may include requirement for teaching certification for a particular practice setting), ASHA offers Certification of Clinical Competency in Audiology (CCC-A).	American Speech-Language-Hearing Association (ASHA) 1080 Rockville Pike Rockville, MD 20852 800-498-2071 American Academy of Audiology (AAA) 11730 Plaza America Dr., Suite 300 Reston, VA 20190 800-AAA-2336
Blood bank technologist Collects, types, and prepares blood and its components for transfusions and laboratory tests.	Baccalaureate degree in clinical laboratory science or other physical science degree, plus a 12-month program in blood bank technology. Some programs also offer master's degrees.	Certification through Board of Registry of the American Society of Clinical Pathologists (ASCP) (www.ascp.org).	American Association of Blood Banks (AABB) 8101 Glenbrook Road Bethesda, MD 20814 301-215-6482
Chiropractor Treats health problems associated with the muscular, nervous, and skeletal systems, especially the spine.	College degree plus 4 years of resident instruction in a college of chiropractic.	Must pass the National State Board Exam.	American Chiropractic Association (ACA) Public Information Department 1702 Clarenden Blvd. Arlington, VA 22209 703-276-8880
Clinical laboratory technologist (CLT) (also see *Medical laboratory technologist*) (CLT, CLS, MLT, MLS) Performs tests to examine and analyze body fluids, tissues and cells.	2-year associate's degree or 12-month certificate program.	Certification available through the following: Board of Registry of the American Society for Clinical Pathology, American Medical Technologists Association, the National Credentialing Agency for Laboratory Personnel, and Board of Registry of the American Association of Bioanalysts.	American Medical Technologists Association (AMTA) 710 Higgins Road Park Ridge, IL 60068 847-823-5169

Title/Description	Education Requirements	Certification or Licensure Requirements	National Association or Additional Information
Dental assistant Assists a dentist with dental procedures.	Typically, 9- to 11-month program at a community college, vocational school, or career school. It is also possible to work as a dental assistant without attending a program and learn on the job.	In most states, certification is optional. Person is eligible to take exam if a graduate of an accredited dental assisting program or has 2 years of work experience. Exam for Certified Dental Assistant (CDA) is administered by the American Dental Assistants Association.	American Dental Assistants Association (ADAA) 35 E. Wacker Dr., Suite 1730 Chicago, IL 60601 312-541-1550
Dental hygienist Provides preventive dental care and teaches the practice of good oral hygiene.	2-year associate's degree or 4-year baccalaureate degree.	State requirements vary. In most states, the person must graduate from an accredited dental hygiene program, pass the state-authorized licensure exam, and pass the comprehensive written exam. On passing the exam, the dental hygienist becomes a Registered Dental Hygienist (RDH).	American Dental Hygienists Association (ADHA) 444 N. Michigan Ave., Suite 3400 Chicago, IL 60611 312-440-8900
Dental laboratory technician Prepares materials (crowns, bridges) for use by a dentist.	A 2-year program at a community, vocational, or technical college, either an associate's degree or certificate. The person also can work as a dental laboratory technician with on-the-job training.	In most states, certification to become a Certified Dental Technician (CDT) is optional.	National Board of Certification for Dental Laboratory Technicians (NBCDLT) 1530 Metropolitan Blvd. Tallahassee, FL 32308 850-224-0711
Diagnostic medical sonographer Performs diagnostic ultrasound procedures.	From 1 to 4 years for certificate, associate's degree, or baccalaureate degree.	Optional certification exam through American Registry of Diagnostic Medical Sonographers, with the designation Registered Diagnostic Medical Sonographer (RDMS).	Society of Diagnostic Medical Sonographers (SDMS) 2745 Dallas Pkwy., Suite 350 Plano, TX 75093 214-473-8057

Title/Description	Education Requirements	Certification or Licensure Requirements	National Association or Additional Information
Dietitian/ nutritionist Plans nutrition programs and supervises the preparation and serving of meals.	2-year component within a baccalaureate or master's degree program, plus internship of 6 months to 2 years.	National certification exam to become a Certified Registered Dietitian (CRD) through the Commission on Dietetic Registration.	American Dietetic Association (ADA) 120 S. Riverside Plaza, Suite 2000 Chicago, IL 60606 312-899-0400, ext 5500
ECG technician (cardiovascular technician) Operates an electro-cardiograph to record ECGs and for Holter monitoring and stress tests.	Training often done on the job in 8- to 16-week programs. Longer programs are also available.	Optional	Alliance of Cardiovascular Professionals (ACP) P.O. Box 2007 Midlothian, VA 23113 804-632-0078
Emergency medical technician 1. First responder 2. Basic (EMT-B) 3. Intermediate (EMT-I) 4. Paramedic (EMT-P) Gives immediate care and transports sick or injured to medical facilities.	Four levels: *First responder*: 40 hours *EMT Basic*: 120 hours *EMT Intermediate*: 200 to 400 hours *EMT Paramedic*: 1000+ hours	Administered by the National Registry of Emergency Medical Technicians (NREMT) for each level from EMT-B, EMT-I, and EMT-Paramedic.	National Association of Emergency Medical Technicians (NAEMT) P.O. Box 1400 Clinton, MS 39060 800-34-NAEMT
Health information management professional 1. Health information technician (HIT) 2. Health information administrator (HIA) Designs, manages, and administers the use of health care data and information.	Two levels: *Health Information Technician (HIT):* 2-year associate's degree *Health Information Administrator (HIA):* 4-year baccalaureate degree	On completion of the education program, a test is required through the national association (AHIMA) to become a Registered Health Information Technician (RHIT) or Registered Health Information Administrator (RHIA).	American Health Information Management Association (AHIMA) 233 N. Michigan Ave., Suite 2150 Chicago, IL 60601 312-233-1100

Title/Description	Education Requirements	Certification or Licensure Requirements	National Association or Additional Information
Home health aide Cares for elderly, disabled, and ill persons in their own homes, helping them live there instead of in an institution.	Often on-the-job training or technical/career college.	National Association for Home Care & Hospice offers optional certification.	National Association for Home Care & Hospice (NAHCH) (www.nahc.org) 202-547-7424
Licensed practical nurse (LPN) Cares for sick, injured, convalescing, and handicapped persons, under the direct supervision of physicians and registered nurses; provides basic bedside care.	Approximately 1-year program, with 36 to 28 semester hours.	Must pass the National Council Licensure Examination for Practical Nurses (NCLEX-PN).	National Federation for Licensed Practical Nurses (NFLPN) 1418 Aversboro Road Garner, NC 27529 919-779-0046
Medical assistant Helps physicians examine and treat patients and performs tasks to keep offices running smoothly.	Associate's degree, certificate and diploma programs available. Medical assistants can focus on either administrative or clinical duties or both.	Optional certifications available. Exam to become a Certified Medical Assistant (CMA) through the AAMA or a Registered Medical Assistant (RMA) through American Medical Technologists Association (see next entry).	American Association of Medical Assistants (AAMA) 20 N. Wacker Dr., Suite 1575 Chicago, IL 60606 800-228-2262
Medical laboratory technologist (also see *Clinical laboratory technologist [CLT]*) Performs routine tests and laboratory procedures.	A 2-year associate's degree or a 12-month certificate program.	Certification available through the following: Board of Registry of the American Society for Clinical Pathology, the American Medical Technologists Association, the National Credentialing Agency for Laboratory Personnel, and the Board of Registry of the American Association of Bioanalysts.	American Medical Technologists Association (AMTA) 710 Higgins Road Park Ridge, IL 60068 847-823-5169 American Society of Clinical Laboratory Science (ASCLS) 6701 Democracy Blvd., Suite 300 Bethesda, MD 20817 301-657-2768

Title/Description	Education Requirements	Certification or Licensure Requirements	National Association or Additional Information
Nuclear medicine technologist Performs radioactive tests and procedures under the supervision of a nuclear medicine physician, who interprets the results.	Professional portion of the program is 1-2 years within an associate's or baccalaureate degree program.	On completion of an accredited program, certification exam is available through the Nuclear Medicine Technology Certification Board.	Society of Nuclear Medicine— Technologist Section (SNMTS) 1850 Samuel Morse Dr. Reston, VA 22090 703-708-9000 American Society of Radiologic Technologists (ASRT) 1500 Central Ave. SE Albuquerque, NM 87123
Nurse anesthetist Aids in the delivery of anesthesia during surgery.	RN with baccalaureate degree plus 24-month anesthesiology training course (leading to a master's degree).	Required exam by the Council on Certification for Nurse Anesthetists, to become a Certified Registered Nurse Anesthetist (CRNA).	Association of Nurse Anesthetists (ANA) 222 S. Prospect Ave. Park Ridge, IL 60068 847-692-7050 Additional information: National League of Nursing
Nursing aide (nursing assistant, orderly, hospital attendant) Helps care for physically or mentally ill, injured, or disabled patients confined to nursing, hospital, or residential care facilities; also known as nursing assistants or hospital attendants.	Often on-the-job training or technical/career college.	Optional certification is available through state nursing registries for Certified Nursing Assistant (CNA).	National Association of Health Care Assistants (NAHCA) 1201 L St. Washington, DC 20005 202-454-1288

Title/Description	Education Requirements	Certification or Licensure Requirements	National Association or Additional Information
Occupational therapist (OT) Helps people with mentally, physically, developmentally, or emotionally disabling conditions to develop, recover, or maintain daily living and working skills.	Two levels: *Baccalaureate degree*: 4- to 5-year program *Master's degree*: additional 2.5 years	National certification exam through National Board for Certification of Occupational Therapy (NBCOT). All states also regulate occupational therapists. Upon passing the exam, the occupational therapist becomes an Occupational Therapist Registered (OTR).	American Occupational Therapy Association (AOTA) 4720 Montgomery Lane P.O. Box 31220 Bethesda, MD 20824 301-652-2682
Occupational therapy assistant (OTA) Under the direction of an occupational therapist, the OTA works with patients to restore or enhance activities of daily living.	2-year associate's degree or 1-year certificate program.	National certification exam for OTA administered by: National Board for Certification of Occupational Therapy (NBCOT). Many states also regulate occupational therapy assistants.	American Occupational Therapy Association (AOTA) 4720 Montgomery Lane P.O. Box 31220 Bethesda, MD 20824 301-652-2682
Ophthalmic professional 1. Ophthalmic assistant 2. Ophthalmic technician/ technologist Helps ophthalmologists provide medical eye care.	Two levels: *Assistant*: less than 1 year *Technician/ technologist*: 1-2 years	After 1 year on the job, the person may test to become a Certified Ophthalmic Medical Assistant (COMA) through the Joint Commission on Allied Health Professionals in Ophthalmology (JCAHPO).	Association of Technical Personnel in Ophthalmology (ATPO) 2025 Woodland Dr. St. Paul, MN 55125 651-731-7233
Pharmacy technician Under the direction of licensed pharmacists, dispenses, distributes, and administers medications prescribed.	Usually 15 weeks (minimum 600 hours) of training required; can be on the job or through a career, technical, or community college.	Optional through the AAPT and Pharmacy Technician Certification Board, to become a Certified Pharmacy Technologist (CPhT).	American Association of Pharmacy Technologists (AAPT) P.O. Box 1447 Greensboro, NC 27402 877-368-4771

Title/Description	Education Requirements	Certification or Licensure Requirements	National Association or Additional Information
Phlebotomist Draws and tests blood under the supervision of a medical technologist or laboratory manager.	Minimum 100 hours of clinical instruction.	Optional certification available through the following: American Medical Technologists Association, National Credentialing Agency for Laboratory Personnel, and Board of Registry of the American Association of Bioanalysts.	American Medical Technologists Association (AMTA) 710 Higgins Road Park Ridge, IL 60068 847-823-5169 American Society of Phlebotomy Technicians (ASPT) P.O. Box 1831 Hickory, NC 28603 828-294-0078 National Phlebotomy Association (NPA) 1901 Brightseat Road Landover, MD 20785 301-386-4200
Physical therapist (PT) Improves mobility, relieves pain, and prevents or limits permanent physical disabilities of patients suffering from injuries or disease.	Most programs are doctoral degree programs granting a doctorate in physical therapy (DPT); a few master's degree programs are still offered.	On completion of accredited program, national exam is required. Other requirements vary by state.	American Physical Therapy Association (APTA) 111 North Fairfax St. Alexandria, VA 22314 703-684-2782
Physical therapy assistant (PTA) Under the direction of a physical therapist, works with patients to improve mobility.	Most programs are associate's degree programs, 1 year of which is for technical courses and clinical experience.	Most states require physical therapy assistants to be licensed, registered, or certified.	American Physical Therapy Association (APTA) 111 North Fairfax St. Alexandria, VA 22314 703-684-2782

Title/Description	Education Requirements	Certification or Licensure Requirements	National Association or Additional Information
Physician assistant (PA) Examines, diagnoses, and treats patients under the direct supervision of a physician.	Varies, but commonly a 25- to 27-month program in addition to at least 2 years of undergraduate study.	All states require passage of national exam through National Commission on Certification of Physician Assistants (NCCPA). To practice, PAs must also meet any additional state criteria and have a sponsoring physician.	American Association of Physician Assistants (AAPA) 950 N. Washington St. Alexandria, VA 22314 703-836-2272 National Commission on Certification of Physician Assistants (NCCPA) 12000 Findley Road, Suite 200 Duluth, GA 30097 678-417-8100
Radiation therapist Prepares cancer patients for treatment and examinations, and administers medications (this career is a specialty within imaging technology—see next entry).	After becoming a radiographer, 1 to 2 years of training.	Certification through American Registry of Radiologic Technologists (ARRT).	American Society of Radiologic Technologists (ASRT) 1500 Central Ave. SE Albuquerque, NM 87123 505-298-4500 American Registry of Radiologic Technologists (ARRT) 1255 Northland Dr. Mendota Heights, MN 55120 651-687-0048
Radiographer/ radiologic technologist Produces x-ray images of parts of the body for use in diagnosing medical problems.	A 2- to 4-year training program resulting in degree or certificate.	Certification through American Registry of Radiologic Technologists (ARRT).	American Society of Radiologic Technologists (ASRT) 1500 Central Ave. SE Albuquerque, NM 87123 505-298-4500 American Registry of Radiologic Technologists (ARRT) 1255 Northland Dr. Mendota Heights, MN 55120 651-687-0048

Title/Description	Education Requirements	Certification or Licensure Requirements	National Association or Additional Information
Registered nurse (RN) Cares for sick and injured people by assessing and recording symptoms, assisting physicians during treatments and examinations, and administering medications.	ADN—community college or technical school, 2 years Diploma—hospital-based, often 3 years BSN—baccalaureate degree program, 4 years	All registered nurses must pass the NCLEX-RN, administered by the National Council of Licensure Examinations for RN.	American Nursing Association (ANA) 600 Maryland Ave. SW, Suite 100 Washington, DC 20024 800-274-4ANA National League of Nursing (NLN) 61 Broadway, 33rd Floor New York, NY 10006 212-363-5555
Respiratory therapist Evaluates, treats, and cares for patients with breathing disorders.	*Entry level*: 2-year associate's degree program. *Advanced level*: 2- to 4-year program with baccalaureate or graduate degree.	Certification through National Board for Respiratory Care for Certified Respiratory Therapist (CRT).	American Association for Respiratory Care (AARC) 11030 Ables Lane Dallas, TX 75229 972-243-2272
Speech-language pathologist Assesses and treats persons with speech, language, voice, and fluency disorders.	2-year master's degree plus typically 9 to 12 months of clinical experience.	Most states require compliance with state licensure standards and/or a teacher certification. Exam administered by ASHA for Certification of Clinical Competency in Speech-Language Pathology (CCC-SLP).	American Speech-Language-Hearing Association (ASHA) 1080 Rockville Pike Rockville, MD 20852 800-498-2071
Surgical technologist (CST) Assists in operations under the supervision of surgeons or registered nurses.	12- to 24-month associate's degree or certificate program.	Optional certification exam through National Board for Surgical Technologists and Surgical Assistants for Certified Surgical Technician (CST).	Association of Surgical Technologists (AST) 6 West Dry Creek Circle Littleton, CO 80120 800-637-7433

Mini-Dictionary: Glossary of Medical Terms

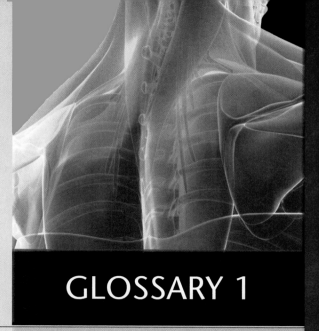

GLOSSARY 1

Pronunciation of each term is given with its meaning. The syllable that gets the accent is in CAPITAL LETTERS. Terms in SMALL CAPITAL LETTERS are defined elsewhere in this glossary.

A

Abdomen (AB-do-men):   Space below the chest that contains organs such as the stomach, liver, intestines, and gallbladder. The abdomen lies between the diaphragm and the pelvis.

Abdominal (ab-DOM-ih-nal):   Pertaining to the abdomen.

Abdominal cavity (ab-DOM-ih-nal KAV-ih-te):   See ABDOMEN.

Ablation (ab-LA-shun):   Removal of abnormal tissue by surgical or mechanical means

Abnormal (ab-NOR-mal):   Pertaining to being away (AB-) from the norm; irregular.

Acquired immunodeficiency syndrome (ah-KWIRD im-u-no-deh-FISH-en-se SIN-drom) or AIDS: Suppression or deficiency of the immune response caused by exposure to the HUMAN IMMUNODEFICIENCY VIRUS (HIV).

Acromegaly (ak-ro-MEG-ah-le):   Enlargement of extremities as a result of thickening of the bones and soft tissues; it is caused by excessive secretion of growth hormone from the pituitary gland (after completion of puberty).

Acute (ah-KUT):   Sharp, sudden, and intense for a short period of time.

Acute myocardial ischemia (ah-KUT mi-o-KAR-de-al is-KE-me-ah):   Sudden decrease in blood flow to heart muscle.

Adenectomy (ad-eh-NEK-to-me):   The removal of a gland.

Adenitis (ad-e-NI-tis):   Inflammation of a gland.

Adenocarcinoma (ah-deh-no-kar-sih-NO-mah):   Cancerous tumor derived from glandular cells.

Adenoidectomy (ah-deh-noyd-EK-to-me):   Removal of the adenoids.

Adenoids (AD-eh-noydz):   Enlarged lymphatic tissue in the upper part of the throat near the nasal passageways.

Adenoma (ah-deh-NO-mah):   Benign tumor of glandular cells.

Adenopathy (ah-deh-NOP-ah-the):   Disease of glands. Often this term refers to enlargement of lymph nodes (which are not true glands, but collections of lymphatic tissue).

Adnexa uteri (ad-NEKS-ah U-ter-i):   Accessory structures of the uterus (ovaries and fallopian tubes).

Adrenal cortex (ah-DRE-nal KOR-teks):   Outermost part of the adrenal gland. The adrenal cortex secretes steroid hormones such as GLUCOCORTICOIDS (cortisone).

Adrenal glands (ah-DRE-nal glanz):   Two endocrine glands, each above a kidney. The adrenal glands produce hormones such as adrenaline (epinephrine) and hydrocortisone (cortisol).

Adrenalectomy (ah-dre-nal-EK-to-me):   Removal (excision) of adrenal glands.

Adrenaline (ah-DREN-ah-lin):   Hormone secreted by the adrenal glands. It is released into the bloodstream in response to stress, such as from fear or physical injury. Also called EPINEPHRINE.

Adrenocorticotropic hormone (ah-dre-no-kor-tih-ko-TROP-ic HOR-mone):   Hormone secreted by the pituitary gland. It stimulates the adrenal gland (cortex or outer region) to secrete the hormone cortisone. Also called ACTH.

Adrenopathy (ah-dreh-NOP-a-the):   Disease of ADRENAL GLANDS.

AIDS: See ACQUIRED IMMUNODEFICIENCY SYNDROME.

Air sacs (ayr saks):   Thin-walled sacs within the lung. Inhaled oxygen passes into the blood from the sacs, and carbon dioxide passes out from the blood into the sacs to be exhaled.

Albumin (al-BU-min):   A large-molecule protein found in blood and tissues.

Albuminuria (al-bu-min-U-re-ah):   Albumin (protein) in the urine; it indicates a malfunction of the kidney.

Alkaline phosphatase (AL-kah-line PHOS-fah-tays):   An enzyme present in blood and body tissues, such as bone and liver. Elevated in diseases such as those of bone and liver. Also called alk phos.

Allergist (AL-er-jist):   Medical doctor specializing in identifying and treating abnormal sensitivity to substances such as pollen, dust, foods, and drugs.

Alopecia (ah-lo-PE-shah):   Loss of hair; baldness.

ALT: Alanine transferase, an enzyme normally found in blood and tissues, especially the liver. ALT is elevated in liver disease. (Formerly called SGPT.)

Alveolar (al-VE-o-lar):   Pertaining to air sacs (alveoli) within the lungs.

Alveolus (al-ve-O-lus):   An air sac within the lung (*plural:*   alveoli).

Alzheimer disease (ALTZ-hi-mer di-ZEEZ):   Deterioration of mental capacity (irreversible dementia) marked by intellectual deterioration, disorganization of personality, and difficulties in carrying out tasks of daily living.

Amenorrhea (a-men-o-RE-ah):   Absence of menstrual periods.

Amniocentesis (am-ne-o-sen-TE-sis):   Surgical puncture to remove fluid from the amnion (sac surrounding the developing fetus).

Anal (A-nal):   Pertaining to the anus (opening of the rectum to the outside of the body).

Analgesic (an-al-JE-zik):   Medication that reduces or eliminates pain.

Analysis (ah-NAL-ih-sis):   Separating a substance into its component parts.

Anastomosis (ah-nah-sto-MO-sis):   New surgical connection between two previously unconnected bowel parts, vessels, or ducts.

Androgen (AN-dro-jen):   Hormone that controls the development of masculine characteristics. An example is TESTOSTERONE.

Anemia (ah-NE-me-ah):   Deficiency of hemoglobin and/or in number of red blood cells, which results in reduced oxygen to body cells. Literally, *anemia* means lacking (AN-) in blood (-EMIA).

Anemic (ah-NE-mik):   Pertaining to ANEMIA.

Anesthesiologist (an-es-the-ze-OL-o-jist):   Medical doctor specializing in administering agents capable of bringing about loss of sensation and consciousness.

Anesthesiology (an-es-the-ze-OL-o-je):   Study of how to administer agents capable of bringing about loss of sensation and consciousness.

Aneurysm (AN-u-rizm):   Localized widening of the wall of an artery, of a vein, or of the heart. From the Greek *aneurysma,* meaning "widening."

Angina (an-JI-nah):   Sharp pain in the chest resulting from a decrease in blood supply to heart muscle. Also called angina pectoris (PECT/O means chest).

Angiography (an-je-OG-rah-fe):   X-ray recording of blood vessels after contrast is injected.

Angioplasty (AN-je-o-plas-te):   Surgical repair of a blood vessel. A tube (catheter) is placed in a clogged artery and a balloon at the end of the tube is inflated to flatten the clogged material against the wall of the artery. This enlarges the opening of the artery so that more blood can pass through. Also called balloon angioplasty.

Angiotensin (an-je-o-TEN-sin):   Hormone that is a powerful vasoconstrictor and raises blood pressure.

Ankylosing spondylitis (ang-kih-LO-sing spon-dih-LI-tis):   Chronic inflammation of the vertebrae (backbones) with stiffening of spinal joints so that movement becomes increasingly painful.

Ankylosis (ang-kih-LO-sis):   Stiffening and immobility of a joint caused by injury, disease, or a surgical procedure.

Anomaly (ah-NOM-ah-le):   Irregularity; a deviation from the normal. A congenital anomaly (irregularity) is present at birth.

Antenatal (an-teh-NA-tal):   Before birth.

Antepartum (an-teh-PAR-tum):   Before birth.

Anterior (an-TE-re-or):   Located in the front (of the body or of a structure).

Antiandrogen (an-tih-AN-dro-jen):   Substance that inhibits the effects of androgens (male hormones).

Antiarrhythmic (an-te-ah-RITH-mik):   Pertaining to a drug that works against or prevents abnormal heartbeats (arrhythmias).

Antibiotic (an-tih-bi-OT-ik):   A chemical substance produced by various microorganisms or fungi (immature plants) that inhibits or destroys bacteria or other small organisms. Examples of antibiotics are penicillin and streptomycin. They are used in the treatment of infectious diseases.

Antibody (AN-tih-bod-e):   A substance that works against (ANTI-) germs ("bodies" of infection). Antibodies are produced by white blood cells when germs (antigens) enter the bloodstream.

Anticoagulant (an-tih-ko-AG-u-lant):   Drug that prevents clotting (coagulation). Anticoagulants are given when there is danger of clot formation in blood vessels, as may happen after a heart attack.

Anticonvulsant (an-tih-kon-VULS-ent):   Drug that prevents or relieves convulsions (involuntary muscular contractions).

Antidepressant (an-tih-de-PRES-ent):   Drug used to prevent or treat depression.

Antidiabetic (an-tih-di-ah-BET-ik):   Drug that prevents or relieves symptoms of diabetes.

Antiestrogen (an-tih-ES-tro-jen):   Substance that inhibits the effects of estrogens (female hormones).

Antifungal (an-tih-FUNG-al):   Drug that destroys or inhibits the growth of fungi (organisms such as yeasts, molds, and mushrooms).

Antigen (AN-tih-jen):   Foreign protein (such as on a bacterium or virus) that stimulates white blood cells to make antibodies. Antigens are then destroyed by the antibodies.

Antihistamine (an-tih-HIS-tah-meen):   Drug used to counteract the effects of histamine production in allergic reactions and colds.

Antihypertensive (an-te-hi-per-TEN-siv):   Drug that reduces high blood pressure.

Antitubercular (an-tih-too-BER-ku-lar):   Agent or drug used to treat tuberculosis.

Antiviral (an-tih-VI-ral):   Agent that inhibits and prevents the growth and reproduction of viruses.

Anuria (an-U-re-ah):   Lack of urine formation by the kidney.

Anus (A-nus):   Opening of the rectum to the surface of the body; solid wastes (feces) leave the body through the anus.

Aorta (a-OR-tah):   Largest artery, which leads from the lower left chamber of the heart to arteries all over the body.

Aortic stenosis (a-OR-tik steh-NO-sis):   Narrowing of the aorta.

Apex (A-peks):   Pointed end of an organ (*plural:* apices [A-pih-seez]).

Aphakia (ah-FA-ke-ah):   Absence of the lens of the eye.

Aphasia (ah-FA-ze-ah):   Absence or impairment of communication through speech.

Apnea (AP-ne-ah):   Not (A-) able to breathe (-PNEA); temporary stoppage of breathing. In *sleep apnea,* during sleep, a person is momentarily unable to contract respiratory muscles and maintain air flow through the nose and mouth.

Appendectomy (ap-en-DEK-to-me):   Removal of the appendix.

Appendicitis (ap-en-dih-SI-tis):   Inflammation of the appendix.

Appendix (ah-PEN-dikz):   Small sac that hangs from the juncture of the small and large intestines in the right lower quadrant of the abdomen. Its function is unknown.

Arachnoid membrane (ah-RAK-noyd MEM-brayn): The middle membrane of the MENINGES (coverings around the brain and spinal cord).

Areola (ah-RE-o-lah): Dark, pigmented area around the nipple of the breast.

Arrhythmia (a-RITH-me-ah): Abnormal heart rhythm.

Arteriography (ar-teer-e-OG-rah-fe): Process of recording (x-ray) of arteries after injecting contrast material.

Arteriole (ar-TEER-e-ole): Small artery.

Arteriolitis (ar-teer-e-o-LI-tis): Inflammation of small arteries (arterioles).

Arteriosclerosis (ar-teer-e-o-skleh-RO-sis): Hardening of arteries. The most common form is *atherosclerosis,* which is hardening of arteries caused by collection of fatty, cholesterol-like deposits (plaque) in arteries.

Arteriovenous fistula (ar-teer-e-o-VE-nus FIST-u-lah): An abnormal communication between an artery and a vein. It can also be created surgically to provide access for hemodialysis.

Artery (AR-ter-e): Largest blood vessel. Arteries carry blood away from the heart.

Arthralgia (ar-THRAL-je-ah): Pain in a joint.

Arthritis (ar-THRI-tis): Inflammation of a joint.

Arthrocentesis (ar-thro-sen-TE-sis): Surgical puncture to remove fluid from a joint.

Arthrogram (AR-thro-gram): X-ray record of a joint.

Arthropathy (ar-THROP-ah-the): Disease of joints.

Arthroplasty (AR-thro-plas-te): Surgical repair of a joint, especially to restore mobility in osteoarthritis or rheumatoid arthritis.

Arthroscope (AR-thro-skope): Instrument used to examine the inside of a joint.

Arthroscopy (ar-THROS-ko-pe): Process of visual examination of a joint.

Arthrosis (ar-THRO-sis): Abnormal condition of a joint.

Ascites (ah-SI-teez): Abnormal collection of fluid in the abdomen.

Asphyxia (as-FIK-se-ah): Deficiency of oxygen in the blood and increase in carbon dioxide in blood and tissues. Major symptom is a complete absence of breathing.

AST: Aspartate transferase, an enzyme normally present in blood and tissues such as heart and liver. (Formerly called SGOT.)

Asthma (AZ-mah): Difficult breathing caused by a spasm of the bronchial tubes or a swelling of their mucous membrane lining.

Atelectasis (ah-teh-LEK-tah-sis): Collapsed lung (ATEL-, meaning incomplete; -ECTASIS, meaning widening or dilation).

Atherosclerosis (ah-theh-ro-skle-RO-sis): See ARTERIOSCLEROSIS.

Atrium (A-tre-um): Upper chamber of the heart (*plural:* atria).

Atrophy (AT-ro-fe): Decrease in size of cells within an organ.

Auditory canal (AW-dih-to-re kah-NAL): Passageway leading into the ear from the outside of the body.

Auditory nerve (AW-dih-to-re nurv): Nerve that carries messages from the inner ear to the brain, making hearing possible.

Aura (AW-rah): A strange sensation coming before more definite symptoms of illness. An aura often precedes a migraine headache, warning the patient that an attack is beginning.

Aural discharge (AW-rahl DIS-charj): Fluid or material from the ear.

Autopsy (AW-top-se): Examination of a dead body to determine the cause of death. Also called a POSTMORTEM exam or NECROPSY. Literally, it means "to see" (-OPSY) with "one's own" (AUT-) eyes.

Axial (AKS-e-al): Pertaining to an axis (an imaginary line through the center of a body or about which a structure revolves). Axial (transverse plane) views are seen in CT and MRI scans.

Axillary (AKS-ih-lar-e): Pertaining to the armpit or underarm.

B

Bactericidal (bak-tih-re-SI-dal):   Pertaining to an agent that destroys bacteria.

Bacteriostatic (bak-tih-re-o-STAT-ik):   Pertaining to an agent that inhibits bacterial growth.

Bacterium (bak-TIH-re-um):   Type of one-celled organism whose genetic material (DNA) is not organized within a nucleus (*plural:* bacteria).

Balanitis (bah-lah-NI-tis):   Inflammation of the penis.

Bariatric surgery (bah-re-AH-trik SUR-jer-e):   Surgery on part of the gastrointestinal tract for obesity. BARI/O means weight, and IATR/O means treatment.

Barium (BAH-re-um):   Substance used as a radiopaque (x-rays cannot pass through it) contrast medium for x-ray examination of the digestive tract.

Barium enema (BAH-re-um EN-eh-mah):   X-ray study of the lower digestive tract performed by instilling a solution of barium into the rectum, which highlights structures seen on the x-ray images.

Barium swallow (BAH-re-um SWAH-lo):   X-ray study of the upper digestive tract performed by having the patient swallow a solution of barium, which highlights structures seen on the x-ray images.

Benign (be-NIN):   Not cancerous; a tumor that does not spread and is limited in growth.

Benign prostatic hyperplasia (be-NIN pro-STAH-tik hi-per-PLA-ze-ah):   Nonmalignant enlargement of the prostate gland. Also called benign prostatic hypertrophy (hi-PER-tro-fe).

Benzodiazepine (ben-zo-di-AZ-eh-pin):   Drug used to relieve anxiety, relax muscles, and produce sedation.

Beta blocker (BA-tah BLOK-er):   Drug that is used for the treatment of high blood pressure (hypertension), chest pain (angina), and abnormal rhythms of the heart (arrhythmias).

Bilateral (bi-LAT-er-al):   Pertaining to two (both) sides.

Bile (bil):   A yellow or orange fluid produced by the liver. It breaks up large fat globules and helps in the digestion of fats.

Bile duct (bil dukt):   Tube that carries bile from the liver and gallbladder to the intestine.

Bilirubin (bil-ih-RU-bin):   A red blood cell pigment excreted with bile from the liver into the intestine.

Biology (bi-OL-o-je):   Study of life.

Biopsy (BI-op-se):   Removing living tissue for subsequent viewing under a microscope or other laboratory studies. In a *core (needle) biopsy*, a small sample of tissue is removed using a hollow needle. It is typically performed under imaging guidance such as ULTRASOUND or CT SCAN.

Bladder (BLAH-der):   See URINARY BLADDER.

Bone (bone):   Hard, rigid type of connective tissue that makes up most of the skeleton. It is composed of calcium salts.

Bone marrow (bone MAH-ro):   Soft, sponge-like material in the inner part of bones. Blood cells are made in the bone marrow.

Bradycardia (bra-de-KAR-de-ah):   Slow heartbeat.

Brain (brayn):   Organ in the head that controls the activities of the body.

Breast (brest):   One of two glandular organs in front of the chest. The breasts produce milk after childbirth.

Bronchial tube (BRONG-ke-al toob):   One of two tubes that carry air from the windpipe to the lungs. Also called a bronchus (*plural:* bronchi).

Bronchiole (BRONG-ke-ol):   Small bronchial tube.

Bronchiolitis (brong-ke-o-LI-tis):   Inflammation of bronchioles.

Bronchitis (brong-KI-tis):   Inflammation of bronchial tubes.

Bronchoscope (BRONG-ko-skope):   Instrument used to visually examine bronchial tubes.

Bronchoscopy (brong-KOS-ko-pe):   Visual examination of bronchial tubes by passing an endoscope through the trachea (windpipe) into the bronchi.

Bronchus (BRONG-kus):   See BRONCHIAL TUBE.

Bursa (BUR-sah):   Sac of fluid near a joint (*plural:* bursae [BUR-se]).

Bursitis (bur-SI-tis):   Inflammation of a bursa.

C

Calcaneus (kal-KA-ne-us):   Heel bone.

Calcification (cal-sih-fih-KA-shun):   Accumulation of calcium salts in tissues.

Calcium channel blocker (KAL-se-um CHAH-nel BLOK-er):   Drug that dilates arteries by inhibiting the flow of calcium into muscle cells that line arteries. It is used to treat hypertension (high blood pressure) and angina (chest pain caused by insufficient oxygen to heart muscle).

Calculus (KAL-ku-lus):   Stone (*plural:* calculi [KAL-ku-li]).

Callus (KAL-us):   Bony deposit formed between and around the broken ends of a fractured bone. Also, a painless thickening of skin cells in areas of external pressure or friction.

Capillary (KAP-ih-lar-e):   Smallest blood vessel (*plural:* capillaries).

Carbon dioxide (KAR-bon di-OK-side):   Odorless, colorless gas formed in tissues and eliminated by the lungs.

Carcinoma (kar-sih-NO-mah):   Cancerous tumor. Carcinomas form from epithelial cells, which line the internal organs and cover the outside of the body.

Cardiac (KAR-de-ak):   Pertaining to the heart.

Cardiac catheter ablation (KAR-de-ak KAH-theh-ter ab-LA-shun):   Procedure to correct an ARRHYTHMIA by advancing a flexible tube (catheter) through blood vessels into the heart. High-frequency electrical impulses then destroy the abnormal tissue that is causing the arrhythmia.

Cardiologist (kar-de-OL-o-jist):   Physician specializing in the study of the heart and heart disease.

Cardiology (kar-de-OL-o-je):   Study of the heart.

Cardiomegaly (kar-de-o-MEG-ah-le):   Enlargement of the heart.

Cardiomyopathy (kar-de-o-mi-OP-ah-the):   Disease of heart muscle.

Cardiovascular surgeon (kar-de-o-VAS-ku-lar SUR-jun):   Specialist in operating on the heart and blood vessels.

Cardioversion (KAR-de-o-ver-zhun):   Brief discharges of electricity passing across the chest to stop a cardiac ARRHYTHMIA. Also called DEFIBRILLATION.

Carpals (KAR-palz):   Wrist bones.

Carpal tunnel syndrome (KAR-pal TUN-el SIN-drom):   Group of symptoms resulting from compression of the median nerve in the wrist. Symptoms include tingling, pain, and burning sensations in the hand and wrist.

Cartilage (KAR-tih-laj):   Flexible, fibrous connective tissue, found as part of the nose, ears, voice box, and windpipe and chiefly attached to bones at joints.

Cataract (KAT-ah-rakt):   Clouding of the lens of the eye.

Cathartic (ka-THAR-tik):   Pertaining to a substance that causes the release of feces from the large intestine.

Catheter (KATH-eh-ter):   Flexible or rigid hollow tube used to drain fluids from the body or inject fluids into the body. Catheters are also used to help keep passageways open.

CAT scan (kat skan):   Computerized axial tomography. See CT SCAN.

Cauda equina (KAW-dah eh-KWI-nah):   Bundle of nerve fibers and nerve roots extending from the end of the spinal cord (L3) to the sacral and coccygeal nerves. *Cauda equina* is Latin for "horse's tail," which describes its appearance.

Caudal (KAW-dal):   Pertaining to the tail or the lower portion of the body.

Cell (sel):   Smallest unit or part of an organ.

Cellulitis (sel-u-LI-tis):   Inflammation of soft tissue under the skin; it is marked by swelling, redness, and pain and is caused by bacterial infection.

Cephalgia (seh-FAL-je-ah):   Headache. Shortened form of *cephalalgia*.

Cephalic (seh-FAL-ik):   Pertaining to the head. *Cephalic presentation* refers to a fetal position in which the head of the fetus appears at the uterine cervix as the infant is born.

Cephalosporin (sef-ah-lo-SPOR-in):   Antibiotic similar to penicillin and used to treat infections of the respiratory tract, ear, urinary tract, bones, and blood.

Cerebellar (ser-eh-BEL-ar):   Pertaining to the cerebellum.

Cerebellum (ser-eh-BEL-um):   Lower, back part of the brain that coordinates muscle movement and balance.

Cerebral (seh-RE-bral *or* SER-eh-bral):   Pertaining to the CEREBRUM.

Cerebrospinal fluid (seh-RE-bro SPI-nal FLOO-id):   Fluid surrounding the brain and spinal cord.

Cerebrovascular accident (seh-re-bro-VAS-ku-lar AK-sih-dent):   Disorder of blood vessels within the cerebrum. It results from inadequate blood supply to the brain. See also STROKE.

Cerebrum (seh-RE-brum):   Largest part of the brain. It controls thought processes, hearing, speech, vision, and body movements.

Cervical (SER-vih-kal):   Pertaining to the neck of the body or the neck (cervix) of the uterus.

Cervical region (SER-vih-kal RE-jun):   Seven backbones in the area of the neck.

Cervical vertebra (SER-vih-kal VER-teh-brah):   Backbone in the neck.

Cervix (SER-viks):   Lower, neck-like portion of the uterus opening into the vagina.

Cesarean section (seh-ZAR-re-an SEK-shun):   Incision of the uterus to remove the fetus at birth.

Chlamydial infection (klah-MID-e-al in-FEK-shun):   A bacterial infection commonly transmitted by sexual contact.

Chemotherapy (ke-mo-THER-ah-pe):   Treatment with drugs. Chemotherapy is most often used in the treatment of cancer.

Cholecystectomy (ko-leh-sis-TEK-to-me):   Removal of the gallbladder.

Choledochoduodenostomy (ko-led-oh-ko-doo-o-deh-NOS-to-me):   New surgical attachment of the common bile duct to the duodenum; an anastomosis.

Choledochotomy (ko-led-o-KOT-o-me):   Incision of the common bile duct.

Cholelithiasis (ko-leh-lih-THI-ah-sis):   Abnormal condition of gallstones.

Cholesterol (ko-LES-ter-ol):   Fatty substance made in the liver and found in the bloodstream. It is an important part of all cells and is necessary for creating hormones. It may accumulate in the lining of arteries, such as in the heart, causing heart disease, or in the gallbladder to form gallstones. Normal adult levels are 120 to 200 mg/dL.

Chondroma (kon-DRO-mah):   Benign tumor of CARTILAGE.

Chondrosarcoma (kon-dro-sar-KO-mah):   Malignant tumor of CARTILAGE.

Chronic (KRON-ik):   Lasting a long time.

Chronic obstructive pulmonary disease (KRON-ik ob-STRUK-tiv PUL-mo-na-re dih-ZEEZ):   Chronic limitation in airflow into and out of the body; includes chronic bronchitis, ASTHMA, and EMPHYSEMA. Also called COPD.

Circulatory system (SER-ku-lah-tor-e SIS-tem):   Organs (heart and blood vessels) that carry blood throughout the body.

Cirrhosis (seh-RO-sis):   Liver disease with deterioration of the liver cells. Cirrhosis is often caused by alcoholism and poor nutrition.

Clavicle (KLAV-ih-kul):   Collarbone.

Clinical (KLIN-ih-kal):   Pertaining to the bedside or clinic; involving patient care.

Coccygeal (kok-sih-JE-al):   Pertaining to the tailbone (coccyx).

Coccygeal region (kok-sih-JE-al RE-jun): Four fused (joined-together) bones at the base of the spinal column (backbone).

Coccyx (KOK-siks): Tailbone.

Colectomy (ko-LEK-to-me): Removal of the colon (large intestine).

Colitis (ko-LI-tis): Inflammation of the colon (large intestine).

Colocolostomy (ko-lo-ko-LOS-to-me): New surgical connection between two previously unconnected portions of the colon. This is an anastomosis.

Colon (KO-lon): Large intestine (bowel).

Colonic polyposis (ko-LON-ik pol-ih-PO-sis): Condition of growths or masses protruding from the mucous membrane lining the colon.

Colonoscopy (ko-lon-OS-ko-pe): Visual examination of the colon.

Colorectal surgeon (ko-lo-REK-tal SUR-jun): Physician specializing in operating on the colon and rectum.

Colostomy (ko-LOS-to-me): Opening of the colon to the outside of the body.

Colposcopy (kol-POS-ko-pe): Visual examination of the vagina and cervix.

Computed tomography scan (kom-PU-ted to-MOG-rah-fe skan): X-ray images taken to show the body in cross-sectional views. Also called CT SCAN.

Concussion (kon-KUSH-un): Loss of consciousness resulting from a blow to the head.

Congenital anomaly (con-JEN-ih-tal ah-NOM-ah-le): See ANOMALY.

Congestive heart failure (kon-JES-tiv hart FAIL-ur): Condition in which the heart is unable to pump its required amount of blood, resulting in inadequate oxygen to body cells.

Conization (ko-nih-ZA-shun): Removal of a wedge-shaped piece (cone) of tissue from the cervix in the diagnosis and treatment of early cancer of the cervix.

Conjunctiva (kon-junk-TI-vah): Thin protective membrane over the front of the eye and attached to the eyelids.

Conjunctivitis (kon-junk-ti-VI-tis): Inflammation of the CONJUNCTIVA.

Connective tissue (kon-NEK-tiv TIS-u): Fibrous tissue that supports and connects internal organs, bones, and walls of blood vessels.

Core biopsy (kor BI-op-se): See BIOPSY.

Corium (KOR-e-um): Middle layer of the skin below the epidermis; DERMIS.

Cornea (KOR-ne-ah): Transparent layer over the front of the eye. It bends light to focus it on sensitive cells (retina) at the back of the eye.

Coronal plane (kor-O-nal playn): See FRONTAL PLANE.

Coronary (KOR-on-ayr-e): Pertaining to the heart.

Coronary angiogram (KOR-on-ayr-e AN-je-o-gram): X-ray record of blood vessels surrounding the heart.

Coronary arteries (KOR-on-ayr-e AR-ter-eez): Blood vessels that carry oxygen-rich blood from the aorta to the heart muscle.

Coroner (KOR-oh-ner): A person who determines the cause of death in cases where the death was sudden, unexpected, of suspicious origin, or while under police custody. Generally, coroners have legal and/or medical backgrounds.

Cortex (KOR-teks): Outer part of an organ (*plural:* cortices [KOR-tih-seez]).

Cortisol (KOR-tih-sol): Anti-inflammatory hormone secreted by the adrenal cortex.

Costochondritis (kos-to-kon-DRI-tis): Inflammation of a rib and its cartilage.

Costochondral (kos-to-KON-dral): Pertaining to a rib and its cartilage.

Cranial cavity (KRA-ne-al KAV-ih-te): Space surrounded by the skull and containing the brain and other organs.

Craniotomy (kra-ne-OT-o-me): Incision of the skull.

Cranium (KRA-ne-um): Skull.

Creatinine (kre-AT-tih-nin): Nitrogen-containing waste that is removed from the blood by the kidney and excreted in urine.

Crohn disease (kron dih-ZEEZ): Inflammation of the gastrointestinal tract (often the ileum) marked by bouts of diarrhea, abdominal cramping, and fever. Along with ulcerative colitis, Crohn's is a type of INFLAMMATORY BOWEL DISEASE.

Cross-section (kros SEK-shun): Division of an organ or the body into upper and lower portions; TRANSVERSE PLANE.

Cryotherapy (kri-o-THER-ah-pe): Treatment using cold (CRY/O) temperatures.

Cryptorchism (kript-OR-kizm): Undescended (CRYPT- means hidden) testicle. The testicle is not in the scrotal sac at birth. Also called CRYPTORCHIDISM.

CT colonography (CT ko-lon-OG-ra-fe): CT imaging procedure using x-rays and computer equipment to produce images of the colon and display them on a screen. Also called *virtual colonoscopy*.

CT scan: Computed tomography study; series of x-ray images showing organs in cross-section (transverse view). Also called a CAT SCAN.

Cusp (KUSP): Any one of the small flaps on the valves of the heart. Also, a sharp projection extending from the surface of a tooth.

Cushing syndrome (KOOSH-ing SIN-drom): Clinical signs and symptoms produced by an excess of cortisol from the adrenal cortex. Cushing syndrome is marked by "moon face," fatty swellings, and weakness.

Cyanosis (si-ah-NO-sis): Bluish discoloration of the skin due to deficient OXYGEN in the bloodstream.

Cystitis (sis-TI-tis): Inflammation of the urinary bladder.

Cystoscope (SIS-to-skope): Instrument (endoscope) used to view the urinary bladder.

Cystoscopy (sis-TOS-ko-pe): Visual examination of the urinary bladder.

Cytology (si-TOL-o-je): Study of cells.

Ⓓ

Debridement (de-BREED-ment): Removal of diseased tissue from the skin.

Deep vein thrombosis (deep vane throm-BO-sis): Abnormal condition of clot formation in a deep vein, usually in the leg or pelvic (hip) region.

Defibrillation (de-fib-rih-LA-shun): Brief discharges of electricity applied to the chest to stop an abnormal heart rhythm.

Delusion (deh-LU-zhun): A persistent belief held by a person despite evidence to the contrary.

Dementia (deh-MEN-shah): Loss of memory and mental abilities.

Dermal (DER-mal): Pertaining to the skin.

Dermatitis (der-mah-TI-tis): Inflammation of the skin.

Dermatologist (der-mah-TOL-o-jist): Physician specializing in the skin and its diseases.

Dermatology (der-mah-TOL-o-je): Study of the skin and its diseases.

Dermatosis (der-mah-TO-sis): Any abnormal condition of the skin.

Dermis (DER-mis): Fibrous middle layer of the skin below the epidermis. The dermis contains nerves and blood vessels, hair roots, and oil and sweat glands.

Diabetes mellitus (di-ah-BE-teez MEL-lih-tus): Disorder marked by deficient insulin in the blood, which causes sugar to remain in the blood rather than entering cells. Diabetes is named from a Greek word meaning "siphon" (through which water passes easily). One symptom is frequent urination (polyuria). Type 1 diabetes is marked by lack of insulin, and patients need injections of insulin. In type 2 diabetes, insulin is not adequately or appropriately secreted. Type 2 diabetes has a tendency to develop later in life, and patients can be managed with diet, exercise, and oral antidiabetic drugs.

Diagnosis (di-ag-NO-sis):   Complete knowledge of patient's condition (*plural:*   diagnoses).

Dialysis (di-AL-ih-sis):   Complete separation (-LYSIS) of wastes (urea) from the blood when the kidneys fail. See also HEMODIALYSIS and PERITONEAL DIALYSIS.

Diameter (di-AM-eh-ter):   Length of a straight line passing through the center of a circle when the end points are on the circle.

Diaphragm (DI-ah-fram):   Muscle that separates the chest from the abdomen.

Diarrhea (di-ah-RE-ah):   Discharge of watery wastes from the COLON.

Digestive system (di-JES-tiv SIS-tem):   Organs that bring food into the body and break it down to enter the bloodstream or eliminate it through the rectum and anus.

Dilation (di-LA-shun):   Widening; dilatation.

Dilation and curettage (di-LA-shun and kur-eh-TAZH):   Widening of the opening to the cervix and scraping (curettage) of the inner lining of the uterus; also called D&C.

Disk (disk):   Pad of cartilage that is between each backbone.

Diuretic (di-u-RET-ik):   Drug that causes kidneys to allow more fluid (as urine) to leave the body. Diuretics remove fluid from the blood and are used to treat HYPERTENSION. DI- (from DIA-) means complete, and UR- means urine.

Diverticula (di-ver-TIK-u-lah):   Small pouches or sacs created by herniation of mucous membrane linings, most commonly in the colon (*singular:*   diverticulum).

Diverticulitis (di-ver-tik-u-LI-tis):   Inflammation of diverticula. Penetration of fecal material through thin-walled diverticula causes inflammation and infection in the colon.

Diverticulosis (di-ver-tik-u-LO-sis):   Abnormal condition of small pouches in the lining of the intestines.

Duodenal (do-o-DE-nal):   Pertaining to the duodenum.

Duodenum (do-o-DE-num):   First part of the small intestine.

Dura mater (DU-rah MAH-ter):   Outermost of the three layers of the MENINGES surrounding the brain and spinal cord. The name comes from Latin, meaning "hard mother." It is the toughest of the three layers.

Dysentery (DIS-en-teh-re):   Condition of painful intestines (often caused by bacterial infection).

Dysmenorrhea (dis-men-o-RE-ah):   Painful menstrual flow.

Dyspepsia (dis-PEP-se-ah):   Painful (DYS-) digestion (-PEPSIA).

Dysphagia (dis-FA-jah):   Difficult swallowing.

Dysphasia (dis-FA-zhah):   Difficult (impairment of) speech.

Dysplasia (dis-PLA-zhah):   Abnormality of the development or the formation of cells. Normal cells change in size, shape, and organization.

Dyspnea (disp-NE-ah):   Painful (DYS-) (labored, difficult) breathing (-PNEA).

Dysuria (dis-U-re-ah):   Painful or difficult urination.

E

Ear: Organ that receives sound waves and transmits them to nerves leading to the brain.

Eardrum (EAR-drum):   Membrane separating the outer and middle parts of the ear; the tympanic membrane.

Ectopic pregnancy (ek-TOP-ik PREG-nan-se):   Development of the zygote (early product of conception) in a place outside the uterus. The FALLOPIAN TUBES are the most common ectopic site.

Edema (eh-DE-mah):   Swelling in tissues. Edema is often caused by retention (holding back) of fluid and salt by the kidneys.

Ejaculation (e-jak-ku-LA-shun):   Release of semen from the male urethra.

Electrocardiogram (e-lek-tro-KAR-de-o-gram):   Record of the electricity in the heart.

Electroencephalogram (e-lek-tro-en-SEF-ah-lo-gram):   Record of the electricity in the brain.

Electroencephalography (e-lek-tro-en-sef-ah-LOG-rah-fe):   Process of recording the electricity in the brain.

Electrolyte (eh-LEK-tro-lite):   Substance that conducts an electrical current and is found in blood (serum) and body cells. Examples are sodium (Na^+), potassium (K^+), calcium (Ca^{2+}), and chloride (Cl^-).

Embolization (em-bo-lih-ZA-shun):   Use of a substance to block or reduce blood flow in a vessel.

Embolus (EM-bo-lus):   Foreign object (air, tissue, tumor, or clot) that circulates in the bloodstream until it lodges in a vessel.

Embryo (EM-bre-o):   A new organism in an early stage of development (2 to 6 weeks). From 6 to 38 weeks, the developing infant is a FETUS.

Emergency medicine (e-MER-jen-se MED-ih-sin):   Care of patients requiring immediate action.

Emphysema (em-fih-SE-mah):   Lung disorder in which air becomes trapped in the air sacs and bronchioles, making breathing difficult. Emphysema is marked by the accumulation of mucus and the loss of elasticity in lung tissue.

Encephalitis (en-sef-ah-LI-tis):   Inflammation of the brain.

Encephalopathy (en-sef-ah-LOP-ah-the):   Disease of the brain.

Endocarditis (EN-do-kar-DI-tis):   Inflammation of the inner lining of the heart (ENDOCARDIUM).

Endocardium (en-do-KAR-de-um):   Inner lining of the heart.

Endocrine glands (EN-do-krin glanz):   Organs that produce (secrete) hormones.

Endocrine system (EN-do-krin SIS-tem):   Endocrine glands. Examples are the pituitary, thyroid, and adrenal glands and the pancreas.

Endocrinologist (en-do-krih-NOL-o-jist):   Specialist in the study of endocrine glands and their disorders.

Endocrinology (en-do-krih-NOL-o-je):   Study of ENDOCRINE GLANDS.

Endodontist (en-do-DON-tist):   Dentist who specializes in diagnosis and treatment of the inner parts of a tooth (root canal therapy).

Endometriosis (en-do-me-tre-O-sis):   An abnormal condition in which tissue from the inner lining of the uterus is found outside the uterus, usually in the pelvic cavity.

Endometrium (en-do-ME-tre-um):   Inner lining of the uterus.

Endoscope (EN-do-skope):   Instrument used to view a hollow organ or body cavity; a tube fitted with a lens system that allows viewing in different directions.

Endoscopic retrograde cholangiopancreatography (en-do-SKOP-ik RET-tro-grade kol-an-je-o-pan-kre-ah-TOG-rah-fe):   X-ray images of bile ducts and pancreas after injection of contrast through a catheter from the mouth, esophagus, and stomach into bile and pancreatic ducts.

Endoscopy (en-DOS-ko-pe):   Process of viewing the inside of hollow organs or cavities with an endoscope.

Enteric (en-TER-ik):   Pertaining to the small intestine.

Enteritis (en-teh-RI-tis):   Inflammation of the small intestine.

Epidermis (ep-ih-DER-mis):   Outer (EPI-) layer of the skin (-DERMIS).

Epidural hematoma (ep-ih-DUR-al he-mah-TO-mah):   Pathologic mass of blood above the dura mater (outermost layer of membranes surrounding the brain and spinal cord).

Epiglottis (ep-ih-GLOT-tis):   Flap of cartilage that covers the mouth of the trachea when swallowing occurs so that food cannot enter the airway.

Epiglottitis (ep-ih-gloh-TI-tis):   Inflammation of the EPIGLOTTIS.

Epilepsy (EP-ih-lep-se):   Condition in which abnormal electrical activity in the brain results in sudden, fleeting disturbances in nerve cell functioning. An attack of epilepsy is called a SEIZURE.

Epinephrine (eh-pih-NEF-rin):   Hormone secreted by the adrenal gland in response to stress and physical injury. It is a drug used to treat hypersensitivity reactions (severe allergy), asthma, bronchial spasm, and nasal congestion. Also called ADRENALINE.

Epithelial (ep-ih-THE-le-al):   Pertaining to skin cells. This term originally described cells upon (EPI-) the breast nipple (THELI-). Now, it indicates cells lining the inner part of internal organs and covering the outside of the body.

Epithelium (ep-ih-THE-le-um):   Covering of the internal and external tissues of the body (skin, vessels, body cavities, glands, and organs).

Erythrocyte (eh-RITH-ro-site):   Red blood cell.

Erythrocytosis (eh-rith-ro-si-TO-sis):   Abnormal condition (slight increase in numbers) of red blood cells.

Erythromycin (eh-rith-ro-MI-sin):   An antibiotic that is produced from a red (ERYTHR/O-) mold (-MYCIN).

Esophageal (eh-sof-ah-JE-al):   Pertaining to the esophagus.

Esophagitis (eh-sof-ah-JI-tis):   Inflammation of the esophagus.

Esophagoscopy (eh-sof-ah-GOS-ko-pe):   Visual examination of the esophagus.

Esophagus (eh-SOF-ah-gus):   Tube leading from the throat to the stomach.

Estrogen (ES-tro-jen):   Hormone that promotes the development of female secondary sex characteristics. Examples are estradiol, estriol, and conjugated estrogen.

Eustachian tube (u-STA-she-an tube):   Channel connecting the middle part of the ear with the throat.

Exacerbation (eg-zas-er-BA-shun):   Increase in the seriousness of a disease, with greater intensity in the signs or symptoms.

Excision (ek-SIZH-un):   Act of cutting out, removing, or resecting.

Exocrine glands (EK-so-krin glanz):   Glands that produce (secrete) chemicals that leave the body through tubes (ducts). Examples are tear, sweat, and salivary glands.

Exophthalmic goiter (ek-sof-THAL-mik GOY-ter):   Enlargement of the thyroid gland accompanied by high levels of thyroid hormone in the blood and protrusion of the eyeballs (EXOPHTHALMOS).

Exophthalmos (ek-sof-THAL-mos):   Abnormal protrusion of eyeballs usually caused by HYPERTHYROIDISM.

Extracranial (eks-tra-KRA-ne-al):   Pertaining to outside the skull.

Extrahepatic (eks-tra-heh-PAT-ik):   Pertaining to outside the liver.

Extrapulmonary (eks-trah-PUL-mo-nah-re):   Outside the lungs.

Eye (i):   Organ that receives light waves and transmits them to the brain.

Fallopian tubes (fah-LO-pe-an toobz):   Two tubes that lead from the ovaries to the uterus. They transport egg cells to the uterus; also called uterine tubes.

Family medicine (FAM-ih-le MED-ih-sin):   Primary care of all members of the family on a continuing basis.

Family practitioner (FAM-ih-le prak-TIH-shan-er):   Medical doctor responsible for primary care and treatment of patients on a continuing basis.

Fatigue (fah-TEEG):   State of exhaustion or loss of strength.

Feces (FEE-seez):   Waste material from the digestive tract that is expelled from the body through the rectum and anus.

Fellowship training (FEL-o-ship TRA-ning):   Postgraduate training for doctors in specialized fields. The training may include CLINICAL and RESEARCH (laboratory) work.

Female reproductive system (FE-male re-pro-DUK-tiv SIS-tem):   Organs (OVARIES) that produce and transport (FALLOPIAN TUBES) egg cells and secrete female hormones (ESTROGEN and PROGESTERONE). The system includes the uterus, where the embryo and fetus grow.

Femur (FE-mer):   Thigh bone.

Fetus (FE-tus):   Unborn offspring in the uterus after 8 weeks of pregnancy until birth.

Fibrillation (fih-brih-LA-shun):   Rapid, irregular, involuntary muscular contraction. Atrial and ventricular fibrillation are cardiac (heart) ARRHYTHMIAS.

Fibroid (FI-broyd):   Benign growth of muscle tissue in the uterus.

Fibrosarcoma (fi-bro-sar-KO-mah):   Malignant tumor of fibrous tissue.

Fibula (FIB-u-lah):   Smaller lower leg bone.

Fistula (FIS-tu-lah):   Abnormal passageway from an internal organ to the body surface or between two internal organs.

Fixation (fik-SA-shun):   Act of holding, sewing, or fastening a part in a fixed position.

Flutter (FLUT-er):   Rapid but regular, abnormal heart muscle contraction. Atrial and ventricular flutter are heart ARRHYTHMIAS.

Follicle-stimulating hormone (FOL-ih-kl STIM-u-la-ting HOR-mone):   A hormone secreted by the pituitary gland to stimulate the egg cells in the ovaries.

Fracture (FRAK-chur):   Breaking of a bone.

Frontal (FRUN-tal):   Pertaining to the front; anterior.

Frontal plane (FRUN-tal playn):   A vertical plane that divides the body or an organ into front and back portions; the CORONAL PLANE.

Functional disorder (FUNG-shih-nal dis-OR-der):   A condition in which there are clinical signs and symptoms but no evidence of structural or biochemical cause.

G

Gadolinium (gad-o-LIN-e-um):   A chemical element that is used as a contrast agent in MRI studies. Symbol is Gd.

Gallbladder (GAWL-blah-der):   Sac below the liver that stores bile and delivers it to the small intestine.

Ganglion (GANG-le-on):   Benign cyst near a joint (wrist); also, a group of nerve cells (*plural:* ganglia [GANG-le-ah]).

Gastralgia (gas-TRAL-jah):   Stomach pain.

Gastrectomy (gas-TREK-to-me):   Excision (removal) of the stomach.

Gastric (GAS-trik):   Pertaining to the stomach.

Gastritis (gas-TRI-tis):   Inflammation of the stomach.

Gastroenteritis (gas-tro-en-teh-RI-tis):   Inflammation of the stomach and intestines.

Gastroenterologist (gas-tro-en-ter-OL-o-jist):   Specialist in the treatment of stomach and intestinal disorders.

Gastroenterology (gas-tro-en-ter-OL-o-je):   Study of the stomach and intestines.

Gastroesophageal reflux disease (gas-tro-eh-sof-ah-JE-al RE-flux dih-ZEEZ):   A condition marked by backflow (reflux) of contents of the stomach into the esophagus. Abbreviation is GERD.

Gastrojejunostomy (gas-tro-jeh-joo-NOS-to-me):   New surgical opening between the stomach and the jejunum (second part of the small intestine). This procedure is an anastomosis.

Gastroscope (GAS-tro-skope):   Instrument used to view the stomach. It is passed down the throat and esophagus into the stomach.

Gastroscopy (gas-TROS-ko-pe):   Visual examination of the stomach.

Gastrotomy (gas-TROT-o-me):   Incision of the stomach.

GERD: See GASTROESOPHAGEAL REFLUX DISEASE.

Geriatric (jer-e-AH-trik):   Pertaining to treatment of older people.

Geriatrician (jer-e-ah-TRISH-an):   Specialist in the treatment of diseases of old age.

Geriatrics (jer-e-AH-triks):   Treatment of disorders of old age.

Gestation (jes-TA-shun):   Growth of the fetus that occurs during pregnancy.

Gland: Group of cells that secretes chemicals to the outside of the body (EXOCRINE GLANDS) or hormones directly into the bloodstream (ENDOCRINE GLANDS).

Glaucoma (glaw-KO-mah):   Increase of fluid pressure within the eye. Fluid is formed more rapidly than it is removed. The increased pressure damages sensitive cells in the back of the eye, and vision is disturbed.

Glial cells (GLI-al selz):   Supporting cells of nervous tissue in the brain. Examples are astrocytes and microglial and oligodendroglial cells. These cells are the source of primary brain tumors.

Glioblastoma (gli-o-blas-TO-mah):   Malignant brain tumor composed of immature (-BLAST) glial (supportive nervous tissue) cells.

Glucocorticoid (gloo-ko-KOR-tih-koyd):   Hormone secreted by the adrenal gland (cortex) to raise blood sugar levels. Examples are cortisone and cortisol.

Glycosuria (gli-ko-SU-re-ah):   Abnormal condition of sugar in the urine.

Goiter (GOY-ter):   Enlargement of the thyroid gland.

Gonorrhea (gon-oh-RE-ah):   Sexually transmitted disease most often affecting the reproductive and urinary tracts and caused by infection with the bacterium *Neisseria gonorrhoeae.*

Gout (gout):   See GOUTY ARTHRITIS.

Gouty arthritis (GOW-te arth-RI-tis):   Deposits of uric acid crystals in joints and other tissues that cause swelling and inflammation of joints. Also called GOUT.

Graves disease (grayvz dih-ZEEZ):   See HYPERTHYROIDISM.

Growth hormone (groth HOR-mone):   Hormone secreted by the pituitary gland to stimulate the growth of bones and the body in general. Also called somatotropin.

Gynecologist (gi-neh-KOL-o-jist):   Specialist in the medical and surgical treatment of female disorders.

Gynecology (gi-neh-KOL-o-je):   Study of female disorders.

H

Hair follicle (hayr FOL-ih-k'l):   Pouch-like depression in the skin in which a hair develops.

Hair root (hahr root):   Part of the hair from which growth occurs.

Hallucination (hah-loo-sih-NA-shun):   False sensory perception, such as hearing voices when none are present.

HDL: See HIGH-DENSITY LIPOPROTEIN.

Heart (hart):   Hollow, muscular organ in the chest that pumps blood throughout the body.

Heart attack (hart ah-TAK):   See MYOCARDIAL INFARCTION.

Hemangioma (he-man-je-O-mah):   Tumor (benign) of blood vessels.

Hematemesis (he-mah-TEM-eh-sis):   Vomiting (-EMESIS) of blood (HEMAT/O-).

Hematologist (he-mah-TOL-o-jist):   Specialist in blood and blood disorders.

Hematology (he-mah-TOL-o-je):   Study of the blood.

Hematoma (he-mah-TO-mah):   Mass or collection of blood under the skin. Commonly called a bruise or "black-and-blue" mark.

Hematuria (he-mah-TUR-e-ah):   Abnormal condition of blood in the urine.

Hemigastrectomy (heh-me-gas-TREK-to-me):   Removal of half of the stomach.

Hemiglossectomy (heh-me-glos-EK-to-me):   Removal of half of the tongue.

Hemiplegia (hem-ih-PLE-jah):   Paralysis of one side of the body.

Hemoccult test (he-mo-KULT test):   A standardized test to look for hidden (occult) blood in stool. It is a screening test for colon and rectal cancer. See also STOOL GUAIAC.

Hemodialysis (he-mo-di-AL-ih-sis):   Use of a kidney machine to filter blood to remove waste materials such as urea. Blood leaves the body, enters the machine, and is carried back to the body through a catheter (tube).

Hemoglobin (HE-mo-glo-bin):   Oxygen-carrying protein found in red blood cells.

Hemoptysis (he-MOP-tih-sis):   Spitting up (-PTYSIS) of blood (HEM/O-).

Hemorrhage (HEM-or-ij):   Bursting forth of blood.

Hemothorax (he-mo-THOR-aks):   Collection of blood in the chest (pleural cavity).

Hepatic (heh-PAT-ik):   Pertaining to the liver.

Hepatitis (hep-ah-TI-tis):   Inflammation of the liver. Viral hepatitis is an acute infectious disease caused by at least three different viruses: hepatitis A, B, and C viruses.

Hepatocellular carcinoma (hep-ah-to-SEL-u-lar kar-sih-NO-mah):   Malignant tumor of the liver.

Hepatoma (hep-ah-TO-mah):   Tumor (malignant) of the liver; hepatocellular carcinoma.

Hepatomegaly (hep-ah-to-MEG-ah-le):   Enlargement of the liver.

Hernia (HER-ne-ah):   Bulge or protrusion of an organ or part of an organ through the wall of the cavity that usually contains it. In an INGUINAL hernia, part of the wall of the abdomen weakens and the intestine bulges outward or into the SCROTAL sac (in males).

Herpes genitalis (HER-peez jen-ih-TAL-is):   Chronic sexually transmitted disease caused by type 2 herpes simplex virus.

Hiatal hernia (hi-A-tal HER-ne-ah):   Upward protrusion of the wall of the stomach into the lower part of the esophagus.

High-density lipoprotein (hi DEN-sih-te li-po-PRO-teen):   Combination of fat and protein in the blood. It carries cholesterol to the liver, which is beneficial.

Hilum (HI-lum):   Depression at that part of an organ where blood vessels and nerves enter.

HIV: See HUMAN IMMUNODEFICIENCY VIRUS.

Hodgkin disease (HOJ-kin di-ZEEZ):   Malignant tumor of lymph nodes.

Hormone (HOR-mone):   Chemical made by a gland and sent directly into the bloodstream, not to the outside of the body. ENDOCRINE GLANDS produce hormones.

Hospitalist (HOS-pih-tah-list):   A physician whose primary focus is hospital medicine. This includes patient care, teaching, and research related to hospital care.

Human immunodeficiency virus (HYOO-man im-u-no-deh-FISH-en-se VI-rus):   Virus that infects white blood cells (T cell lymphocytes), causing damage to the patient's immune system. It is the cause of AIDS. Abbreviated HIV.

Humerus (HYOO-mer-us):   Upper arm bone.

Hydrocele (HI-dro-seel):   Swelling of the SCROTUM caused by a collection of fluid within the outermost covering of the TESTIS.

Hyperbilirubinemia (hi-per-bil-ih-roo-bin-E-me-ah):   High levels of bilirubin (pigment released from hemoglobin breakdown and processed in the liver) in the bloodstream. See JAUNDICE.

Hyperglycemia (hi-per-gli-SE-me-ah):   Higher-than-normal levels of sugar in the blood.

Hyperparathyroidism (hi-per-par-ah-THI-royd-ism):   Higher-than-normal level of parathyroid hormone in the blood.

Hyperplastic (hi-per-PLAS-tik):   Pertaining to excessive growth of normal cells in an organ.

Hypersecretion (hi-per-se-KRE-shun):   Abnormally high production of a substance.

Hypertension (hi-per-TEN-shun):   High blood pressure. *Essential hypertension* has no known cause, but contributing factors are age, obesity, smoking, and heredity. *Secondary hypertension* is a sign of other disorders such as kidney disease.

Hyperthyroidism (hi-per-THI-royd-izm):   Excessive activity of the thyroid gland.

Hypertrophy (hi-PER-tro-fe):   Enlargement or overgrowth of an organ or part of the body as a result of an increase in size of individual cells.

Hypochondriac (hi-po-KON-dre-ak):   Pertaining to lateral regions of the upper abdomen beneath the lower ribs. Also, the term describes a person who has chronic concern about his or her health and body functions.

Hypodermic (hi-po-DER-mik):   Pertaining to under or below the skin.

Hypoglycemia (hi-po-gli-SE-me-ah):   Blood condition of decreased sugar (lower-than-normal levels).

Hypophyseal (hi-po-FIZ-e-al):   Pertaining to the pituitary gland.

Hypopituitarism (hi-po-pih-TOO-ih-tah-rizm):   Decrease or stoppage of hormonal secretion by the pituitary gland.

Hypoplastic (hi-po-PLAS-tik):   Pertaining to underdevelopment of a tissue or organ in the body.

Hyposecretion (hi-po-se-KRE-shun):   Abnormally low production of a substance.

Hypotensive (hi-po-TEN-siv):   Pertaining to low blood pressure or to a person with abnormally low blood pressure.

Hypothyroidism (hi-po-THI-royd-izm):   Lower-than-normal activity of the thyroid gland.

Hysterectomy (his-teh-REK-to-me):   Excision of the uterus, either through the abdominal wall (abdominal hysterectomy) or through the vagina (vaginal hysterectomy).

Hysteroscopy (his-ter-OS-ko-pe):   Visual examination of the uterus with an endoscope inserted through the vagina and uterine cervix.

Iatrogenic (i-ah-tro-JEN-ik):   Pertaining to a patient's abnormal condition that results unexpectedly from a specific treatment.

Ileostomy (il-e-OS-to-me):   New opening of the ILEUM to the outside of the body.

Ileum (IL-e-um):   Third part of the small intestine.

Ilium (IL-e-um):   Side, high portion of the hip bone (pelvis).

Incision (in-SIZH-un):   Cutting into the body or into an organ.

Infarction (in-FARK-shun):   Area of dead tissue (necrosis) caused by decreased blood flow to that part of the body. Also called *infarct*.

Infectious disease specialist (in-FEK-shus dih-ZEEZ SPESH-ah-list):   Physician who treats disorders caused and spread by microorganisms such as bacteria.

Infiltrate (IN-fil-trat):   Material that accumulates in an organ. The term infiltrate often describes solid material or fluid collection in the lungs.

Inflammatory bowel disease (in-FLAM-ah-tor-e BOW-el dih-ZEEZ):   Disorder marked by inflammation of the small and large intestines with bouts of diarrhea, abdominal cramping, and fever. Inflammatory bowel diseases include CROHN DISEASE and ULCERATIVE COLITIS.

Inguinal (IN-gwih-nal):   Pertaining to the groin or the area where the legs meet the body. Inguinal lymph nodes are located in the groin.

Insulin (IN-su-lin):   Hormone produced by the pancreas and released into the bloodstream. Insulin allows sugar to leave the blood and enter body cells.

Insulin pump (IN-su-lin pump):   Portable, battery-powered device that delivers insulin through the abdominal wall in measured amounts.

Internal medicine (in-TER-nal MED-ih-sin):   Branch of medicine specializing in the diagnosis of disorders and treatment with drugs.

Intervertebral (in-ter-VER-teh-bral):   Pertaining to lying between two backbones. A disk (disc) is an intervertebral structure.

Intra-abdominal (in-trah-ab-DOM-ih-nal):   Pertaining to within the abdomen.

Intracranial (in-trah-KRA-ne-al):   Pertaining to within the skull.

Intrauterine (in-trah-U-ter-in):   Pertaining to within the uterus.

Intravenous (in-trah-VE-nus):   Pertaining to within a vein.

Intravenous pyelogram (in-trah-VE-nus PI-eh-lo-gram):   X-ray record of the kidney (PYEL/O- means renal pelvis) after contrast is injected into a vein.

Intravesical (in-trah-VES-ih-kal):   Pertaining to within the urinary bladder.

Iris (I-ris):   Colored (pigmented) portion of the eye.

Irritable bowel syndrome (IR-ih-tah-bl BOW-el SIN-drom):   A FUNCTIONAL DISORDER of the bowel marked by abdominal pain, discomfort, and bloating, but without evidence of detectable lesions or cause.

Ischemia (is-KE-me-ah):   Deficiency of blood flow to a part of the body, caused by narrowing or obstruction of blood vessels.

J

Jaundice (JAWN-dis):   Orange-yellow coloration of the skin and other tissues. A symptom caused by accumulation of BILIRUBIN (pigment) in the blood.

Jejunum (jeh-JOO-num):   Second part of the small intestine.

Joint (joynt):   Place where two or more bones come together (articulate).

K

Kidney (KID-ne):   One of two organs located behind the abdomen that produce urine by filtering wastes from the blood.

L

Laminectomy (lah-mih-NEK-to-me):   Removal of a piece of backbone (lamina) to relieve pressure on nerves from a herniating disk (disc).

Laparoscope (LAP-ah-ro-skope):   Instrument to visually examine the abdomen. An endoscope is inserted through a small incision in the abdominal wall.

Laparoscopic appendectomy (lap-ah-ro-SKOP-ik ah-pen-DEK-to-me):   Removal of the appendix through a small incision in the abdomen and with the use of a laparoscope.

Laparoscopic cholecystectomy (lap-ah-ro-SKOP-ik ko-leh-sis-TEK-to-me):   Removal of the gallbladder through a small incision in the abdomen and with the use of a laparoscopic instrument.

Laparoscopy (lap-ah-ROS-ko-pe):   Visual examination of the abdomen. A small incision is made near the navel, and an instrument (endoscope) is inserted to view abdominal organs.

Laparotomy (lap-ah-ROT-o-me):   Incision of the abdomen. A surgeon makes a large incision across the abdomen to examine and operate on its organs.

Large intestine (larj in-TES-tin):   Part of the intestine that receives undigested material from the small intestine and transports it out of the body; the COLON.

Laryngeal (lah-rin-JE-al):   Pertaining to the larynx (voice box).

Laryngectomy (lah-rin-JEK-to-me):   Removal of the larynx (voice box).

Laryngitis (lah-rin-JI-tis):   Inflammation of the larynx.

Laryngoscopy (lar-in-GOS-ko-pe):   Visual examination of the interior of the voice box (larynx) with an endoscope.

Laryngotracheitis (lah-ring-o-tra-ke-I-tis):   Inflammation of the larynx and the trachea (windpipe).

Larynx (LAR-inks):   Voice box; located at the top of the trachea and containing vocal cords.

Lateral (LAT-er-al):   Pertaining to the side.

LDL: See LOW-DENSITY LIPOPROTEIN.

Leiomyoma (li-o-mi-O-mah):   Benign tumor derived from smooth (involuntary or visceral) muscle, most often of the uterus (leiomyoma uteri). LEIOMY/O- means smooth muscle.

Leiomyosarcoma (li-o-mi-o-sar-KO-mah):   Malignant tumor of smooth (involuntary) muscle.

Lens (lenz):   Structure behind the pupil of the eye. The lens bends light rays so that they are properly focused on the RETINA at the back of the eye.

Lesion (LE-zhun):   Abnormal tissue, usually damaged by disease or trauma. From the Latin *laesio,* meaning injury.

Leukemia (loo-KE-me-ah):   Increase in malignant (cancerous) white blood cells in blood and bone marrow.

Leukocyte (LOO-ko-site):   White blood cell.

Leukocytosis (loo-ko-si-TO-sis):   Slight increase in the numbers of normal white blood cells as a response to infection.

Ligament (LIG-ah-ment):   Connective tissue that joins bones to other bones.

Ligamentous (lig-ah-MEN-tus):   Pertaining to a LIGAMENT.

Liposarcoma (li-po-sar-KO-mah):   Malignant tumor of fatty tissue.

Lithotripsy (LITH-o-trip-se):   Process of crushing a stone in the urinary tract using ultrasonic vibrations. Also called extracorporeal shock-wave lithotripsy (ESWL).

Liver (LIV-er):   Organ in the right upper quadrant of the abdomen. The liver produces BILE, stores sugar, and produces blood-clotting proteins.

Lobe (lobe):   Part of an organ, especially of the brain, lungs, or glands.

Low-density lipoprotein (lo DEN-sih-te li-po-PRO-teen):   Combination of lipid (fat) and protein. It has a high CHOLESTEROL content and is associated with formation of plaques in arteries.

Lower gastrointestinal (GI) series (LO-er gas-tro-in-TES-tin-al SER-eez):   Barium is injected into the anus and rectum and x-rays are taken of the colon (large intestine).

Lumbar (LUM-bar):   Pertaining to the loins; part of the back and sides between the chest and the hip.

Lumbar puncture (LUM-bar PUNK-cher):   Removal of cerebrospinal fluid (CSF) for diagnostic analysis or occasionally as treatment to relieve increased intracranial pressure.

Lumbar region (LUM-bar RE-jun):   Pertaining to the backbones that lie between the thoracic (chest) and sacral (lower back) vertebrae.

Lumbar vertebra (LUM-bar VER-teh-brah):   A backbone in the region between the chest and lower back.

Lung (lung):   One of two paired organs in the chest through which oxygen enters and carbon dioxide leaves the body.

Lung capillaries (lung KAP-ih-layr-eez):   Tiny blood vessels surrounding lung tissue and through which gases pass into and out of the bloodstream.

Lupus erythematosus: See SYSTEMIC LUPUS ERYTHEMATOSUS.

Lymph (limf):   Clear fluid that is found in lymph vessels and produced from fluid surrounding cells. Lymph contains white blood cells (lymphocytes) that fight disease.

Lymphadenectomy (limf-ah-deh-NEK-to-me):   Removal of LYMPH NODES.

Lymphadenopathy (lim-fad-eh-NOP-ah-the):   Disease of lymph nodes (glands).

Lymphangiectasis (limf-an-je-EK-tah-sis):   Dilation (-ECTASIS) of small lymph vessels; often resulting from obstruction in large lymph vessels.

Lymphatic system (lim-FAT-ik SIS-tem):   Group of organs (lymph vessels, lymph nodes, spleen, thymus) composed of lymphatic tissue that produce lymphocytes to defend the body against foreign organisms.

Lymphatic vessels (lim-FAT-ik VES-elz):   Tubes that carry lymph from tissues to the bloodstream (into a vein in the neck region); lymph vessels.

Lymphedema (limf-ah-DE-mah):   Accumulation of fluid in tissue spaces, causing swelling. Lymphedema is caused by the obstruction of lymph nodes or vessels.

Lymph node (limf node):   Stationary collection of lymph cells, found all over the body. Lymph nodes are sometimes called lymph "glands."

Lymphocyte (LIMF-o-site):   White blood cell that is found within lymph and lymph nodes. T cells and B cells are types of lymphocytes.

Lymphoid (LIM-foid):   Resembling or pertaining to lymphatic tissue.

Lymphoma (lim-FO-mah):   Malignant tumor of lymphatic tissue. Previously called lymphosarcoma. There are several types, including Hodgkin disease and non-Hodgkin lymphoma.

Magnetic resonance imaging (mag-NET-ik REZ-o-nans IM-aj-ing):   Image of the body with magnetic and radio waves. Organs are seen in three planes: coronal (front to back), sagittal (side to side), and transverse (cross-section). Also called MRI.

Male reproductive system (male re-pro-DUK-tiv SIS-tem):   Organs that produce sperm cells and male hormones.

Malignant (mah-LIG-nant):   Tending to become progressively worse. The term *malignant* describes cancerous tumors that invade and spread to distant organs.

Mammary (MAM-er-e):   Pertaining to the breast.

Mammogram (MAM-o-gram):   X-ray record of the breast.

Mammography (mam-MOG-ra-fe):   Process of making an x-ray recording of the breast.

Mammoplasty (MAM-o-plas-te):   Surgical repair (reconstruction) of the breast.

Mastectomy (mas-TEK-to-me):   Removal (excision) of the breast.

Mastitis (mas-TI-tis):   Inflammation of the breast.

Mediastinal (me-de-ah-STI-nal):   Pertaining to the MEDIASTINUM.

Mediastinoscopy (me-de-ah-sti-NOS-ko-pe):   Visual examination of the mediastinum with an endoscope.

Mediastinum (me-de-ah-STI-num):   Space between the lungs in the chest. The mediastinum contains the heart, large blood vessels, trachea, esophagus, thymus gland, and lymph nodes.

Medulla oblongata (meh-DUL-ah ob-lon-GAh-tah):   Lower part of the brain near the spinal cord. The medulla oblongata controls breathing and heartbeat.

Medullary (MEH-du-lar-e):   Pertaining to the inner, or soft, part of an organ.

Melanoma (meh-lah-NO-mah):   Malignant tumor arising from pigmented cells (melanocytes) in the skin. A melanoma usually develops from a NEVUS (mole).

Meninges (meh-NIN-jeez):   Membranes surrounding the brain and spinal cord.

Meningitis (men-in-JI-tis):   Inflammation of the meninges (membranes around the brain and spinal cord).

Menorrhagia (men-or-RA-jah):   Excessive bleeding from the uterus during the time of MENSTRUATION.

Menorrhea (men-o-RE-ah):   Normal discharge of blood and tissue from the uterine lining during MENSTRUATION.

Menses (MEN-seez):   Menstruation; menstrual period.

Menstruation (men-stroo-A-shun):   Breakdown of the lining of the uterus that occurs every 4 weeks during the active reproductive period of a female.

Mesothelioma (mez-o-the-le-O-mah):   Malignant tumor of the lining tissue (mesothelium) of the pleura. A mesothelioma is associated with exposure to asbestos.

Metacarpals (met-ah-KAR-palz):   Bones of the hand between the wrist bones (carpals) and the finger bones (phalanges).

Metastasis (meh-TAS-tah-sis):   Spread of a cancerous tumor to a distant organ or location. Metastasis literally means change (META-) of place (-STASIS). *Metastatic* means pertaining to a metastasis.

Metatarsals (meh-tah-TAR-salz):   Foot bones.

Migraine (MI-grayn):   Attack of headache, usually on one side of the head, caused by changes in blood vessel size and accompanied by nausea, vomiting, and sensitivity to light (photophobia). Migraine is a term from the French word *migraine,* meaning "severe head pain."

Minimally invasive surgery (MIN-ih-mah-le in-VA-siv SUR-jer-e):   Removal and repair of organs and tissues with small incisions for an endoscope and instruments. Examples are laparoscopic cholecystectomy (gallbladder removal), laparoscopic appendectomy (appendix removal), laparoscopic herniorrhaphy (repair of a hernia), and laparoscopic colectomy (removal of a portion of the colon).

Mitral valve prolapse (MI-tral valv PRO-laps):   Protrusion of one or both cusps of the mitral valve back into the left atrium when the ventricles contract.

Monocyte (MON-o-site):   White blood cell with one large nucleus.

Mononucleosis (mon-o-nu-kle-O-sis):   An acute infectious disease with excess monocytes in the blood and usually associated with extreme fatigue. Mononucleosis is caused by the Epstein-Barr virus and is transmitted by direct oral (mouth) contact.

Mouth (mowth):   The opening that forms the beginning of the digestive system.

MRI: See MAGNETIC RESONANCE IMAGING.

Mucus (MU-kus):   Sticky secretion from mucous membranes and glands.

Multiple myeloma (MUL-tih-pul mi-eh-LO-mah):   Malignant tumor of the bone marrow.

Multiple sclerosis (MUL-tih-pul skleh-RO-sis):   Chronic neurologic disease in which there are patches of demyelination (loss of myelin sheath covering on nerve cells) throughout the brain and spinal cord. Weakness, abnormal sensations, incoordination, and speech and visual disturbances are symptoms.

Muscle (MUS-el):   Connective tissue that contracts to make movement possible.

Muscular (MUS-ku-lar):   Pertaining to muscles.

Muscular dystrophy (MUS-ku-lar DIS-tro-fe):   Group of degenerative muscle diseases that cause crippling because muscles are gradually weakened and eventually ATROPHY (shrink).

Musculoskeletal system (mus-ku-lo-SKEL-eh-tal SIS-tem):   Organs that support the body and allow it to move, including the muscles, bones, joints, and connective tissues.

Myalgia (mi-AL-jah):   Pain in a muscle or muscles.

Myelin sheath (MI-eh-lin sheath):   Fatty covering around part (axon) of nerve cells. The myelin sheath insulates the nerve, helping to speed the conduction of nerve impulses.

Myelodysplasia (mi-eh-lo-dis-PLA-ze-ah):   Abnormal development of bone marrow, a premalignant condition leading to leukemia.

Myelogram (MI-eh-lo-gram):   X-ray image of the spinal cord after contrast is injected within the membranes surrounding the spinal cord in the lumbar area of the back.

Myelography (mi-eh-LOG-rah-fe):   X-ray imaging of the spinal cord after injection of contrast material.

Myeloma (mi-eh-LO-mah):   Malignant tumor originating in the bone marrow (MYEL/O-). Also called MULTIPLE MYELOMA.

Myocardial (mi-o-KAR-de-al):   Pertaining to the muscle of the heart.

Myocardial infarction (mi-o-KAR-de-al in-FARK-shun):   Death of tissue in heart muscle; also known as a heart attack or an MI.

Myocardial ischemia (mi-o-KAR-de-al is-KE-me-ah):   Decrease in the blood supply to the heart muscle.

Myoma (mi-O-mah):   Tumor (benign) of muscle.

Myomectomy (mi-o-MEK-to-me):   Removal of a benign muscle tumor (fibroid).

Myosarcoma (mi-o-sar-KO-mah):   Tumor (malignant) of muscle. SARC- means flesh, indicating that the tumor is of connective or "fleshy" tissue origin.

Myositis (mi-o-SI-tis):   Inflammation of a muscle.

Myringotomy (mir-in-GOT-o-me):   Incision of the eardrum.

N

Nasal (NA-zl):   Pertaining to the nose.

Nausea (NAW-se-ah):   Unpleasant sensation in the upper abdomen, often leading to vomiting. The term comes from the Greek *nausia,* meaning "sea sickness."

Necropsy: See POSTMORTEM.

Necrosis (neh-KRO-sis):   Death of cells.

Necrotic (neh-KRO-tik):   Pertaining to death of cells.

Needle biopsy (NE-dl BI-op-se):   Removal of living tissue for microscopic examination by inserting a hollow needle through the skin.

Neonatal (ne-o-NA-tal):   Pertaining to new birth; the first 4 weeks after birth.

Neoplasm (NE-o-plazm):   Any new growth of tissue; a tumor.

Neoplastic (ne-o-PLAS-tik):   Pertaining to a new growth, or NEOPLASM.

Nephrectomy (neh-FREK-to-me):   Removal (excision) of a kidney.

Nephritis (neh-FRI-tis):   Inflammation of kidneys.

Nephrolithiasis (neh-fro-lih-THI-ah-sis):   Condition of kidney stones.

Nephrologist (neh-FROL-o-jist):   Specialist in the diagnosis and treatment of kidney diseases.

Nephrology (neh-FROL-o-je):   Study of the kidney and its diseases.

Nephropathy (neh-FROP-ah-the):   Disease of the kidney.

Nephrosis (neh-FRO-sis):   Abnormal condition of the kidney. Nephrosis is often associated with a deterioration of the kidney tubules.

Nephrostomy (neh-FROS-to-me):   Opening from the kidney to the outside of the body.

Nervous system (NER-vus SIS-tem):   Organs (brain, spinal cord, and nerves) that transmit electrical messages throughout the body.

Neural (NU-ral):   Pertaining to nerves.

Neuralgia (nu-RAL-jah):   Nerve pain.

Neuritis (nu-RI-tis):   Inflammation of a nerve.

Neuroglial cells (nu-ro-GLE-al selz):   See GLIAL CELLS.

Neurologist (nu-ROL-o-jist):   Specialist in the diagnosis and treatment of nervous disorders.

Neurology (nu-ROL-o-je):   Study of the nervous system and nerve disorders.

Neuropathy (nu-ROP-ah-the):   Disease of nervous tissue.

Neurosurgeon (nu-ro-SUR-jun):   Physician who operates on the organs of the nervous system (brain, spinal cord, and nerves).

Neurotomy (nu-ROT-o-me):   Incision of a nerve.

Nevus (NE-vus):   Pigmented lesion on the skin; a mole.

Nitroglycerin (ni-tro-GLIS-er-in):   Drug that relaxes muscle and opens blood vessels.

Nocturia (nok-TU-re-ah):   Excessive urination at night.

Nose (noz):   Structure that is the organ of smell and permits air to enter and leave the body.

Nosocomial (nos-o-KO-me-al):   Pertaining to or originating in a hospital. A *nosocomial infection* is acquired during hospitalization.

O

Obstetric (ob-STEH-trik):   Pertaining to pregnancy, labor, and delivery of a baby.

Obstetrician (ob-steh-TRISH-an):   Specialist in the delivery of a baby and care of the mother during pregnancy and labor.

Obstetrics (ob-STET-riks):   Practice or branch of medicine concerned with the management of women during pregnancy, childbirth, and the period just after delivery of the infant.

Ocular (OK-u-lar):   Pertaining to the eye.

Oncogenic (ong-ko-JEN-ik):   Pertaining to producing (-GENIC) tumors.

Oncologist (ong-KOL-o-jist):   Physician specializing in the study and treatment of tumors.

Oncology (ong-KOL-o-je):   Study of tumors.

Onycholysis (on-ih-KOL-ih-sis):   Separating (-LYSIS) of a nail (ONYCH/O) from its foundation (bed).

Oocyte (o-o-site):   Egg cell (ovum).

Oophorectomy (o-of-o-REK-to-me *or* oo-fo-REK-to-me):   Removal of an ovary or ovaries.

Oophoritis (o-of-o-RI-tis *or* oo-pho-RI-tis):   Inflammation of an ovary.

Ophthalmologist (of-thal-MOL-o-jist):   Specialist in the study of the eye and the treatment of eye disorders.

Ophthalmology (of-thal-MOL-o-je):   Study of the eye; the diagnosis and treatment of eye disorders.

Ophthalmoscope (of-THAL-mo-scope):   Instrument used to visually examine the eye.

Optic nerve (OP-tik nerv):   Nerve in the back of the eye that transmits light waves to the brain.

Optician (op-TISH-an):   Nonmedical specialist trained to provide eyeglasses by filling prescriptions.

Optometrist (op-TOM-eh-trist):   Nonmedical specialist trained to examine and test eyes and prescribe corrective lenses.

Oral (OR-al):   Pertaining to the mouth.

Orchidectomy (or-kih-DEK-to-me):   Removal (excision) of a testicle or testicles.

Orchiectomy (or-ke-EK-to-me):   Removal (excision) of a testicle or testicles.

Orchiopexy (or-ke-o-PEK-se):   Surgical fixation of the testicle (testis) into its proper location within the scrotum. This surgery corrects CRYPTORCHISM.

Orchitis (or-KI-tis):   Inflammation of a testicle.

Organ (OR-gan):   Independent part of the body composed of different tissues working together to do a specific job.

Orthodontist (or-tho-DON-tist):   Dentist specializing in straightening teeth.

Orthopedist (or-tho-PE-dist):   Specialist in the surgical correction of musculoskeletal disorders. This physician was originally concerned with straightening (ORTH/O) bones in the legs of children (PED/O) with deformities.

Osteitis (os-te-I-tis):   Inflammation of a bone.

Osteoarthritis (os-te-o-ar-THRI-tis):   Inflammation of bones and joints. Osteoarthritis is a disease of older people and is marked by stiffness, pain, and degeneration of joints.

Osteogenic sarcoma (os-te-o-JEN-ik sar-KO-mah):   Malignant (cancerous) tumor of bone (-GENIC means produced in).

Osteoma (os-te-O-mah):   Tumor (benign) of bone.

Osteomyelitis (os-te-o-mi-eh-LI-tis):   Inflammation of bone and bone marrow. Osteomyelitis is caused by a bacterial infection.

Osteopenia (os-te-o-PE-ne-ah):   Deficiency (-PENIA) of bone tissue.

Osteoporosis (os-te-o-po-RO-sis):   Decrease in bone mass with formation of pores or spaces in normally mineralized bone tissue. This condition is more serious than osteopenia.

Osteotomy (os-te-OT-o-me):   Incision of a bone.

Otalgia (o-TAL-jah):   Pain in an ear.

Otitis (o-TI-tis):   Inflammation of an ear.

Otolaryngologist (o-to-lah-rin-GOL-o-jist):   Specialist in the treatment of diseases of the ear, nose, and throat.

Ovarian (o-VAYR-e-an):   Pertaining to an ovary or ovaries.

Ovarian cancer (o-VAYR-e-an KAN-ser):   Malignant condition of the ovaries.

Ovarian cyst (o-VAYR-e-an sist):   Sac containing fluid or semisolid material in or on the ovary.

Ovary (O-vah-re):   One of two organs in the female abdomen that produces egg cells and female hormones.

Ovum (O-vum):   Egg cell (*plural:*   ova [O-vah]).

Oxygen (OK-sih-jen):   Colorless, odorless gas that is essential to sustaining life.

P

Pancreas (PAN-kre-us):   Gland that produces digestive juices (exocrine function) and the hormone INSULIN (endocrine function).

Pancreatectomy (pan-kre-ah-TEK-to-me):   Removal of the pancreas.

Pancreatitis (pan-kre-ah-TI-tis):   Inflammation of the pancreas.

Paralysis (pah-RAL-ih-sis):   Loss or impairment of movement in a part of the body.

Paraplegia (par-ah-PLE-jah):   Impairment or loss of movement in the lower part of the body, primarily the legs and in some cases bowel and bladder function.

Parathyroid glands (par-ah-THI-royd glanz):   Four endocrine glands behind the thyroid gland. These glands are concerned with maintaining the proper levels of calcium in the blood and bones.

Parathyroid hormone (par-ah-THI-roid HOR-mone):   Hormone secreted by the parathyroid glands to maintain a constant concentration of calcium in the blood and bones. Also called PTH.

Patella (pah-TEL-ah):   Kneecap.

Pathogen (PATH-o-jen):   Disease-producing organism (such as a bacterium or virus).

Pathologist (pah-THOL-o-jist):   Specialist in the study of disease using microscopic examination of tissues and cells and autopsy examination.

Pathology (pah-THOL-o-je):   Study of disease.

Pediatric (pe-de-AT-rik):   Pertaining to treatment of a child.

Pediatrician (pe-de-ah-TRISH-un):   Specialist in the treatment of childhood diseases.

Pediatrics (pe-de-AT-riks):   Branch of medicine specializing in the treatment of children.

Pedodontist (ped-o-DON-tist):   Dentist specializing in the diagnosis and treatment of children's dental problems.

Pelvic (PEL-vik):   Pertaining to the bones of the hip area.

Pelvic cavity (PEL-vik KAV-ih-te):   Space contained within the hip bones (front and sides) and the lower part of the backbone (sacrum and coccyx).

Pelvic inflammatory disease (PEL-vik in-FLAM-ah-to-re dih-ZEEZ):   Inflammation of the pelvic region in females, usually involving the FALLOPIAN TUBES.

Pelvis (PEL-vis):   Lower part of the trunk of the body including the hip bone, tailbone, and sacrum (lower backbones).

Penicillin (pen-ih-SIL-in):   Substance, derived from certain molds, that can destroy bacteria; an ANTIBIOTIC.

Penis (PE-nis):   External male organ containing the urethra, through which both urine and semen (sperm cells and fluid) leave the body.

Peptic ulcer (PEP-tik UL-ser):   Sore (lesion) of the mucous membrane lining the first part of the small intestine (duodenum) or lining the stomach.

Percutaneous (per-ku-TA-ne-us):   Pertaining to through the skin.

Percutaneous transhepatic cholangiography (per-ku-TA-ne-us trans-heh-PAT-ik kol-an-je-OG-rah-fe):   Bile vessels are imaged after injection of contrast material through the skin into the liver.

Perianal (per-e-A-nal):   Pertaining to surrounding the ANUS.

Pericardium (per-e-KAR-de-um):   Membrane surrounding the heart.

Periodontist (per-e-o-DON-tist):   Dentist specializing in the treatment of gum disease (surrounding a tooth).

Periosteum (per-e-OS-te-um):   Membrane that surrounds bone.

Peritoneal (per-ih-to-NE-al):   Pertaining to the PERITONEUM.

Peritoneal dialysis (per-ih-to-NE-al di-AL-ih-sis):   Process of removing wastes from the blood by introducing a special fluid into the abdomen (peritoneal cavity). The wastes pass into the fluid from the bloodstream, and then the fluid is drained from the body.

Peritoneal fluid (per-ih-to-NE-al FLOO-id):   Fluid produced in the abdominal cavity.

Peritoneoscopy (per-ih-to-ne-OS-ko-pe):   Visual examination of the peritoneal cavity with an endoscope. See LAPAROSCOPY.

Peritoneum (per-ih-to-NE-um):   Membrane that surrounds the abdomen and holds the abdominal organs in place.

Peritonitis (per-ih-to-NI-tis):   Inflammation of the peritoneum.

Phalanges (fah-LAN-jeez):   Finger and toe bones.

Pharyngeal (fah-rin-JE-al):   Pertaining to the pharynx (throat).

Pharyngitis (fah-rin-JI-tis):   Inflammation of the pharynx (throat).

Pharynx (FAR-inks):   Organ behind the mouth that receives swallowed food and delivers it into the esophagus. The pharynx (throat) also receives air from the nose and passes it to the trachea (windpipe).

Phenothiazine (fe-no-THI-ah-zeen):   Substance whose derivatives are used as tranquilizers and antipsychotic agents to treat mental illness.

Phlebitis (fleh-BI-tis):   Inflammation of a vein.

Phlebography (fleh-BOG-rah-fe):   X-ray examination of veins after injection of contrast material.

Phlebotomy (fleh-BOT-o-me):   Incision of a vein.

Photoselective vaporization of the prostate (fo-to-se-LEK-tiv va-por-ih-ZA-shun of the PROS-tate):   Use of a GreenLight laser to vaporize and remove prostatic tissue to treat benign prostatic hyperplasia.

Phrenic (FREH-nik):   Pertaining to the DIAPHRAGM.

Physical medicine and rehabilitation (FIZ-ih-kal MED-ih-sin and re-hah-bil-ih-TA-shun):   Field of medicine that specializes in restoring the function of the body after illness.

Pilosebaceous (pi-lo-seh-BA-shus):   Pertaining to hair and its associated sebaceous gland.

Pineal gland (pi-NE-al gland):   Small endocrine gland within the brain that secretes the hormone melatonin, whose exact function is unclear. In lower animals, the pineal gland is a receptor for light.

Pituitary gland (pih-TOO-ih-tar-e gland):   Organ at the base of the brain that secretes hormones. These hormones enter the blood to regulate other organs and other endocrine glands.

Platelet (PLAYT-let):   Cell in the blood that aids clotting; a thrombocyte.

Pleura (PLOO-rah):   Double membrane that surrounds the lungs. *Pleural* means pertaining to the pleura.

Pleural cavity (PLOO-ral KAH-vih-te):   Space between each pleura surrounding the lung.

Pleural effusion (PLOO-ral e-FU-zhun):   Collection of fluid between the double membrane surrounding the lungs.

Pleurisy (PLOO-rih-se):   Inflammation of the PLEURA.

Pleuritis (ploo-RI-tis):   Inflammation of the PLEURA.

Pneumoconiosis (noo-mo-ko-ne-O-sis):   Group of lung diseases resulting from inhalation of particles of dust such as coal, with permanent deposition of such particles in the lung.

Pneumonectomy (noo-mo-NEK-to-me):   Removal of a lung.

Pneumonia (noo-MO-ne-ah):   Abnormal condition of the lungs marked by inflammation and collection of material within the air sacs of the lungs.

Pneumonitis (noo-mo-NI-tis):   Inflammation of a lung or lungs.

Pneumothorax (noo-mo-THOR-aks):   Abnormal accumulation of air in the space between the pleurae.

Polycythemia (pol-e-si-THE-me-ah):   Increase in red blood cells. One form of polycythemia is polycythemia vera, in which the bone marrow produces an excess of erythrocytes and hemoglobin level is elevated.

Polydipsia (pol-e-DIP-se-ah):   Excessive thirst.

Polyneuropathy (pol-e-nu-ROP-ah-the):   Disease of many nerves.

Polyp (POL-ip):   A growth or mass (benign) protruding from a mucous membrane.

Polyuria (pol-e-UR-e-ah):   Excessive urination.

Posteroanterior (pos-ter-o-an-TEER-e-or):   Pertaining to direction from back to front.

Postmortem (post-MOR-tem):   After death.

Postpartum (post-PAR-tum):   After birth.

Posterior (pos-TEER-e-or):   Located in the back portion of a structure or of the body.

Precancerous (pre-KAN-ser-us):   Pertaining to a condition that may come before a cancer; a condition that tends to become malignant.

Prenatal (pre-NA-tal):   Pertaining to before birth.

Proctologist (prok-TOL-o-jist):   Physician who specializes in the study of the anus and rectum.

Proctoscopy (prok-TOS-ko-pe):   Inspection of the anus and rectum with a proctoscope (ENDOSCOPE). Proctoscopy is often performed before rectal surgery.

Proctosigmoidoscopy (prok-to-sig-moyd-OS-ko-pe):   Visual examination of the anus, rectum, and sigmoid colon with an endoscope.

Progesterone (pro-JES-teh-rone):   Hormone secreted by the ovaries to prepare to maintain the uterine lining during pregnancy.

Prognosis (prog-NO-sis):   Prediction as to the outcome of an illness or treatment. Prognosis literally means before (PRO-) knowledge (-GNOSIS).

Prolapse (pro-LAPS):   Falling down or drooping of a part of the body. Prolapse literally means sliding (-LAPSE) forward (PRO-).

Prostate gland (PROS-tayt gland):   Male gland that surrounds the base of the urinary bladder. It produces fluid (semen) that leaves the body with sperm cells.

Prostatectomy (pros-tah-TEK-to-me):   Removal of the prostate gland.

Prostatic (pros-TAH-tik):   Pertaining to the prostate gland.

Prostatic carcinoma (pros-TAH-tik kar-si-NO-mah):   Malignant tumor arising from the PROSTATE GLAND. Also called *prostate cancer.*

Prostatic hyperplasia (pros-TAH-tik hi-per-PLA-zhah):   Abnormal increase in growth (benign) of the prostate gland.

Prosthesis (pros-THE-sis):   Artificial substitute for a missing part of the body. Prosthesis literally means to place (-THESIS) before (PROS-).

Prosthodontist (pros-tho-DON-tist):   Dentist specializing in artificial appliances to replace missing teeth.

Proteinuria (pro-teen-U-re-ah):   Abnormal condition of protein in the urine (albuminuria).

Psychiatrist (si-KI-ah-trist):   Specialist in the treatment of the mind and mental disorders.

Psychiatry (si-KI-ah-tre):   Treatment (IATR/O-) of disorders of the mind (PSYCH/O).

Psychology (si-KOL-o-je):   Study of the mind, especially in relation to human behavior.

Psychosis (si-KO-sis):   Abnormal condition of the mind; a serious mental disorder that involves loss of normal perception of reality (*plural:* psychoses [si-KO-seez]).

Pulmonary (PUL-mo-nair-e):   Pertaining to the lungs.

Pulmonary artery (PUL-mo-nair-e AR-ter-e):   Artery carrying blood from the right ventricle to the lungs.

Pulmonary circulation (PUL-mo-nair-e ser-ku-LA-shun):   Passage of blood from the heart to the lungs and back to the heart.

Pulmonary edema (PUL-mo-nair-e eh-DE-mah):   Abnormal collection of fluid in the lung (within the air sacs of the lung). Fluid backs up into lung tissue commonly from congestive heart failure as the heart weakens and is unable to pump blood effectively.

Pulmonary embolism (PUL-mo-nair-e EM-bo-lizm):   Blockage of blood vessels by foreign matter (clot, tumor, fat, or air). The EMBOLUS frequently arises from the deep veins of the leg.

Pulmonary specialist (PUL-mo-nair-e SPESH-ah-list):   Physician trained to treat lung disorders.

Pupil (PU-pil):   Black center of the eye through which light enters.

Pyelitis (pi-eh-LI-tis):   Inflammation of the renal pelvis (central section of the kidney).

Pyelogram (PI-eh-lo-gram):   Record of the renal pelvis after injection of contrast.

Q

Quadriplegia (kwad-rih-PLE-jah):   Paralysis of all four extremities and usually the trunk of the body caused by injury to the spinal cord in the cervical region of the spine.

R

Radiation oncologist (ra-de-A-shun ong-KOL-o-jist):   Physician trained in the treatment of disease (cancer) with high-energy x-rays or particles.

Radiation therapy (ra-de-A-shun THER-a-pe):   Treatment of disease (cancer) with high-energy x-rays or particles (photons and protons). Also called radiotherapy.

Radioisotope (ra-de-o-I-so-tope):   See RADIONUCLIDE.

Radiologist (ra-de-OL-o-jist):   Physician trained in the use of x-rays (such as computed tomography and also including ultrasound) to diagnose illness.

Radiology (ra-de-OL-o-je):   Science of using x-rays in the diagnosis of disease.

Radionuclide (ra-de-o-NOO-klid):   A chemical substance that emits radioactivity; radioisotope. Radionuclides are used in nuclear medicine to image parts of the body.

Radiotherapist (ra-de-o-THER-ah-pist):   Physician trained to treat disease (cancer) with high-energy x-rays or particles. See RADIATION ONCOLOGIST.

Radiotherapy (ra-de-o-THER-ah-pe):   Treatment of disease (cancer) with high-energy x-rays or particles such as photons and protons. Also called radiation therapy.

Radius (RA-de-us):   One of two lower arm bones. The radius is located on the thumb side of the hand.

Rectal resection (REK-tal re-SEK-shun):   Excision (resection) of the RECTUM.

Rectocele (REK-to-seel):   Hernia (protrusion) of the rectum into the vagina.

Rectum (REK-tum):   End of the colon. The rectum delivers wastes (feces) to the anus for elimination.

Relapse (RE-laps):   Return of disease after its apparent termination.

Remission (re-MISH-un):   Lessening or absence of signs and symptoms of a disease.

Renal (RE-nal):   Pertaining to the kidney.

Renal calculus (RE-nal KAL-ku-lus):   Kidney stone.

Renal failure (RE-nal FAIL-ur):   Condition in which the kidneys no longer function.

Renal pelvis (RE-nal PEL-vis):   Central section of the kidney, where urine collects.

Reproductive (re-pro-DUK-tiv):   Pertaining to the process by which living things produce offspring.

Research (RE-surch):   Laboratory investigation of a medical problem.

Resection (re-SEK-shun):   Removal (excision) of an organ or a structure.

Residency training (RES-i-den-se TRAY-ning):   Period of hospital work involving the care of patients after the completion of four years of medical school.

Respiratory system (RES-pir-ah-tor-e SIS-tem):   Organs that control breathing, allowing air to enter and leave the body.

Retina (RET-ih-nah):   Layer of sensitive cells at the back of the eye. Light is focused on the retina and then is transmitted to the optic nerve, which leads to the brain.

Retinopathy (reh-tih-NOP-ah-the):   Disease of the RETINA.

Retrogastric (reh-tro-GAS-trik):   Pertaining to behind the stomach.

Retroperitoneal (reh-tro-per-ih-to-NE-al):   Pertaining to behind the PERITONEUM.

Rhabdomyosarcoma (rab-do-mi-o-sar-KO-mah):   A malignant tumor of muscle cells (skeletal, voluntary muscle) that occurs most frequently in the head and neck, extremities, body wall, and area behind the abdomen.

Rheumatoid arthritis (ROO-mah-toyd arth-RI-tis):   Chronic inflammatory disease of the joints and connective tissue that leads to deformed joints.

Rheumatologist (roo-mah-TOL-o-jist):   Specialist in the treatment of diseases of connective tissues, especially the joints. RHEUMAT/O- comes from the Greek *rheuma*, meaning "that which flows, as a stream or a river." Inflammatory disorders of joints are often marked by a collection of fluid in joint spaces.

Rheumatology (roo-mah-TOL-o-je):   Branch of medicine dealing with inflammation, degeneration, or chemical changes in connective tissues, such as joints and muscles. Pain, stiffness, or limitation of motion are often characteristics of rheumatologic disorders.

Rhinitis (ri-NI-tis):   Inflammation of the nose.

Rhinoplasty (RI-no-plas-te):   Surgical repair of the nose.

Rhinorrhea (ri-no-RE-ah):   Discharge from the nose.

Rhinotomy (ri-NOT-o-me):   Incision of the nose.

Rib (rib):   One of twelve paired bones surrounding the chest. Seven ribs (true ribs) attach directly to the breastbone, three (false ribs) attach to the seventh rib, and two (floating ribs) are not attached at all.

S

Sacral (SA-kral):   Pertaining to the SACRUM.

Sacral region (SA-kral RE-jun):   Five fused bones in the lower back, below the lumbar bones and wedged between two parts of the hip (ilium).

Sacrum (SA-krum):   Triangular bone in the lower back, below the lumbar bones and formed by five fused bones.

Sagittal plane (SAJ-ih-tal playn):   An imaginary plane that divides an organ or the body into right and left portions. The *midsagittal* plane divides a structure equally into right and left halves.

Sagittal section (SAJ-ih-tal SEK-shun):   Cut (section) through the body, dividing it into a right and a left portion.

Salpingectomy (sal-pin-JEK-to-me):   Removal of a fallopian (uterine) tube.

Salpingitis (sal-pin-JI-tis):   Inflammation of a fallopian (uterine) tube.

Sarcoidosis (sahr-koy-DO-sis):   Chronic, progressive disorder of cells in connective tissue, spleen, liver, bone marrow, lungs, and lymph nodes. Small collections of cells (granulomas) form in affected organs and tissues. The cause is unknown but may involve malfunction of the immune system.

Sarcoma (sar-KO-mah): Cancerous (malignant) tumor of connective tissue, such as bone, muscle, fat, or cartilage.

Scapula (SKAP-u-lah): Shoulder bone.

Sclera (SKLE-rah): White, outer coat of the eyeball.

Scotoma (sko-TO-mah): Defect in vision in a defined area (blind spot).

Scrotal (SKRO-tal): Pertaining to the scrotum.

Scrotum (SKRO-tum): Sac on the outside of the body that contains the testes.

Sebaceous gland (seh-BA-shus gland): Oil-producing (sebum-producing) gland in the skin.

Section (SEK-shun): An act of cutting; a segment or subdivision of an organ.

Seizure (SE-zhur): Convulsion (involuntary contraction of muscles) or attack of epilepsy. A seizure can also indicate a sudden attack or recurrence of a disease.

Sella turcica (SEL-ah TUR-sih-kah): Cup-like depression at the base of the skull that holds the pituitary gland.

Semen (SE-men): Fluid composed of sperm cells and secretions from the prostate gland and other male exocrine glands.

Seminoma (sem-ih-NO-mah): Malignant tumor of the testis.

Sense organs (sens OR-ganz): Parts of the body that receive messages from the environment and relay them to the brain so that we see, hear, and feel sensations. Examples of sense organs are the eye, the ear, and the skin.

Septic (SEP-tik): Pertaining to infection.

Septicemia (sep-tih-SE-me-ah): Infection in the blood. Septicemia is commonly called blood poisoning and is associated with the presence of bacteria or their toxins in the blood.

Sexually transmitted infection (SEK-shoo-ah-le trans-MIT-ed in-FEK-shun): Contagious disease acquired through sexual intercourse or genital contact.

Shock (shok): Group of symptoms (pale skin, rapid pulse, shallow breathing) that indicate poor oxygen supply to tissue and insufficient return of blood to the heart.

Sigmoid colon (SIG-moyd KO-len): S-shaped lower portion of the colon.

Sigmoidoscopy (sig-moyd-OS-ko-pe): Visual examination of the sigmoid colon with an endoscope inserted through the anus and rectum.

Sinus (SI-nus): A cavity or space, such as in a bone. Also, refers to the sinoatrial node or pacemaker of the heart.

Skin (skin): Outer covering that protects the body.

Skull (skul): Bone that surrounds the brain and other organs in the head.

Sleep apnea (SLEEP AP-nee-ah): See APNEA.

Small intestine (smal in-TES-tin): Organ that receives food from the stomach. The small intestine is divided into three sections: duodenum, jejunum, and ileum.

Sonogram (SON-o-gram): Record of sound waves after they bounce off organs in the body; an ULTRASOUND or echogram.

Spasm (SPAZ-um): Involuntary, sudden muscle contraction.

Spermatozoon (sper-mah-to-ZO-on): Sperm cell (*plural:* spermatozoa [sper-mah-to-ZO-ah]).

Spinal (SPI-nal): Pertaining to the spine (backbone).

Spinal cavity (SPI-nal KAV-ih-te): Space in the back that contains the spinal cord and is surrounded by the backbones.

Spinal column (SPI-nal KOL-um): Backbones; vertebrae.

Spinal cord (SPI-nal kord): Bundle of nerves that extends from the brain down the back. Spinal nerves carry electrical messages to and from the spinal cord.

Spinal nerves (SPI-nal nervz): Nerves that transmit messages to and from the spinal cord.

Spinal tap (SPI-nal TAP): See LUMBAR PUNCTURE.

Spirometer (spi-ROM-eh-ter): An instrument for testing lung function by measuring the volume of inspired and expired air.

Spleen (spleen):   Organ in the left upper quadrant of the abdomen. The spleen stores blood cells and destroys red blood cells while producing white blood cells called LYMPHOCYTES.

Splenectomy (splehn-EK-to-me):   Removal of the spleen.

Splenomegaly (splehn-o-MEG-ah-le):   Enlargement of the spleen.

Spondylitis (spon-dih-LI-tis):   Chronic, serious inflammatory disorder of backbones involving erosion and collapse of vertebrae. See ANKYLOSING SPONDYLITIS.

Spondylosis (spon-dih-LO-sis):   Abnormal condition of a vertebra or vertebrae.

Sputum (SPU-tum):   Material expelled from the lungs and expelled through the mouth.

Staging of tumors (STA-ging of TOO-morz):   A system that describes the severity of a patient's cancer based on the extent of the original primary tumor and whether it has spread in the body.

Stent (stent):   A tube inserted into an artery, blood vessel, or duct to keep it open.

Sternum (STER-num):   Breast bone.

Stomach (STUM-ak):   Organ that receives food from the esophagus and sends it to the small intestine. Enzymes in the stomach break down food particles during digestion.

Stomatitis (sto-mah-TI-tis):   Inflammation of the mouth.

Stool culture (stool KUL-tur):   Feces (stools) are placed in a growth medium (culture medium), which is later examined microscopically for evidence of microorganisms (such as bacteria).

Stool guaiac (stool GWI-ak) [test]:   Examination of a small sample of stool for hidden traces of blood; HEMOCCULT TEST.

Stroke (strok):   Trauma to or blockage of blood vessels within the brain, leading to a reduction in the blood supply to brain tissue. This causes nerve cells in the brain to die and results in loss of function to the part of the body controlled by those nerve cells.

Stye (sti):   Infection of a gland in the eyelid, often caused by bacteria (staphylococci). Also spelled *sty*.

Subcostal (sub-KOS-tal):   Pertaining to below the ribs.

Subcutaneous tissue (sub-ku-TA-ne-us TIS-u):   Lower layer of the skin composed of fatty tissue.

Subdural hematoma (sub-DUR-al he-mah-TO-mah):   Collection of blood under the dura mater (outermost layer of the membranes surrounding the brain).

Subgastric (sub-GAS-trik):   Pertaining to below the stomach.

Subhepatic (sub-heh-PAT-ik):   Pertaining to under the liver.

Subscapular (sub-SKAP-u-lar):   Pertaining to under the shoulder bone.

Subtotal (sub-TO-tal):   Less than total; often just under the total amount.

Subungual (sub-UN-gwal):   Pertaining to under (SUB-) a nail (UNGU/O).

Suprarenal glands (soo-prah-RE-nal glanz):   Two endocrine glands, each located above a kidney. See ADRENAL GLANDS.

Surgery (SUR-jer-e):   Branch of medicine that treats disease by manual (hand) or operative methods.

Sweat gland (swet gland):   Organ in the skin that produces a watery substance containing salts.

Syncope (SING-koh-pe):   Fainting; sudden loss of consciousness.

Syndrome (SIN-drom):   Set of symptoms and signs that occur together to indicate a disease condition.

Syphilis (SIF-ih-lis):   Sexually transmitted infection caused by spirochete (type of bacterium).

System (SIS-tem):   Group of organs working together to do a job in the body. For example, the digestive system includes the mouth, throat, stomach, and intestines, all of which help to bring food into the body, break it down, and deliver it to the bloodstream.

Systemic circulation (sis-TEM-ik ser-ku-LA-shun):   Passage of blood from the heart to the tissues of the body and back to the heart.

Systemic lupus erythematosus (sis-TEM-ik LOO-pus er-ih-the-mah-TO-sus):   Chronic inflammatory disease affecting many systems of the body (joints, skin, kidneys, and nerves). A red (erythematous) rash over the nose and cheeks is characteristic.

T

Tachycardia (tak-eh-KAR-de-ah):   Condition of fast, rapid heartbeat.

Tachypnea (tak-ip-NE-ah):   Condition of rapid breathing.

Tendinitis (ten-dih-NI-tis):   Inflammation of a tendon.

Tendon (TEN-don):   Connective tissue that joins muscles to bones.

Tenorrhaphy (ten-OR-ah-fe):   Suture of a tendon.

Testicle (TES-tih-kl):   See TESTIS.

Testicular carcinoma (tes-TIK-u-lar kar-sih-NO-mah):   Malignant tumor originating in a testis. An example is a SEMINOMA.

Testis (TES-tis):   One of two paired male organs in the scrotal sac. The testes (*plural*) produce sperm cells and male hormone (testosterone). Also called a testicle.

Testosterone (tes-TOS-teh-rone):   A hormone that produces male secondary sex characteristics; an ANDROGEN.

Thoracentesis (tho-rah-sen-TE-sis):   Surgical puncture of the chest to remove fluid; thoracocentesis.

Thoracic (tho-RAS-ik):   Pertaining to the chest.

Thoracic cavity (tho-RAS-ik KAV-ih-te):   Space above the abdomen that contains the heart, lungs, and other organs; the chest cavity.

Thoracic region (tho-RAS-ik RE-jun):   Backbones attached to the ribs and located in the region of the chest, between the neck and the waist.

Thoracic surgeon (tho-RAS-ik SUR-jun):   Physician who operates on organs in the chest.

Thoracic vertebra (tho-RAS-ik VER-teh-brah):   A backbone in the region of the chest.

Thoracotomy (tho-rah-KOT-o-me):   Incision of the chest.

Throat (throt):   See PHARYNX.

Thrombocyte (THROM-bo-site):   Clotting cell; a platelet.

Thrombolytic therapy (throm-bo-LIT-ik THER-ah-pe):   Treatment with drugs such as streptokinase and tPA (tissue plasminogen activator) to dissolve clots that may cause a heart attack.

Thrombophlebitis (throm-bo-fleh-BI-tis):   Inflammation of a vein accompanied by formation of a clot.

Thrombosis (throm-BO-sis):   Abnormal condition of clot formation.

Thrombus (THROM-bus):   Blood clot.

Thymoma (thi-MO-mah):   Tumor (malignant) of the thymus gland.

Thymus gland (THI-mus gland):   Endocrine gland in the middle of the chest that produces the hormone *thymosin*. A much larger gland in children, the thymus aids the immune system by stimulating the production of white blood cells (lymphocytes).

Thyroadenitis (thi-ro-ah-deh-NI-tis):   Inflammation of the thyroid gland.

Thyroidectomy (thi-roy-DEK-to-me):   Removal of the thyroid gland.

Thyroid gland (THI-royd gland):   Endocrine gland in the neck that produces hormones that act on cells all over the body. The hormones increase the activity of cells by stimulating metabolism and the release of energy.

Thyroid-stimulating hormone (THI-royd STIM-u-la-ting HOR-mone):   Hormone secreted by the pituitary gland to stimulate the thyroid gland to produce its hormones, such as thyroxine. Also called TSH.

Thyroxine (thi-ROK-sin):   Hormone secreted by the thyroid gland. Also known as T$_4$.

Tibia (TIB-e-ah):   Larger of the two lower leg bones; the shin bone.

Tinnitus (TIN-ih-tus):   Noise in the ears, such as ringing, roaring, or buzzing.

Tissue (TISH-u):   Groups of similar cells that work together to do a job in the body. Examples are muscle tissue, nerve tissue, and epithelial (skin) tissue.

Tissue capillaries (TISH-u KAP-ih-lar-eez):   Tiny blood vessels that lie near cells and through whose walls gases, food, and waste materials pass.

Tomography (to-MOG-rah-fe):   Series of x-ray images that show an organ in depth by producing images of single tissue planes.

Tonsillectomy (ton-sih-LEK-to-me):   Removal (excision) of a tonsil or TONSILS.

Tonsillitis (ton-sih-LI-tis):   Inflammation of the TONSILS.

Tonsils (TON-silz):   Lymphatic tissue in the back of the mouth near the throat.

Trachea (TRA-ke-ah):   Tube that carries air from the throat to the BRONCHIAL TUBES; the windpipe.

Tracheitis (tra-ke-I-tis):   Inflammation of the trachea.

Tracheostomy (tra-ke-OS-to-me):   Opening of the trachea to the outside of the body.

Tracheotomy (tra-ke-OT-o-me):   Incision of the trachea.

Transabdominal (trans-ab-DOM-ih-nal):   Pertaining to across the abdomen.

Transdermal (tranz-DER-mal):   Pertaining to through the skin.

Transgastric (trans-GAS-trik):   Pertaining to across (through) the stomach.

Transhepatic (tranz-he-PAH-tik):   Pertaining to across or through the liver.

Transurethral (trans-u-RE-thral):   Pertaining to across (through) the urethra. TURP is transurethral resection of the prostate by surgery through the urethra.

Transvaginal ultrasound (tranz-VAH-jin-al UL-trah-sownd):   A sound probe is placed in the vagina and ultrasound images are made of the pelvic organs (uterus and ovaries).

Transverse plane (trans-VERS playn):   Imaginary plane that divides an organ or the body into an upper and a lower portion; a cross-sectional view.

Trichophagia (trik-o-FA-jah):   Habit of eating hair; abnormal craving for nonfood substances (dirt, clay, glue, and the like).

Tricuspid valve (tri-KUS-pid valv):   Fold of tissue between the upper and lower chambers on the right side of the heart. It has three cusps or points and prevents backflow of blood into the right ATRIUM when the heart is pumping blood.

Triglyceride (tri-GLIS-eh-ride):   Fat consisting of three molecules of fatty acid and glycerol. It makes up most animal and vegetable fats and is the major lipid (fat) in blood.

Tuberculosis (too-ber-ku-LO-sis):   Infectious, inflammatory disease that commonly affects the lungs, although it can occur in any part of the body. It is caused by the tubercle bacillus (type of bacterium).

Tympanic membrane (tim-PAN-ik MEM-brayn):   See EARDRUM.

Tympanoplasty (tim-pan-o-PLAS-te):   Surgical repair of the eardrum.

U

Ulcer (UL-ser):   Sore or defect in the surface of an organ. Ulcers (hollowed-out spaces) are produced by destruction of tissue.

Ulcerative colitis (UL-seh-rah-tiv ko-LI-tis):   Recurrent inflammatory disorder marked by ulcers in the large bowel. Along with Crohn disease, ulcerative colitis is an INFLAMMATORY BOWEL DISEASE.

Ulna (UL-nah):   One of two lower arm bones. The ulna is located on the little finger side of the hand.

Ultrasonography (ul-trah-so-NOG-rah-fe):   Recording of internal body structures with sound waves.

Ultrasound (UL-tra-sownd):   Sound waves with greater frequency than can be heard by the human ear. This energy is used to detect abnormalities by beaming the waves into the body and recording echoes that reflect off tissues.

Unilateral (u-nih-LAT-er-al):   Pertaining to one side.

Upper gastrointestinal (GI) series (UP-er gas-tro-in-TES-tin-al SEER-eez):   Barium is swallowed and x-ray images are taken of the esophagus, stomach, and small intestine.

Urea (u-RE-ah):   Chief nitrogen-containing waste that the kidney removes from the blood and eliminates from the body in urine.

Uremia (u-RE-me-ah):   Abnormal condition of excessive amounts of urea in the bloodstream.

Ureter (YOOR-eh-ter *or* u-RE-ter):   One of two tubes that lead from the kidney to the urinary bladder.

Ureterectomy (u-re-ter-EK-to-me):   Removal (excision) of a ureter.

Urethra (u-RE-thrah):   Tube that carries urine from the urinary bladder to the outside of the body. In males, the urethra, which is within the penis, also carries sperm from the VAS DEFERENS to the outside of the body when sperm are discharged (ejaculation).

Urethral stricture (u-RE-thral STRIK-shur):   Narrowing of the urethra.

Urethritis (u-re-THRI-tis):   Inflammation of the urethra.

Urinalysis (u-rih-NAL-ih-sis):   Examination of urine to determine its contents.

Urinary bladder (UR-in-air-e BLA-der):   Muscular sac that holds urine and then releases it to leave the body through the urethra.

Urinary catheterization (UR-in-air-e kath-eh-ter-ih-ZA-shun):   Catheter (tube) is passed through the urethra into the urinary bladder for short-term or long-term drainage of urine.

Urinary retention (UR-in-air-e re-TEN-shun):   Condition in which urine is unable to leave the urinary bladder.

Urinary system (UR-in-air-e SIS-tem):   Organs that produce and send urine out of the body. These organs are the kidneys, ureters, bladder, and urethra.

Urinary tract (UR-in-air-e trakt):   Tubes and organs that carry urine from the kidney to the outside of the body.

Urine (UR-in):   Fluid that is produced by the kidneys, passed through the ureters, stored in the bladder, and released from the body through the urethra.

Urologist (u-ROL-o-jist):   Specialist in operating on the urinary tract in males and females and on the reproductive tract in males.

Urology (u-ROL-o-je):   Study of the urinary system in males and females and the reproductive tract in males.

Uterine (U-ter-in):   Pertaining to the uterus.

Uterine artery embolization (U-ter-in AR-ter-e em-bo-lih-ZA-shun):   Blockage of blood flow in the uterine artery to slow the growth of uterine fibroids.

Uterine tubes (U-ter-in toobz):   See FALLOPIAN TUBES.

Uterus (U-ter-us):   Muscular organ in a female that holds and provides nourishment for the developing fetus; the WOMB.

Vagina (vah-JI-nah):   Muscular passageway from the uterus to the outside of the body.

Vaginitis (vah-jih-NI-tis):   Inflammation of the vagina.

Valve (valv):   Natural structure or artificial device that prevents backward flow of fluid (such as blood).

Varicocele (VAR-ih-ko-seel):   Swollen, twisted veins within the spermatic cord, above the testes. It produces a swelling in the scrotum that feels like a "bag of worms."

Varix (VAH-riks):   Enlarged, swollen, tortuous veins (*plural:*   varices [VAH-ri-seez]).

Vas deferens (vas DEF-er-enz):   One of two tubes that carry sperm from the testes to the urethra for ejaculation.

Vascular (VAS-ku-lar):   Pertaining to blood vessels.

Vasculitis (vas-ku-LI-tis):   Inflammation of blood vessels.

Vasectomy (vas-EK-to-me):   Removal of the vas deferens or a portion of it so that sperm cells are prevented from becoming part of SEMEN.

Vasoconstrictor (vas-o-kon-STRIK-tor):   Drug that narrows blood vessels, especially small arteries.

Vasodilator (vas-o-DI-la-tor):   Agent that widens blood vessels.

Vein (van):   Blood vessel that carries blood back to the heart from tissues of the body.

Ventricle (VEN-trih-kl):   One of the two lower chambers of the heart. The right ventricle receives blood from the right atrium (upper chamber) and sends it to the lungs. The left ventricle receives blood from the left atrium and sends it to the body through the aorta.

Ventricular arrhythmia (ven-TRIK-u-lar ah-RITH-me-ah):   Abnormal heart rhythm originating in the lower chambers of the heart.

Venule (VEN-ul):   Small vein.

Venulitis (ven-u-LI-tis):   Inflammation of a small vein.

Vertebra (VER-teh-brah):   A backbone.

Vertebrae (VER-teh-bray):   Backbones.

Vertebral (VER-teh-bral):   Pertaining to a backbone.

Vertebroplasty (ver-teh-bro-PLAS-te):   Surgical repair of backbone fractures by injecting cement into vertebrae to strengthen them and relieve pain.

Vesical (VES-ih-kal):   Pertaining to the urinary bladder (VESIC/O).

Virtual colonoscopy (VER-chu-al ko-lon-OS-ko-pe):   See CT COLONOGRAPHY.

Virus (VI-rus):   Small infectious agent that can reproduce itself only when it is inside another living cell (host).

Visceral (VIS-er-al):   Pertaining to internal organs.

Womb (woom):   See UTERUS.

Wound (woond):   Any physical injury involving a break in the skin (chest wound, gunshot wound, puncture wound, and so on).

Glossary of Word Parts

GLOSSARY 2

*Also appears on the Student Evolve Resources.

Section I of this glossary is a list of **medical terminology** word parts and their **English** meanings. **Section II** is the reverse of that list, giving **English** meanings and their corresponding **medical terminology** word parts. If you wish to identify various combining forms, suffixes, and prefixes for the corresponding English term, check Section II.

Section I: Medical Terminology → English

WORD PART	MEANING
a-, an-	no, not
ab-	away from
abdomin/o	abdomen; *see also* lapar/o
-ac	pertaining to
ad-	toward
aden/o	gland
adenoid/o	adenoids
adren/o	adrenal gland
-al	pertaining to
-algia	pain; *see also* -dynia
alveol/o	alveolus (air sac within the lung)
amni/o	amnion (sac that surrounds the embryo)
-an	pertaining to
ana-	up, apart
an/o	anus
angi/o	vessel (blood)
ante-	before, forward
anter/o	front
anti-	against
aort/o	aorta
append/o, appendic/o	appendix
-ar	pertaining to
arteri/o	artery
arteriol/o	small artery
arthr/o	joint
-ary	pertaining to
ather/o	fatty plaque
-ation	process, condition
aur/o	ear; *see also* ot/o
aut-	self
axill/o	armpit
balan/o	penis
bari/o	weight
bi-	two
bi/o	life
blephar/o	eyelid
brady-	slow
bronch/o	bronchial tube
bronchiol/o	small bronchial tube

calcane/o	calcaneus (heel bone)
capillar/o	capillary
carcin/o	cancer, cancerous
cardi/o	heart
carp/o	wrist bones (carpals)
-cele	hernia
-centesis	surgical puncture to remove fluid
cephal/o	head
cerebell/o	cerebellum (posterior part of the brain)
cerebr/o	cerebrum (largest part of the brain)
cervic/o	neck
chem/o	drug, chemical
cholecyst/o	gallbladder
choledoch/o	common bile duct
chondr/o	cartilage
chron/o	time
-cision	process of cutting
cis/o	to cut
clavicul/o	clavicle (collarbone)
-coccus	bacterium (berry-shaped); *plural:* -cocci
coccyg/o	tailbone
col/o	colon (large intestine)
colon/o	colon
colp/o	vagina
comi/o	to care for
con-	with, together
coni/o	dust
-coniosis	abnormal condition of dust
coron/o	heart
cost/o	rib
crani/o	skull
crin/o	secrete
-crine	secretion
-crit	separation
cry/o	cold
cutane/o	skin
cyan/o	blue
cyst/o	urinary bladder
-cyte	cell
cyt/o	cell
dactyl/o	fingers or toes
dent/i	tooth
dermat/o, derm/o	skin
dia-	thorough, complete
-dipsia	thirst
duoden/o	duodenum
dur/o	dura mater (outermost meningeal layer)
-dynia	pain
dys-	abnormal, bad, difficult, painful

-eal	pertaining to
ec-	out, outside
-ectasia, -ectasis	dilation, stretching, widening
ecto-	out, outside
-ectomy	excision (resection, removal); process of cutting out
electr/o	electricity
-emesis	vomiting
-emia	blood condition
en-	in, inner, within
encephal/o	brain
endo-	within, in, inner
endocrin/o	endocrine glands
endometr/o, endometri/o	endometrium (inner lining of the uterus)
enter/o	intestines (usually small intestine)
epi-	above, upon
epiglott/o	epiglottis
epitheli/o	skin (surface tissue)
erythr/o	red
esophag/o	esophagus
esthesi/o	sensation
ex-, exo-, extra-	out, outside
femor/o	femur, thigh bone
fibr/o	fibrous tissue
fibul/o	fibula (smaller lower leg bone)
gastr/o	stomach
gen/o	to produce
-gen	production, formation
-genesis	producing, forming
-genic	pertaining to producing, produced by
ger/o	old age
-globin	protein
glyc/o	sugar
gnos/o	knowledge
-gram	record
-graph	instrument to record
-graphy	process of recording, to record
gynec/o	woman, female
hemat/o, hem/o	blood
hepat/o	liver
humer/o	humerus (upper arm bone)
hydr/o	water
hyper-	above, excessive, more than normal, too much
hypo-	below, deficient, less than normal, too little
hypophys/o	pituitary gland
hyster/o	uterus
-ia	condition
-ian	practitioner

iatr/o	treatment
-ic, -ical	pertaining to
ile/o	ileum (third part of small intestine)
ili/o	ilium (upper part of hip bone)
in-	in, into
-ine	pertaining to
infra-	below
inguin/o	groin
inter-	between
intra-	within
-ior	pertaining to
isch/o	to hold back
-ism	condition, process
-ist	specialist
-itis	inflammation
jejun/o	jejunum
lapar/o	abdomen
-lapse	slide
laryng/o	larynx (voice box)
later/o	side
ligament/o	ligament
leiomy/o	smooth muscle
leuk/o	white
lip/o	fat
-listhesis	sliding
lith/o	stone
-lith	stone
-logist	one who specializes in study of
-logy	process of study, study of
lumb/o	loin, waist region
lymph/o	lymph
lymphaden/o	lymph nodes
lymphangi/o	lymph vessel
lys/o	breakdown, destruction, separation
-lysis	breakdown, destruction, separation
mal-	bad
-malacia	softening
mamm/o	breast
mast/o	breast
mediastin/o	mediastinum
medull/o	medulla oblongata (lower part of the brain)
-megaly	enlargement
men/o	menstruation
mening/o	meninges (membranes covering brain and spinal cord)
meta-	beyond, change
metacarp/o	metacarpals (hand bones)
metatars/o	metatarsals (foot bones)
-meter	measure

metr/o, metri/o	uterus; to measure
-metry	measurement
-mortem	death
-motor	movement
muscul/o	muscle
my/o	muscle
myel/o	bone marrow (with -blast,-cyte, -genous, -oma)
myel/o	spinal cord (with -cele, -gram, -itis)
myos/o	muscle
myring/o	eardrum
nas/o	nose
nat/i	birth
necr/o	death
neo-	new
nephr/o	kidney
neur/o	nerve
norm/o	rule, order
nos/o	disease
obstetr/o	midwife
ocul/o	eye
odont/o	tooth
-oid	pertaining to, resembling
-oma	tumor, mass, swelling
onc/o	tumor
onycho/o	nail
o/o	egg
oophor/o	ovary
ophthalm/o	eye
-opsy	process of viewing
opt/o, optic/o	eye
or/o	mouth
orch/o	testicle, testis
orchi/o	testicle, testis
orchid/o	testicle, testis
orth/o	straight
-osis	abnormal condition
osm/o	smell
oste/o	bone
ot/o	ear
-ous	pertaining to
ovari/o	ovary
pancreat/o	pancreas
para-	along the side of, beside, near
parathyroid/o	parathyroid gland
-partum	birth
path/o	disease
-pathy	disease condition
ped/o	child

pelv/o	hip bone
-penia	deficiency
per-	through
peri-	surrounding
peritone/o	peritoneum (membrane around abdominal organs)
perone/o	fibula
-pexy	fixation (surgical)
phak/o	lens of the eye
phalang/o	phalanges (finger and toe bones)
pharyng/o	pharynx, throat
-phasia	speech
-philia	attraction to
phleb/o	vein
phren/o	diaphragm
phren/o	mind
pituitar/o	pituitary gland
plas/o	development, formation, growth
-plasm	development, formation, growth
-plasia	formation, growth
-plasty	surgical repair
-plegia	paralysis
pleur/o	pleura (membranes surrounding the lungs)
-pnea	breathing
pneum/o	air, lung
pneumon/o	lung
-poiesis	formation
poly-	many, much
post-	after, behind
poster/o	back, behind
pre-	before
pro-, pros-	before, forward
prosth/o	artificial replacement
proct/o	anus and rectum
prostat/o	prostate gland
psych/o	mind
-ptosis	prolapse, sagging
-ptysis	spitting
pulmon/o	lung
pyel/o	renal pelvis (central section of the kidney)
radi/o	x-ray; radius (lateral lower arm bone)
re-, retro-	behind, back
rect/o	rectum
ren/o	kidney
retin/o	retina of the eye
rhabdomy/o	striated (skeletal) muscle
rheumat/o	flow, fluid
rhin/o	nose
-rrhage	excess flow of blood
-rrhagia	excess flow of blood
-rrhaphy	suture
-rrhea	discharge, flow

sacr/o	sacrum
salping/o	fallopian (uterine) tube; eustachian tube
-salpinx	fallopian (uterine) tube; eustachian tube
sarc/o	flesh
scapul/o	shoulder blade (bone)
-sclerosis	hardening
-scope	instrument to view or visually examine
-scopy	process of visual examination
scrot/o	scrotal sac, scrotum
-section	process of cutting into
sept/o	infection
septic/o	infection
-sis	condition
-somatic	pertaining to the body
son/o	sound
-spasm	constriction
spin/o	backbone, spine, vertebra
splen/o	spleen
spondyl/o	backbone, vertebra
-stasis	control, stop; place, to stand
-stat	stop, control
-stenosis	narrowing
stern/o	sternum (breastbone)
stomat/o	mouth
-stomy	opening
sub-	below, under
supra-	above
sym-	with, together (use before b, p, and m)
syn-	with, together
tachy-	fast
tendin/o, ten/o	tendon
-tension	pressure
theli/o, thel/o	nipple
-therapy	treatment
-thesis	put, place
thorac/o	chest
thromb/o	clot
thym/o	thymus gland
thyr/o, thyroid/o, thyroaden/o	thyroid gland
tibi/o	tibia or shin bone (larger lower leg bone)
-tic	pertaining to
-tomy	incision, process of cutting into
tonsill/o	tonsils
top/o	to put, place
trache/o	trachea, windpipe
trans-	across, through
tri-	three
troph/o	development, nourishment

-trophy	development, nourishment
tympan/o	eardrum
uln/o	ulna (medial lower arm bone)
ultra-	beyond
-um	structure
ungu/o	nail
uni-	one
ureter/o	ureter
urethr/o	urethra
ur/o	urine, urinary tract
-uria	urine condition
uter/o	uterus
vagin/o	vagina
vas/o	vas deferens, vessel
vascul/o	blood vessel
ven/o	vein
venul/o	venule
vertebr/o	backbone, vertebra
vesic/o	urinary bladder
-y	condition, process

Section II: English → Medical Terminology

MEANING	WORD PART
abdomen	abdomin/o (*use with* -al, -centesis)
	lapar/o (*use with* -scope, -scopy, -tomy)
abnormal	dys-
abnormal condition	-osis
abnormal condition of dust	-coniosis
above	epi-, hyper-, supra-
across	trans-
adenoids	adenoid/o
adrenal gland	adren/o
after	post-
against	anti-
air	pneum/o
air sac	alveol/o
along the side of	para-
alveolus	alveol/o
amnion	amni/o
anus	an/o
anus and rectum	proct/o
aorta	aort/o
apart	ana-
appendix	append/o (*use with* -ectomy)
	appendic/o (*use with* -itis)
armpit	axill/o
artery	arteri/o
artificial replacement	prosth/o
attraction to	-philia
away from	ab-
back	poster/o, re-, retro-
backbone	spin/o (*use with* -al)
	spondyl/o (*use with* -itis, -listhesis, -osis, -pathy)
	vertebr/o (*use with* -al)
bacterium (berry-shaped)	-coccus (*plural:* -cocci)
bad	dys-, mal-
before	ante-, pre-, pro-, pros-
behind	post-, poster/o, re-, retro-
below	hypo-, infra-, sub-
beside	para-
between	inter-
beyond	meta-, ultra-
birth	nat/i, -partum
bladder (urinary)	cyst/o (*use with* -ic, -itis, -cele, -gram, -scopy)
	vesic/o (*use with* -al, -stomy, -tomy)
blood	hem/o (*use with* -cyte, -dialysis, -globin, -lysis, -philia, -ptysis, -rrhage, -stasis, -stat)
	hemat/o (*use with* -crit, -emesis, -logist, -logy, -oma, -poiesis, -salpinx, -uria)

blood condition	-emia
blood flow, excess	-rrhage, -rrhagia
blood vessel	angi/o (*use with* -ectomy, -dysplasia, -genesis, -gram, -graphy, -oma, -plasty, -spasm)
	vas/o (*use with* -constriction, -dilatation, -motor)
	vascul/o (*use with* -ar, -itis)
blue	cyan/o
body	-somatic
bone	oste/o
bone marrow	myel/o
brain	encephal/o
breakdown	-lysis, lys/o
breast	mamm/o (*use with* -ary, -gram, -graphy, -plasty)
	mast/o (*use with* -algia, -ectomy, -itis)
breastbone	stern/o
breathing	-pnea
bronchial tube	bronch/o
bronchiole	bronchiol/o
calcaneus	calcane/o
cancer	carcin/o
cancerous	carcin/o
capillary	capillar/o
care for (to)	comi/o
carpals	carp/o
cartilage	chondr/o
cell	-cyte, cyt/o
cerebellum	cerebell/o
cerebrum	cerebr/o
change	meta-
chemical	chem/o
chest	thorac/o
child	ped/o
clavicle	clavicul/o
clot	thromb/o
cold	cry/o
collarbone	clavicul/o
colon	col/o (*use with* -ectomy, -itis, -stomy)
	colon/o (*use with* -pathy, -scope, -scopy)
common bile duct	choledoch/o
complete	dia-
condition	-ation, -ia, -ism, -osis, -sis, -y
condition of blood	-emia
constriction	-spasm
control	-stasis, -stat
cut	-cision, cis/o, -section, -tomy
death	-mortem, necr/o
deficiency	-penia
deficient	hypo-
destruction	lys/o, -lysis

development	plas/o, -plasm, troph/o, -trophy
dilation	-ectasia, -ectasis
diaphragm	phren/o
difficult	dys-
discharge	-rrhea
disease	nos/o; path/o, -pathy
drug	chem/o
duodenum	duoden/o
dura mater	dur/o
dust	coni/o
dust condition	-coniosis
ear	aur/o, ot/o
eardrum	myring/o (*use with* -ectomy, -itis, -tomy)
	tympan/o (*use with* -ic, -metry, -plasty)
egg	o/o
electricity	electr/o
endocrine gland	endocrin/o
endometrium	endometri/o
enlargement	-megaly
epiglottis	epiglott/o
esophagus	esophag/o
eustachian tube	salping/o, -salpinx
excessive	hyper-
excision	-ectomy
eye	ocul/o (*use with* -ar, -facial, -motor)
	ophthalm/o (*use with* -ia, -ic, -logist, -logy, -pathy, -plasty, -plegia, -scope, -scopy)
	opt/o (*use with* -ic, -metrist)
	optic/o (*use with* -ian)
eyelid	blephar/o
fallopian tube	salping/o, -salpinx
fast	tachy-
fat	lip/o
fatty plaque	ather/o
female	gynec/o
femur	femor/o
fibrous tissue	fibr/o
fibula	fibul/o, perone/o
fingers	dactyl/o
fixation (surgical)	-pexy
flesh	sarc/o
flow	-rrhea, rheumat/o
fluid	rheumat/o
foot bones	metatars/o
formation	-genesis, -plasia, plas/o, -plasm, -poiesis
forward	ante-, pro-, pros-
front	anter/o

gallbladder	cholecyst/o
gland	aden/o
groin	inguin/o
growth	plas/o, -plasm
hand bones	metacarp/o
hardening	-sclerosis
head	cephal/o
heart	cardi/o (*use with* -ac, -graphy, -logy, -logist, -megaly, -pathy, -vascular)
	coron/o (*use with* -ary)
heel bone	calcane/o
hernia	-cele
hip bone	pelv/o
hold back (to)	isch/o
humerus	humer/o
ileum	ile/o
ilium	ili/o
in, into	in-, en-, endo-
incision	-section, -tomy
infection	sept/o, septic/o
inflammation	-itis
inner	en-, endo-
instrument to record	-graph
instrument to visually examine	-scope
intestines (small)	enter/o
jejunum	jejun/o
joint	arthr/o
kidney	nephr/o (*use with* -algia, -ectomy, -ic, -itis, -lith, -megaly, -oma, -osis, -pathy, -ptosis, -sclerosis, -stomy, -tomy)
	ren/o (*use with* -al, -gram)
kidney (central section)	pyel/o
knowledge	gnos/o
larynx	laryng/o
lens of the eye	phak/o
less than normal	hypo-
life	bi/o
ligament	ligament/o
liver	hepat/o
loin	lumb/o
lung	pneum/o (*use with* -coccus, -coniosis, -thorax)
	pneumon/o (*use with* -ectomy, -ia, -ic, -itis, -pathy)
	pulmon/o (*use with* -ary)
lymph	lymph/o
lymph node	lymphaden/o
lymph vessel	lymphangi/o

mass	-oma
many	poly-
measure (to)	meter, metr/o, metry
mediastinum	mediastin/o
medulla oblongata	medull/o
meninges	mening/o
menstruation	men/o
metacarpals	metacarp/o
metatarsals	metatars/o
midwife	obstetr/o
mind	psych/o, phren/o
more than normal	hyper-
mouth	or/o (*use with* -al)
	stomat/o (*use with* -itis)
movement	-motor
much	poly-
muscle	muscul/o (*use with* -ar, -skeletal)
	myos/o (*use with* -itis)
	my/o (*use with* -algia, -ectomy, -oma, -gram, -neural)
nail	onych/o (*use with* -lys), ungu/o (*use with* -al)
narrowing	-stenosis
near	para-
neck	cervic/o
nerve	neur/o
new	neo-
nipple	thel/o, theli/o
no, not	a-, an-
nose	nas/o (*use with* -al)
	rhin/o (*use with* -itis, -rrhea, -plasty)
nourishment	troph/o, -trophy
old age	ger/o
one	uni-
opening	-stomy
order	norm/o
out, outside	ec-, ecto-, ex-, exo- extra-
ovary	oophor/o (*use with* -itis, -ectomy, -pexy, -plasty, -tomy)
	ovari/o (*use with* -an)
pain	-algia, -dynia
painful	dys-
pancreas	pancreat/o
paralysis	-plegia
parathyroid gland	parathyroid/o
pelvis	pelv/o
pelvis (renal)	pyel/o
penis	balan/o
peritoneum	peritone/o
pertaining to	-ac, -al, -an, -ar, -ary, -eal, -ic, -ine, -ior, -oid, -ous, -tic
pertaining to the body	-somatic

phalanges	phalang/o
pharynx	pharyng/o
pituitary gland	hypophys/o, pituitar/o
place	top/o, -stasis
pleura	pleur/o
practitioner	-ian
pressure	-tension
process	-ation, -ism, -y
process of cutting into	-cision, -tomy, -section
process of cutting out	-ectomy
process of recording	-graphy
process of viewing	-opsy
produce (to)	-gen, gen/o
produced by	-genic
producing	-genic, -genesis
prolapse	-ptosis
prostate gland	prostat/o
puncture to remove fluid	-centesis
put, place (to)	-thesis, top/o
radius (lower arm bone)	radi/o
record	-gram
recording (process)	-graphy
rectum	rect/o
red	erythr/o
removal	-ectomy
renal pelvis	pyel/o
repair	-plasty
resection	-ectomy
resembling	-oid
retina of the eye	retin/o
rib	cost/o
rule	norm/o
sacrum	sacr/o
sagging	-ptosis
scapula	scapul/o
scrotum, scrotal sac	scrot/o
secrete, secretion	-crine, crin/o
self	aut-
sensation	esthesi/o
separation	-crit, -lysis, lys/o
shin bone	tibi/o
shoulder blade	scapul/o
side	later/o
skin	cutane/o (*use with* -ous)
	derm/o (*use with* -al); dermat/o (*use with* -itis, -logy, -osis)
	epitheli/o (*use with* -al)
skull	crani/o
sliding	-lapse, -listhesis
slip (to)	-listhesis

slow	brady-
small artery	arteriol/o
small bronchial tube	bronchiol/o
small intestine	enter/o
smell	osm/o
smooth muscle	leiomy/o
softening	-malacia
sound	son/o
specialist	-ist
speech	-phasia
spinal cord	myel/o
spine	spin/o
spitting	-ptysis
spleen	splen/o
stand (to)	-stasis
sternum	stern/o
stomach	gastr/o
stone	lith/o, -lith
stop	-stasis, -stat
straight	orth/o
stretching	-ectasia, -ectasis
striated (skeletal) muscle	rhabdomy/o
structure	-um
study of	-logy
sugar	glyc/o
surgical puncture to remove fluid	-centesis
surgical repair	-plasty
surrounding	peri-
suture	-rrhaphy
swelling	-oma
tailbone	coccyg/o
tendon	tendin/o, ten/o
testicle, testis	orch/o, orchi/o, orchid/o
thigh bone	femor/o
thirst	-dipsia
throat	pharyng/o
three	tri-
through	dia-, per-, trans-
thymus gland	thym/o
thyroid gland	thyr/o, thyroid/o, thyroaden/o
tibia	tibi/o
time	chron/o
toes	dactyl/o
together	con-, syn-, sym-
tonsil	tonsill/o
too much	hyper-
too little	hypo-
tooth	dent/i, odont/o
toward	ad-

trachea	trache/o
treatment	iatr/o, -therapy
tumor	-oma, onc/o
two	bi-
ulna	uln/o
under	hypo-, sub-
up	ana-
upon	epi-
ureter	ureter/o
urethra	urethr/o
urinary bladder	cyst/o, vesic/o
urinary tract	ur/o
urine	ur/o
urine condition	-uria
uterus	hyster/o (*use with* -ectomy, -graphy, -gram)
	metr/o (*use with* -itis, -rrhagia)
	metri/o (*use with* -al)
	uter/o (*use with* -ine)
uterus (inner lining)	endometr/o, endometri/o
vagina	colp/o (*use with* -pexy, -plasty, -scope, -scopy, -tomy)
	vagin/o (*use with* -al, -itis)
vas deferens	vas/o
vein	phleb/o (*use with* -ectomy, -itis, -lith, -thrombosis, -tomy)
	ven/o (*use with* -ous, -gram)
venule	venul/o
vertebra	spin/o (*use with* -al)
	spondyl/o (*use with* -itis, -listhesis, -osis, -pathy)
	vertebr/o (*use with* -al)
vessel	angi/o (*use with* -ectomy, -dysplasia, -genesis, -gram, -graphy, -oma, -plasty, -spasm)
	vas/o (*use with* -constriction, -dilation, -motor)
	vascul/o (*use with* -ar, -itis)
view (to)	-opsy
visual examination	-scopy
voice box	laryng/o
vomiting	-emesis
waist region	lumb/o
water	hydr/o
weight	bari/o
white	leuk/o
widening	-ectasia, -ectasis
windpipe	trache/o
with	con-, syn-, sym-
within	en-, endo-, intra-
woman	gynec/o
wrist bones	carp/o
x-ray	radi/o

Glossary of English→ Spanish Terms*

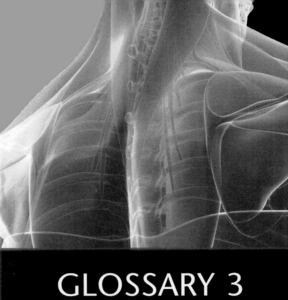

*Diagrams of the body labeled with Spanish terms are on pages 400 and 401.

Here is a list of English → Spanish terms that will help you communicate with Spanish-speaking patients in offices, hospitals, and other medical settings. Included are parts of the body and other medical terms as well.

abdomen	abdomen (ahb-DOH-mehn)
acne	acné (ahk-NEH)
acoustic	acústico (ah-KOOS-tee-ko)
adenoid	adenoide (ah-deh-NOH-ee-deh)
amebic	amébico (ah-MEH-bee-ko)
analgesic	analgésico (ah-nahl-HEH-see-koh)
anemia	anemia (ah-NEH-mee-ah)
anesthesia	anestesia (ah-nehs-TEH-see-ah)
angina	angina (ahn-HEE-na)
angioma	angioma (ahn-hee-OH-mah)
ankle	tobillo (toh-BEE-yoh)
antacid	antiácido (ahn-tee-AH-see-doh)
antiarrhythmic	antiarrítmico (ahn-tee-ah-RREET-mee-koh)
antibiotic	antibiótico (ahn-tee-bee-OH-tee-koh)
anticonvulsant	anticonvulsivante (ahn-tee-kohn-bool-SEE-ban-teh)
antidiarrheal	antidiarrético (ahn-tee-dee-ah-RREH-tee-koh)
antiemetic	antiemético (ahn-tee-eh-MEH-tee-koh)
antiepileptic	antiepiléptico (ahn-tee-eh-pee-LEHP-tee-koh)
antihistamine	antihistamínico (ahn-tee-ees-tah-MEE-nee-koh)
antiviral	antivirus (ahn-tee-BEE-roos)
anus	ano (AH-no)
appendix	apéndice (ah-PEHN-dee-seh)
arm	brazo (BRAH-soh)
armpit	axila (ahk-SEE-lah)
arteriogram	arteriograma (ahr-teh-ree-oh-GRAH-mah)
arthritis	artritis (ahr-TREE-tees)
asthma	asma (AHS-mah)
bacteria	bacteria (bahk-TEH-ree-ah)
barbiturates	barbitúricos (bahr-bee-TOO-ree-kohs)
birthmark	lunar (loo-NAHR)
bleeding	sangrado (sahn-GRAH-doh)
blood	sangre (SAHN-greh)
blood count	biometría hemática (bee-oh-meh-TREE-ah eh-MAH-tee-kah)
bradycardia	bradicardia (brah-dee-KAHR-dee-ah)
brain	cerebro (seh-REH-bro)
breast/chest	seno (SEH-noh), pecho (PEH-choh)
bronchial tube	bronquio (BROHN-kee-oh)
bronchitis	bronquitis (brohn-KEE-tees)
bruises	moretónes (moh-reh-TOH-nehs)
burn	quemadura (keh-mah-DOO-rah)
buttocks	nalgas (NAHL-gahs)
calf	pantorrilla (pahn-toh-RREE-yah)
callus	callo (KAH-yoh)
calm	calma (KAHL-mah)
cardiac	cardiaco (kahr-DEE-ah-koh)

cataract	catarata (kah-tah-RAH-tah)
cervix	cuello uterino (KOO-eh-yoh) (oo-teh-REE-noh), cerviz (SERH-bees)
chancre	chancro (CHAHN-kroh)
cheek	mejilla (meh-HEE-yah)
chemotherapy	quimioterapia (kee-mee-oh-teh-RAH-pee-ah)
chin	barbilla (bar-BEE-yah)
cholesterol	colesterol (koh-lehs-teh-ROHL)
cirrhosis	cirrosis (see-RROH-sees)
claustrophobia	claustrofobia (klah-oos-troh-FOH-bee-ah)
coagulation	coagulación (koh-ah-goo-lah-see-OHN)
collar bone	clavícula (klah-VEE-kuh-la)
colon	colon (KOH-lohn)
constipation	estreñimiento (ehs-treh-nyee-mee-EHN-toh)
cortisone	cortisona (kohr-tee-SOH-nah)
cough	tos (tohs)
cyanotic	cianótico (see-ah-NOH-tee-ko)
decongestants	descongestionantes (dehs-kohn-hehs-tee-oh-NAHN-tehs)
dehydrated	deshidratado (deh-see-drah-TAH-doh)
delirious	delirio (deh-LEE-ree-oh)
depressed	deprimido (deh-pree-MEE-doh)
diabetes	diabetes (dee-ah-BEH-tehs)
diarrhea	diarrea (dee-ah-RREH-ah)
digitalis	digital (dee-hee-TAHL)
ear (inner)	oído (oh-EE-do)
ear (outer)	oreja (oh-REH-hah)
ecchymosis	equimosis (eh-kee-MOH-sees)
eczema	eccema (ehk-SEH-mah)
elbow	codo (KOH-doh)
embolism	embolia (ehm-boh-LEE-ah)
emetic	emético (eh-MEH-tee-koh)
enteritis	enteritis (ehn-teh-REE-tees)
epilepsy	epilepsia (eh-pee-LEHP-see-ah)
euphoric	eufórico (eh-oo-FOH-ree-koh)
exudate	exudado (ehk-soo-DAH-doh)
eye	ojo (OH-hoh)
eyebrow	ceja (SEH-hah)
eyelash	pestaña (pehs-TAH-nyah)
eyelids	párpados (PAHR-pah-dohs)
fibroid	-fibroma (fee-BROH-mah)
finger	dedo (DEH-doh)
fingernail	uña (OO-nyah)
fist	puño (POO-nyoh)
fistula	fístula (FEES-too-lah)
foot	pie (pee-EH)
forearm	antebrazo (an-teh-BRAH-zoh)
forehead	frente (FREN-teh)
fungus	hongo (OHN-goh)

gallbladder	vesícula biliar (beh-SEE-koo-lah bee-lee-AHR)
gangrene	gangrena (gahn-GREH-nah)
gastroenteritis	gastroenteritis (gahs-troh-ehn-teh-REE-tees)
gastroenterology	gastroenterología (gahs-troh-ehn-teh-roh-loh-HEE-ah)
genital organs	órganos genitales (ORH-gah-nohs heh-nee-TAH-lehs)
glaucoma	glaucoma (glah-oo-KOH-mah)
groin	ingle (EEN-gleh)
gums	encías (ehn-SEE-ahs)
gynecologist	ginecólogo (hee-neh-KOH-loh-goh)
hair	cabello (kah-BEH-yoh)
hand	mano (MAH-noh)
head	cabeza (kah-BEH-sah)
heart	corazón (koh-rah-SOHN)
heel	talón (tah-LOHN)
hematology	hematología (eh-mah-toh-loh-HEE-ah)
hematoma	hematoma (eh-mah-TOH-mah)
hemolysis	hemólisis (eh-MOH-lee-sees)
hemorrhage	hemorragia (eh-moh-RRAH-hee-ah)
hepatitis	hepatitis (eh-pah-TEE-tees)
hernia	hernia (EHR-nee-ah)
hip	cadera (kah-DEH-rah)
hypertension	hipertensión (ee-pehr-tehn-see-OHN)
icteric	ictérico (eek-TEH-ree-koh)
infection	infección (een-fehk-see-OHN)
inflammation	inflamación (een-flah-mah-see-OHN)
insulin	insulina (een-soo-LEE-nah)
intestine	intestino (een-tes-TEE-noh)
intramuscular	intramuscular (een-trah-moos-koo-LAHR)
intravenous	intravenoso (een-trah-beh-NOH-soh)
irradiate	irradiar (ee-rrhah-dee-AHR)
jaw	mandíbula (mahn-DEE-boo-lah)
kidney	riñón (ree-NYON)
knee	rodilla (ro-DEE-yah)
laparoscopy	laparoscopia (lah-pah-rohs-KOH-pee-ah)
laryngitis	laringitis (lah-reen-HEE-tees)
laxative	laxante (lahk-SAHN-teh)
left	izquierdo (ees-kee-EHR-doh)
leg	pierna (pee-EHR-nah)
ligament	ligamento (lee-gah-MEHN-toh)
lingual	lingual (leen-GUAHL)
lip	labio (LAH-bee-oh)
lithium	litio (LEE-tee-oh)
liver	hígado (EE-gah-doh)
low cholesterol	bajo colesterol (bah-hoh koh-lehs-teh-ROHL)
low fat	bajo grasa (bah-hoh GRAH-sah)
low sodium	bajo sodio (bah-hoh soh-dee-oh)
lung	pulmón (pool-MOHN)

meningitis	meningitis (meh-neen-HEE-tees)
morphine	morfina (mohr-FEE-nah)
mouth	boca (BOH-kah)
muscle	músculo (MOOS-koo-loh)
narcotics	narcóticos (nahr-KOH-tee-kohs)
nasal	nasal (nah-SAHL)
nausea	náusea (NAH-oo-seh-ah)
navel	ombligo (ohm-BLEE-goh)
neck	cuello (koo-EH-yoh)
neonatal	neonatal (neh-oh-nah-TAHL)
nephrologist	nefrólogo (neh-PHROH-lo-goh)
nephrology	nefrología (neh-phroh-lo-HEE-ah)
nervous	nervioso (nehr-bee-OH-soh)
neurotic	neurótico (neh-oo-ROH-tee-koh)
nipple	pezón (peh-SOHN)
nitroglycerin	nitroglicerina (nee-troh-glee-seh-REE-nah)
nose	nariz (nah-REES)
nostrils	fosas nasales (foh-SAHS na-SAH-lehs)
Novocain	novocaína (noh-boh-kah-EE-nah)
nuclear medicine	medicina nuclear (meh-dee-SEE-nah NOO-kleh-ahr)
obstetrics	obstetricia (ohbs-teh-TREE-see-ah)
oncology	oncología (ohn-koh-loh-HEE-ah)
ophthalmic	oftálmico (ohf-TAHL-mee-koh)
ophthalmology	oftalmología (ohf-tahl-moh-loh-HEE-ah)
optic	óptico (OHP-tee-koh)
orthopedics	ortopedia (ohr-toh-PEH-dee-ah)
orthopedic surgeon	cirujano ortopédico (see-roo-HAH-noh ohr-toh-PEH-dee-koh)
otic	ótico (OH-tee-koh)
ovary	ovario (oh-BAH-ree-oh)
palate	paladar (pah-lah-DAHR)
palpation	palpación (pahl-pah-see-OHN)
palpitation	palpitación (pahl-pee-tah-see-OHN)
pancreas	páncreas (PAHN-kreh-ahs)
pancreatitis	pancreatitis (pahn-kreh-ah-TEE-tees)
paralytic	paralítico (pah-rah-LEE-tee-koh)
pathogen	patógeno (pah-TOH-hen-oh)
pathologic	patológico (pah-toh-LOH-hee-koh)
pathology	patología (pah-toh-loh-HEE-ah)
pediatrics	pediatría (peh-dee-ah-TREE-ah)
pelvis	pelvis (PEHL-bees)
penis	pene (PEH-neh), miembro viril (mee-EHM-broh vee-REEL)
pneumonia	pulmonía/neumonía (pool-moh-NEE-ah/neh-oo-moh-NEE-ah)
pruritic	prurito (proo-REE-toh)
psoriasis	psoriasis (soh-ree-AH-sees)
psychiatrist	psiquiatra (see-kee-AH-trah)
psychiatry	psiquiatría (see-kee-ah- TREE-ah)
psychologist	psicólogo (see-KOH-loh-goh)
pubic	púbico (POO-bee-koh)
pyorrhea	piorrea (pee-oh-RREH-ah)

radiologist	radiólogo (rah-dee-OH-loh-goh)
radiology	radiología (rah-dee-oh-loh-HEE-ah)
rectum	recto (REHK-toh)
rheumatic	reumático (reh-oo-MAH-tee-koh)
rib	costilla (kohs-TEE-yah)
right	derecho (deh-REH-choh)
roseola	roseola (roh-seh-OH-lah)
rubella	rubéola (roo-BEH-oh-lah)
scalp	cuero cabelludo (KOO-eh-roh kah-beh-YOO-doh)
sebaceous	sebáceo (seh-BAH-seh-oh)
sedatives	sedativos/sedantes (seh-dah-TEE-bohs/seh-DAHN-tehs)
shin	espinilla (ehs-pee-NEE-yah), canilla (kah-NEE-yah)
shoulder	hombro (OHM-bro)
skin	piel (pee-EHL)
skull	cráneo (KRAH-ne-oh)
spinal column	columna vertebral (koh-LUHM-nah behr-teh-BRAHL)
spleen	bazo (BAH-soh)
stethoscope	estetoscopio (ehs-teh-tohs-KOH-pee-oh)
stomach	estómago (ehs-TOH-mah-goh)
stool sample	muestra – fecal (moo-EHS-trah -feh-KAHL)
straight	derecho (deh-REH-choh)
subaxillary	subaxilar (soob-AHK-see-lahr)
subcutaneous	subcutáneo (soob-koo-TAH-neh-oh)
sublingual	sublingual (soob-LEEN-goo-ahl)
substernal	subesternal (soob-ehs-TEHR-nahl)
surgeon	cirujano (see-roo-HAH-noh)
surgery	cirugía (see-roo-HEE-ah)
symptoms	síntomas (SEEN-toh-mahs)
syncope	síncope (SEEN-koh-peh)
systole	sístole (SEES-toh-leh)
teeth	dientes (dee-EHN-tehs)
temple	sien (see-EHN)
testicles	testículos (tehs-TEE-koo-lohs)
tetanus	tétano (TEH-tah-noh)
therapy	terapia (teh-RAH-pee-ah)
thigh	muslo (MOOS-loh)
throat	garganta (gahr-GAHN-tah)
thumb	pulgar (POOL-gahr)
thyroid	tiroide (tee-ROY-deh)
toes	dedos (DEH-dos), del pié (dehl PEE-eh)
tongue	lengua (LEHN-goo-ah)
tonsillitis	tonsilitis/amigdalitis (tohn-see-LEE-tees/ah-meeg-dah-LEE-tees)
tonsils	amígdalas (ah-MEEG-da-las)
ulcer	úlcera (OOL-seh-rah)
ulnar	ulnar (OOL-nahr)
ultrasound	ultrasonido (ool-trah-soh-NEE-doh)
uremia	uremia (oo-REH-mee-ah)
urinary bladder	vejiga (beh-HEE-gah)

urine	orina (oh-REE-nah)
urticaria	urticaria (oor-tee-KAH-ree-ah)
uterus	útero (OO-teh-roh)
uvula	úvula (OO-boo-lah)
vaginitis	vaginitis (bah-hee-NEE-tees)
vagus	vago (BAH-goh)
valve	válvula (BAHL-boo-lah)
varicocele	varicocele (bah-ree-koh-SEH-leh)
vertigo	vértigo (BEHR-tee-goh)
waist	cintura (sin-TOO-rah)
womb	vientre (bee-EHN-treh)
wrist	muñeca (moo-NYEH-kah)
x-rays	rayos equis (rah-YOHS EH-kees)
zygomatic	cigomático (see-goh-MAH-tee-koh)

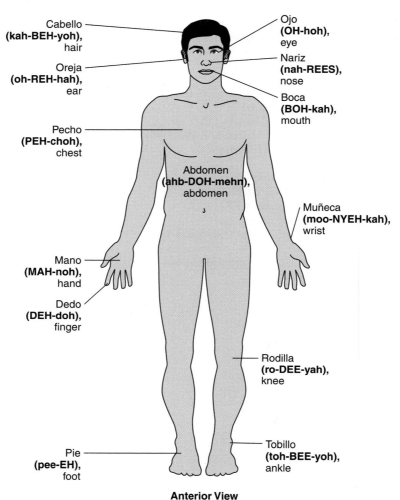

Cabello
(kah-BEH-yoh),
hair

Ojo
(OH-hoh),
eye

Oreja
(oh-REH-hah),
ear

Nariz
(nah-REES),
nose

Boca
(BOH-kah),
mouth

Pecho
(PEH-choh),
chest

Abdomen
(ahb-DOH-mehn),
abdomen

Muñeca
(moo-NYEH-kah),
wrist

Mano
(MAH-noh),
hand

Dedo
(DEH-doh),
finger

Rodilla
(ro-DEE-yah),
knee

Pie
(pee-EH),
foot

Tobillo
(toh-BEE-yoh),
ankle

Anterior View

The body/El cuerpo (ehl KWEHR-poh).

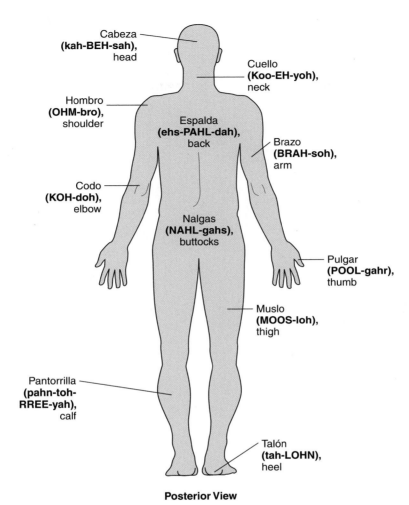

Cabeza
(kah-BEH-sah),
head

Cuello
(Koo-EH-yoh),
neck

Hombro
(OHM-bro),
shoulder

Espalda
(ehs-PAHL-dah),
back

Brazo
(BRAH-soh),
arm

Codo
(KOH-doh),
elbow

Nalgas
(NAHL-gahs),
buttocks

Pulgar
(POOL-gahr),
thumb

Muslo
(MOOS-loh),
thigh

Pantorrilla
**(pahn-toh-
RREE-yah),**
calf

Talón
(tah-LOHN),
heel

Posterior View

The body/El cuerpo (ehl KWEHR-poh).

Index

Page numbers in italics denote figures; those followed by t denote tables.